COMPLICATIONS IN NEUROANESTHESIA

Dedication

This book is dedicated to my parents, my family, my teachers and the ones who mean everything to me – Amyra, Anavi, Anav, Avi and Aishwarya

COMPLICATIONS IN NEUROANESTHESIA

Edited by

HEMANSHU PRABHAKAR

Department of Neuroanaesthesiology and Critical Care, All India Institute of Medical Sciences, New Delhi, India

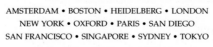

AMSTERDAM • BOSTON • HEIDELBERG • LONDON
NEW YORK • OXFORD • PARIS • SAN DIEGO
SAN FRANCISCO • SINGAPORE • SYDNEY • TOKYO

Academic Press is an imprint of Elsevier

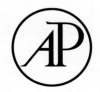

Academic Press is an imprint of Elsevier
125 London Wall, London EC2Y 5AS, UK
525 B Street, Suite 1800, San Diego, CA 92101-4495, USA
50 Hampshire Street, 5th Floor, Cambridge, MA 02139, USA
The Boulevard, Langford Lane, Kidlington, Oxford OX5 1GB, UK

Notices
Knowledge and best practice in this field are constantly changing. As new research and
experience broaden our understanding, changes in research methods, professional practices,
or medical treatment may become necessary.

Practitioners and researchers must always rely on their own experience and knowledge
in evaluating and using any information, methods, compounds, or experiments described
herein. In using such information or methods they should be mindful of their own safety
and the safety of others, including parties for whom they have a professional responsibility.

To the fullest extent of the law, neither the Publisher nor the authors, contributors, or editors,
assume any liability for any injury and/or damage to persons or property as a matter
of products liability, negligence or otherwise, or from any use or operation of any methods,
products, instructions, or ideas contained in the material herein.

British Library Cataloguing-in-Publication Data
A catalogue record for this book is available from the British Library

Library of Congress Cataloging-in-Publication Data
A catalog record for this book is available from the Library of Congress

ISBN: 978-0-12-804075-1

For information on all Academic Press publications
visit our website at https://www.elsevier.com/

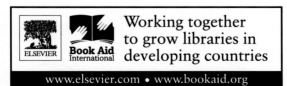

Working together
to grow libraries in
developing countries

www.elsevier.com • www.bookaid.org

Typeset by TNQ Books and Journals
www.tnq.co.in

Contents

I

COMPLICATIONS RELATED TO THE BRAIN

II

COMPLICATIONS RELATED TO SPINAL CORD

III

COMPLICATIONS RELATED TO CARDIO-VASCULAR SYSTEM

IV

COMPLICATIONS RELATED TO COAGULATION

V

COMPLICATIONS RELATED TO RESPIRATORY SYSTEM

VI

COMPLICATIONS RELATED TO AIRWAY

VII

COMPLICATIONS RELATED TO FLUID AND ELECTROLYTE DISTURBANCES

VIII

POSTOPERATIVE PAIN

IX

MISCELLANEOUS

X

CLINICAL SCENARIOS

List of Contributors

Richa Aggarwal Department of Neuroanaesthesiology and Critical Care, All India Institute of Medical Sciences, New Delhi, India

Zulfiqar Ali Division of Neuroanesthesiology, Department of Anesthesiology, SKIMS, Srinagar, Jammu and Kashmir, India

Federico Bilotta Department of Anaesthesia and Intensive Care, University of Rome "Sapienza", Rome, Italy

Parmod K. Bithal Department of Neuroanaesthesiology and Critical Care, All India Institute of Medical Sciences, New Delhi, India

Matthew T.V. Chan Department of Anaesthesia and Intensive Care, The Chinese University of Hong Kong, Hong Kong Special Administrative Region, China

Mandy H.M. Chu Department of Anaesthesia, Pamela Youde Nethersole Eastern Hospital, Chai Wan, Hong Kong Special Administrative Region, China

Melissa Ehlers Associate Professor of Anesthesiology, Albany Medical Center, Albany, NY, USA

Neus Fabregas Servicio de Anestesiología, Hospital Clínic, Universitat de Barcelona, Barcelona, Spain

Juan Fernández-Candil Servicio de Anestesiología, Parc de Salut Mar, Barcelona, Spain

Vinod K. Grover Department of Anaesthesia and Intensive Care, Postgraduate Institute of Medical Education and Research, Chandigarh, India

Nidhi Gupta Department of Neuroanaesthesia, Indraprastha Apollo Hospital, New Delhi, India

Kiran Jangra Department of Anaesthesia and Intensive Care, Postgraduate Institute of Medical Education and Research, Chandigarh, India

Kavitha Jayaram Department of Anesthesia and Intensive Care, Nizam's Institute of Medical Sciences, Hyderabad, India

Patricia K.Y. Kan Department of Anaesthesia and Intensive Care, Prince of Wales Hospital, Hong Kong Special Administrative Region, China

Indu Kapoor Department of Neuroanaesthesiology and Critical Care, All India Institute of Medical Sciences, New Delhi, India

Emily G.Y. Koo Department of Anaesthesia, Pamela Youde Nethersole Eastern Hospital, Chai Wan, Hong Kong Special Administrative Region, China

Laura Leduc Department of Anesthesiology, Albany Medical Center, Albany, NY, USA

Ankur Luthra Department of Neuroanaesthesia and Intensive Care, Medanta, The Medicity, Gurgaon, Haryana, India

Giuseppina Magni   Department of Anaesthesia and Intensive Care, University of Rome "Sapienza", Rome, Italy

Charu Mahajan   Department of Neuroanaesthesiology and Critical Care, All India Institute of Medical Sciences, New Delhi, India

Pirjo H. Manninen   Department of Anesthesia, Toronto Western Hospital, University Health Network, University of Toronto, Toronto, ON, Canada

Eckhard Mauermann   Anesthesiology, University Hospital Basel, Basel, Switzerland

Ranadhir Mitra   Department of Neuroanaesthesiology and Critical Care, All India Institute of Medical Sciences, New Delhi, India

Hemanshu Prabhakar   Department of Neuroanaesthesiology and Critical Care, All India Institute of Medical Sciences, New Delhi, India

M.V.S. Satya Prakash   Department of Anaesthesiology and Critical Care, JIPMER, Puducherry, India

Shobana Rajan   Department of Anesthesiology, Cleveland Clinic, Cleveland, OH, USA

Bernhard J. Schaller   University of Southampton, Southampton, UK

Vasudha Singhal   Department of Neuroanaesthesia and Intensive Care, Medanta, The Medicity, Gurgaon, Haryana, India

Gyaninder P. Singh   Department of Neuroanaesthesiology and Critical Care, All India Institute of Medical Sciences, New Delhi, India

M. Srilata   Department of Anesthesia and Intensive Care, Nizam's Institute of Medical Sciences, Hyderabad, India

Luzius A. Steiner   Anesthesiology, University Hospital Basel, Basel, Switzerland

Prasanna Udupi Bidkar   Department of Anaesthesiology and Critical Care, JIPMER, Puducherry, India

Zoe M. Unger   Department of Anesthesia, Toronto Western Hospital, University Health Network, University of Toronto, Toronto, ON, Canada

Foreword

Until about two decades ago, neuroanesthesia practice was not deemed any different from general anesthesia practice. Neuroanesthesia has of recent emerged as a challenging subspecialty of anesthesia because of the absence of leeway to its practitioners. Therefore, the anesthesia provider has to be extra vigilant during the intraoperative and postoperative periods. Owing to the vulnerability of the brain to suffer from irreversible damage following an even innocuous looking insult, failure to anticipate complication/s could make or mar the outcome of a neurosurgical patient. How to recognize complications quickly and manage them efficiently, therefore, is central to the practice of neuroanesthesia.

There are quite a few popular textbooks on neurosurgical anesthesia practice by eminent authors from the Western world but they all have mentioned complications in a perfunctory manner. The editor of this book realized this shortcoming and took it upon himself to write comprehensively in *Complications in Neuroanesthesia*.

The editor has ensured this book is written in a very simple language, which readers will find easy to read and assimilate. Under his guidance, he has compiled the various topics penned by distinguished neuroanesthesiologists. He has tried to include all the possible complications that a practitioner of neuroanesthesia may come across at some point in time. This book is meant for both the occasional neuroanesthesiologist and those physicians who are regular providers of neuroanesthesia. Furthermore, this book will be handy not only for students of neuroanesthesia but also for the consultants of neuroanesthesia too because, it is a kind of ready reckoner. The book would prove equally useful for trainees and specialists of allied branches, such as neurointensivists, neurosurgery, neurology and neuroradiology. The simple and easy-to-understand language makes it accessible to technical and nursing staff as well. Efficient management of the complications in neuroanesthesia is not determined entirely by the experience of the anesthesia provider. It requires an in-depth knowledge of pathophysiology behind it and understanding of the surgical procedure. A half-baked knowledge may thus result in irrational management, spelling doom for the patient.

Written in a very comprehensive manner, this book is sure to find its place in the bookshelves of all neuroanesthetists.

Parmod K. Bithal
Department of Neuroanaesthesiology and Critical Care,
All India Institute of Medical Sciences, New Delhi, India

Preface

This book is a compilation of possible complications one can encounter during the practice of neuroanesthesia. Each chapter reviews challenges we face in our day-to-day practice. Readers will get a comprehensive insight of various complications one can possibly confront while managing neurosurgical cases in the operation theater and in the intensive care units. Familiarity with these complexities is essential for successful management and a good outcome of patients.

I am grateful to all the authors who believed in me and my proposed format of this book. Above all, I am also thankful to the patients who actually taught and made us aware of these complications. I'm sure readers will benefit from the cognizance of the renowned neuroanesthetists. The vignettes described toward the end of the book will help readers stimulate their neurons, searching for the right answer and also testing their knowledge.

The purpose of this book will be truly accomplished if we are able to improve the clinical conditions of our patients by providing better care.

Acknowledgments

I wish to acknowledge the support of the administration of the All India Institute of Medical Sciences (AIIMS), New Delhi, in allowing me to conduct this academic task, especially, Prof. M.C. Misra (Director, AIIMS, New Delhi).

Words are not enough to express my gratitude for the constant support and encouragement from Prof. P.K. Bithal (Head of Neuroanaesthesiology and Critical Care, AIIMS, New Delhi). I thank the faculty and staff of the department of Neuroanaesthesiology and Critical Care, for their support.

Acknowledgments are due to Dr. Purva Mathur, Dr. Shilpa Sharma, Prof. Bernhard Schaller, and Dr. Sonu Singh, who showed me the right path.

Special thanks are due to the production team of Elsevier: Melanie Tucker, Kristi Anderson, Kirsten Chrisman, and Unni Kannan.

COMPLICATIONS RELATED TO THE BRAIN

Brain Herniation

Patricia K.Y. Kan[1], Mandy H.M. Chu[2],
Emily G.Y. Koo[2], Matthew T.V. Chan[3]

[1]Department of Anaesthesia and Intensive Care, Prince of Wales Hospital, Hong Kong Special Administrative Region, China; [2]Department of Anaesthesia, Pamela Youde Nethersole Eastern Hospital, Chai Wan, Hong Kong Special Administrative Region, China; [3]Department of Anaesthesia and Intensive Care, The Chinese University of Hong Kong, Hong Kong Special Administrative Region, China

OUTLINE

Complications in Neuroanesthesia
http://dx.doi.org/10.1016/B978-0-12-804075-1.00001-8

3

OVERVIEW

Brain herniation is the displacement of brain tissue through the rigid dural folds (i.e., falx and tentorium) or skull openings (e.g., foramen magnum).[1] Although patients with chronic brain herniation associated with developmental defects, such as Arnold–Chiari malformation, may remain asymptomatic for many years,[2] acute brain herniation following neurosurgery is a catastrophic event that results in mechanical and vascular damage of the brain. In many circumstances, brain herniation is often regarded as a terminal event.

MECHANISM OF BRAIN HERNIATION

From a mechanistic point of view, brain herniation is the result of a pressure gradient that squeezes the vulnerable brain matter from one compartment in the brain to another through various anatomical channels. In general, any pathologic process that increases intracranial pressure provides the driving pressure for brain herniation.[1] It should be clear that the pressure gradient appears to be the most important factor, and brain herniation may occur regardless of the size of the opening.[3] In the perioperative setting, hemorrhage, cerebral swelling associated with perioperative stroke, and hydrocephalus are the common causes for intracranial hypertension after neurosurgery (Table 1). In a systematic review of patients with clinical deterioration following intracranial surgery, 0.8–6.9% of cases were thought to be due to postoperative hemorrhage.[4] In patients who received regular imaging surveillance, up to 50% of cases had evidence of significant intracranial hemorrhage following neurosurgery.[4,5] It is reassuring that few patients with postoperative intracranial hematoma actually end up with brain herniation. However, even a small amount of blood may produce

TABLE 1   Common Causes of Intracranial Hypertension Following Neurosurgery that May Lead to Brain Herniation

1. Postoperative intracranial hemorrhage (extradural, subdural, intracerebral, or intraventricular hematoma) due to surgical bleeding or patients with bleeding tendency.
2. Brain contusion related to primary traumatic brain injury or instrumental damage (e.g., brain retraction injury).
3. Cerebral swelling due to:
   a. Perioperative stroke
   b. Exacerbation of peritumor or periabscess edema
   c. Cerebral venous thrombosis
   d. Hyperemia (e.g., hyperperfusion syndrome following carotid endarterectomy)
   e. Metabolic causes (e.g., diabetic ketoacidosis, hyponatremia, liver failure)
4. Hydrocephalus

sufficient pressure to produce significant brain herniation. This is especially important in patients who already have limited intracranial compliance.

It should be noted that not all cases of brain herniation are related to intracranial hypertension. In patients who had decompressive craniectomy, acute drainage of cerebrospinal fluid, upright posture, or hyperventilation may produce a transient negative pressure gradient between the atmosphere and intracranial compartments. This extra intracranial pressure gradient across the skull defect may be large enough to push the brain matter down into the tentorial notch or the foramen magnum, resulting in a rare phenomenon known as paradoxical brain herniation.[6,7]

CLASSIFICATION OF BRAIN HERNIATION

The brain can be broadly divided into a number of compartments, with boundaries formed by the falx, the tentorium, and the foramen magnum. When the pressure within a compartment is increased, its contents will be pushed toward the adjacent compartments. The directions of displacements are shown in Figure 1.[1] Briefly, the inner part of the temporal lobe (uncal herniation), the entire diencephalon (central/downward transtentorial herniation), and the frontal lobe (cingulate or subfalcine herniation) are common areas for herniation within the supratentorial compartment.

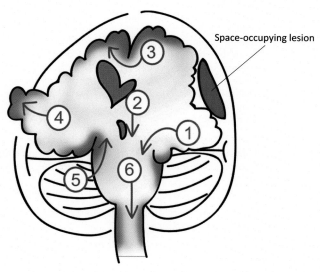

FIGURE 1   Coronal view of brain herniations. (1) uncal herniation, (2) central transtentorial herniation, (3) subfalcine/cingulate herniation, (4) transcalvarial herniation, (5) reverse transtentorial herniation, and (6) tonsillar herniation. Red arrows indicate the direction of brain displacement. Noted that reverse transtentorial herniation is due to the effect of infratentorial lesion and not related to the space occupying lesion shown (red).

In the infratentorial compartment, cerebellar tonsils may be squeezed down through the foramen magnum (tonsillar herniation or coning). In contrast, the cerebellum in the posterior fossa may also be pushed upward when the infratentorial pressure exceeds that in the supratentorial compartment (reverse transtentorial herniation). Finally, the part of brain matter that is adjacent to a craniectomy wound or site of fracture may be herniated out of the skull (transcalvarial herniation).

CLINICAL FEATURES OF BRAIN HERNIATION

The clinical presentation of brain herniation depends largely on the underlying lesion in the brain, the manifestations of intracranial hypertension, and the function of specific part of the brain that is being compressed. Table 2 summarizes the mechanisms and common clinical signs associated with different forms of brain herniations.

TABLE 2   Clinical Presentations of Brain Herniation

Type of herniation	Mechanisms	Clinical presentations
Uncal herniation	1. Compression on parasympathetic followed by somatic component of oculomotor nerve 2. Infarction of ipsilateral visual cortex 3. Lateral displacement of brain stem to compress the contralateral corticospinal tract 4. Distortion of the ascending arousal system 5. Duret hemorrhage	1. Dilated pupils, ptosis, and "down and out position" of the ipsilateral eye 2. Contralateral homonymous hemianopia 3. Ipsilateral hemiparesis or hemiplegia 4. Unconsciousness 5. Decorticate posture, respiratory depression, and death
Central transtentorial herniation	1. Early stage 2. Late stage 3. Compression of pituitary stalk	1. Agitation and drowsiness; pupils are small but reactive 2. Decorticate, decerebrate posture 3. Diabetes insipidus
Subfalcine herniation	Compression of cingulate gyrus and intracranial hypertension	Nonspecific signs
Transcalvarial herniation	Compression against external wound	Physical sign depends on the part and extent of brain herniation
Tonsillar herniation	Brain stem compression	1. Unconsciousness 2. Respiratory depression and cardiovascular instability

Uncal (Transtentorial) Herniation

The uncus is the most medial part of the temporal lobe. When it is squeezed against the tentorium, it exerts pressure on the third cranial (oculomotor) nerve as it leaves the midbrain and travels along the free edge of the tentorium. In addition, there is pressure against the ipsilateral brain stem. Not surprisingly, the earliest clinical signs associated with an uncal herniation are those due to ipsilateral third nerve palsy. It is often suggested that the parasympathetic input to the eye, lying in the outermost part of the nerve, is first affected. This will result in an ipsilateral fixed and dilated pupil. As the pressure on the third cranial nerve is further increased, the somatic component is also affected, leading to complete ptosis and deviation of the eye to a "down and out" position. However, the motor functions of the eye cannot be easily tested in an unconscious patient. Therefore, a fixed and dilated pupil may become the only physical sign of an uncal herniation. As lateral displacement becomes more severe, the brain stem is being compressed against the contralateral tentorium leading to injury of the contralateral corticospinal tract with ipsilateral hemiparesis.[8] This is obviously a false localizing sign. In addition, the contralateral posterior cerebral artery may be compressed leading to ipsilateral visual cortex infarction and giving rise to contralateral homonymous hemianopia.

When both hemispheres are under pressure, the diencephalon and parts of the temporal lobes are squeezed through the tentorial notch, resulting in central transtentorial herniation. In the early stage, the pupils are small and reactive. Interestingly, they dilate briskly in response to pinching of the neck (ciliospinal reflex). Oculocephalic reflexes and plantar responses are intact. In patients who are breathing spontaneously, yawning with occasional pauses are often observed. This may progress to Cheyne–Stokes breathing in the later stage. Further compression on the brain stem will result in decorticate posture, respiratory depression, and death.

Radiologically, one should observe the general features of intracranial hypertension in the computed tomography (CT) scans. These include midline shift, obliteration of ventricles, and effacement of sulci and cisterns. Specifically, uncal herniation produces a duret hemorrhage that appears as flame or linear-shaped hyperintensities in the brain stem. This is due to tearing of small vessels. In addition, notching of the contralateral midbrain (Kernohan's notch)[8] indicates severe lateral displacement of the brain stem (Figure 2).

Subfalcine/Cingulate Herniation

Subfalcine herniation is the displacement of the medial frontal lobe (cingulate gyrus) underneath the free edge of the falx cerebri. Symptoms

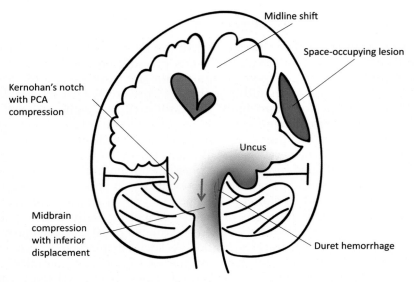

FIGURE 2   Important radiological features seen in uncal and central transtentorial herniation.
Red arrows indicate the direction of brain displacement.

are generally nonspecific. On the axial image of a CT scan, subfalcine shift
can be demonstrated by drawing a straight line from the anterior to the
posterior aspect of the falx, highlighting the deviation of the septum pellucidum from its expected midline position (Figure 3). This may result
in cerebral infarction over the ipsilateral anterior cerebral artery territory.
One may also note the dilatation of the contralateral ventricle due to the
obstruction of the foramen of Monro.

Transcalvarial Herniation

This is also known as "external herniation," where part of the brain is displaced out of the cranium because intracranial pressure is much larger than
that of the atmosphere (Figure 4). Obviously, clinical presentation depends on
the part and extent of brain matter that is herniated through the skull defect.

Reverse Transtentorial Herniation

Reverse transtentorial herniation occurs when pressure in the posterior fossa exceeds that of the supratentorial compartment. The cerebellum
is therefore pushed superiorly between the free edges of the tentorium
(Figure 5). Clinically, bilateral fixed dilated pupils may be the only physical
sign that can be elicited. This is due to injury to the third cranial nerves as
the midbrain is being compressed and the tentorium is stretched. Reverse
transtentorial herniation should be suspected when there is rapid postoperative deterioration in patients with unrelieved pressure in the posterior

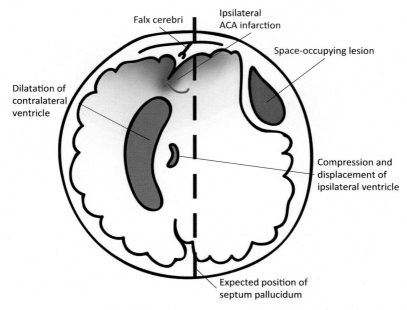

FIGURE 3   Subfalcine/cingulate herniation. Dotted line indicate the expected position of septum pellucidum. Red arrow indicates the direction of brain displacement. ACA, anterior cerebral artery.

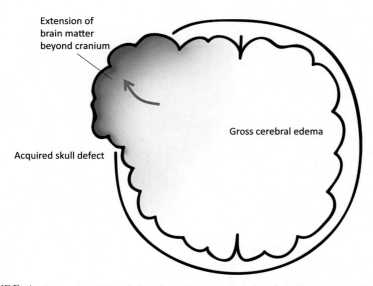

FIGURE 4   Transcalvarial herniation through acquired skull defect. Red arrow indicates the direction of brain displacement.

fossa (e.g., residual cerebellar tumor). In this setting, acute drainage of hydrocephalus produces sufficient negative pressure gradient from infra- to supratentorial compartments for brain herniation.

I. COMPLICATIONS RELATED TO THE BRAIN

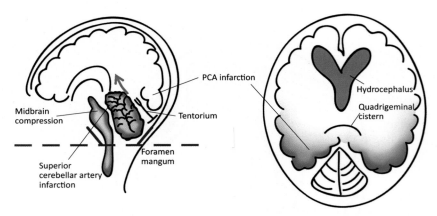

FIGURE 5   Reverse transtentorial herniation. Sagittal view (left) showing upward displacement of cerebellum toward supratentorial compartment. Transverse view (right) showing reverse and flattening of quadrigeminal cistern (frown-shaped appearance). Red arrow indicates the direction of brain displacement. PCA, posterior cerebral artery.

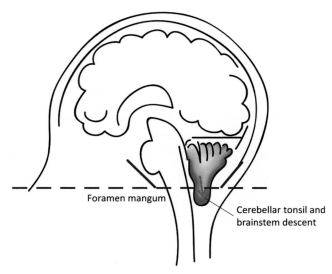

FIGURE 6   Tonsillar herniation—descent of cerebellar tonsils and brain stem beyond foramen magnum. Red arrow indicates the direction of brain displacement.

In the CT scans, flattening of the superior cerebellar cistern may be observed. The usual "smile-shaped" quadrigeminal cistern is reversed to produce a "frown-shaped" appearance (Figure 5). One should also look for infarction in areas supplied by the posterior cerebral and superior cerebellar arteries. Obstructive hydrocephalus due to compression of the cerebral aqueduct may also occur.

Tonsillar Herniation

This is commonly known as coning, when the cerebellar tonsils move downward through the foramen magnum (Figure 6). Tonsillar herniation exerts pressure over the lower brain stem and the upper cervical spinal cord against the narrow foramen magnum. In the postoperative setting, brain stem compression results in unconsciousness, flaccid paralysis, and respiratory and cardiac depression.

In sagittal scans, an inferior descent of the cerebellar tonsils, >5 mm in adults and >7 mm in children, below the foramen magnum is considered significant. The cerebrospinal fluid cisterns around the brain stem may become effaced as well.

PREVENTION OF BRAIN HERNIATION

Little is known about prevention of brain herniation after neurosurgery. Nevertheless, appropriate preoperative preparation for patients with a bleeding diathesis (e.g., desmopressin administration for von Willebrand's disease), stopping aspirin, other antiplatelets, and anticoagulants ahead of scheduled surgery or prior embolization of a vascular tumor may avoid massive bleeding during surgery and may prevent postoperative hematoma.[9] Meticulous surgery to avoid retraction injury and inappropriate coagulation of perforators will prevent postoperative ischemic brain swelling. Other maneuvers include administration of corticosteroid for brain tumor and prophylactic anticonvulsant therapy may also decrease the risk of postoperative malignant brain swelling. Despite success of endovascular treatment for acute stroke in the general population,[10] it is unclear whether the treatment for perioperative stroke could produce a similar benefit after neurosurgery.

TREATMENT OF BRAIN HERNIATION

Brain herniation following neurosurgery is a life-threatening neurosurgical emergency and requires immediate resuscitation to prevent irreversible injury and death. Treatment strategies should be directed to control intracranial pressure, so that an intracranial pressure ≤20 mm Hg and a cerebral perfusion pressure ≥70 mm Hg are the therapeutic targets. General measures include maneuvers to ensure good oxygenation, appropriate head positioning to facilitate cerebral venous drainage, osmotherapy, sedation to decrease cerebral metabolic rate, and hyperventilation to reduce cerebral blood volume (Table 3).[11,12] In addition, it is important to correct any underlying pathology. This may

TABLE 3   General Management for Control of Intracranial Pressure

---

1. Ensure airway patency, adequate breathing, and circulation.
   a. Tracheal intubation for airway protection and invasive mechanical ventilation.
   b. Ensure oxygenation with hemoglobin saturation ≥92%.
   c. Limit positive end-expiratory pressure <12 cm H_2O.
   d. Maintain cerebral perfusion pressure (50–70 mm Hg).
2. Positioning to facilitate cerebral venous drainage with head of bed elevated to 30°–45° in neutral position.
3. Hyperventilation to maintain arterial carbon dioxide tension of 30–35 mm Hg.
4. Correct hyponatremia and maintain normoglycemia.
5. Antipyretics for fever.
6. Use of prophylactic anticonvulsants and treat seizure promptly.
7. Administer sedation and analgesia, when appropriate.
8. Administer dexamethasone for brain tumor–related vasogenic edema.
9. Osmotherapy using mannitol (0.25–2 g/kg over 10–15 min) or hypertonic saline[a] (but keeping plasma sodium <160 mmol/L).
10. Careful drainage of cerebrospinal fluid if an external ventricular drainage device is available.

---

[a] *Common regimens include 3% solution at 5 ml/kg over 15 min; 7.5% solution at 2.5 ml/kg over 15 min; 23.4% solution at 30 ml over 20–30 min.*

include replacement of clotting factors to correct coagulopathy, relief of hydrocephalus, drainage of intracranial hematoma, and surgical excision of contused brain tissue. In patients who suffer from hyperperfusion after neurosurgery, aggressive control of arterial pressure using labetalol or barbiturate infusion to reduce mean flow velocity <120 cm/s of the proximal cerebral artery on transcranial Doppler monitoring may be useful.[13]

In patients with malignant brain swelling following neurosurgery, either due to infarction or hyperemia, early decompressive craniectomy may be lifesaving. Based on the experience from acute ischemic stroke, a large hemicraniectomy performed within 48 h after onset of stroke has been shown to provide survival benefit as well as functional improvement.[14,15]

CONCLUSIONS

Brain herniation is a devastating complication after neurosurgery. Early recognition of brain herniation based on clinical signs, such as failure to arouse and dilated pupils after surgery, should alert clinicians that brain herniation may have occurred. Radiological assessment should be performed to identify the underlying pathology. Timely resuscitation to decrease intracranial pressure is the key to minimize damage.

References

1. Frosch MP, Anthony DC, De Girolami U. The central nervous system. In: Kumar V, Abbas AK, Aster JC, eds. *Robbins and Cotran Pathologic Basis of Disease*. 9th ed. Philadelphia, PA: Elsevier/Saunders; 2015:1251–1318.

2. Meeker J, Amerine J, Kropp D, Chyatte M, Fischbein R. The impact of Chiari malformation on daily activities: a report from the National Conquer Chiari Patient Registry Database. *Disabil Health J*. 2015;8(4):521–526.

3. Battaglia P, Turri-Zanoni M, Castelnuovo P, Prevedello DM, Carrau RL. Brain herniation after endoscopic transnasal resection of anterior skull base malignancies. *Neurosurgery*. 2015;11(suppl 3):457–462.

4. Seifman MA, Lewis PM, Rosenfeld JV, Hwang PY. Postoperative intracranial haemorrhage: a review. *Neurosurg Rev*. 2011;34:393–407.

5. Manninen PH, Raman SK, Boyle K, El-Beheiry H. Early postoperative complications following neurosurgical procedures. *Can J Anaesth*. 1999;46:7–14.

6. Creutzfeldt CJ, Vilela MD, Longstreth Jr WT. Paradoxical herniation after decompressive craniectomy provoked by lumbar puncture or ventriculoperitoneal shunting. *J Neurosurg*. 2015:1–6.

7. Komotar RJ, Mocco J, Ransom ER, et al. Herniation secondary to critical postcraniotomy cerebrospinal fluid hypovolemia. *Neurosurgery*. 2005;57:286–292. discussion 286–292.

8. Panikkath R, Panikkath D, Lim SY, Nugent K. Kernohan's notch: a forgotten cause of Hemiplegia-CT scans are useful in this diagnosis. *Case Rep Med*. 2013;2013:296874.

9. Chan MT, Kan PKY. Blood loss during spine surgery. In: Brambrink A, Kirsch JR, eds. *Essentials of Neurosurgical Anesthesia and Critical Care: Strategies for Prevention, Early Detection, and Successful Management of Perioperative Complications*. Springer; 2012:289–298.

10. Pierot L, Derdeyn C. Interventionalist perspective on the new endovascular trials. *Stroke*. 2015;46:1440–1446.

11. Stocchetti N, Maas AI. Traumatic intracranial hypertension. *N Engl J Med*. 2014;370: 2121–2130.

12. Stevens RD, Huff JS, Duckworth J, Papangelou A, Weingart SD, Smith WS. Emergency neurological life support: intracranial hypertension and herniation. *Neurocrit Care*. 2012;17(suppl 1):S60–S65.

13. van Mook WN, Rennenberg RJ, Schurink GW, van Oostenbrugge RJ, Mess WH, Hofman PA, et al. Cerebral hyperperfusion syndrome. *Lancet Neurol*. 2005;4:877–888.

14. Juttler E, Unterberg A, Woitzik J, Bosel J, Amiri H, Sakowitz OW, et al. Hemicraniectomy in older patients with extensive middle-cerebral-artery stroke. *N Engl J Med*. 2014;370:1091–1100.

15. Vahedi K, Hofmeijer J, Juettler E, et al. Early decompressive surgery in malignant infarction of the middle cerebral artery: a pooled analysis of three randomised controlled trials. *Lancet Neurol*. 2007;6:215–222.

Delayed Emergence

Vasudha Singhal[1], Hemanshu Prabhakar[2]

[1]Department of Neuroanaesthesia and Intensive Care, Medanta, The Medicity, Gurgaon, Haryana, India; [2]Department of Neuroanaesthesiology and Critical Care, All India Institute of Medical Sciences, New Delhi, India

DEFINITION

Emergence from general anesthesia is defined as the return of neuromuscular conduction, airway protective reflexes, and appropriate level of consciousness following discontinuation of anesthetic agents at the end of the surgery or intervention. Failure to regain the expected level of consciousness within 20–30 min of cessation of anesthetic agent administration is termed as delayed emergence.[1]

Time to emergence is variable and depends upon various patient related factors, the type of anesthetic given, and the length of surgery. A pertinent review of the medical and drug history of the patient is important, prior to considering the perioperative anesthetic management, as various medical illnesses predispose a patient to delayed awakening or prolonged paralysis. The differential diagnosis of delayed emergence includes residual drug effects, metabolic derangements, or neurologic disorders. All these should be excluded in a stepwise manner, and supportive ventilation continued till the patient becomes fully responsive.

CAUSES[2]

1. Residual drug effects may be because of several reasons:
   a. Drug overdose: usually hypnotics or opioids: pinpoint pupils and slow, deep respiration are signs of opioid narcosis.
      Patients at extremes of age (pediatric and geriatric patients) show an unusual sensitivity to anesthetic drugs.
      Patients with preoperative cognitive and psychiatric disorders, or patients who were anesthetized while intoxicated with alcohol or recreational drugs, may be more difficult to arouse.
   b. Residual neuromuscular blockade: may occur secondary to overdose, or incomplete reversal of nondepolarising muscle relaxants, or in a patient with suxamethonium apnea (due to an abnormal or absent plasma cholinesterase enzyme), or in patients with myasthenia gravis and muscular dystrophies.
   c. Reduced drug metabolism/excretion: seen in liver disease, renal disease, severe hypothyroidism, hypoalbuminemia. Patients with low cardiac output may have delayed absorption of intramuscular injections.
   d. Potentiation by other drugs[3]:
      - Reserpine and methyldopa decrease minimum alveolar concentration and predispose to anesthetic overdose
      - Acute ethanol intoxication decreases barbiturate metabolism
      - Antiparkinsonian drugs and tricyclic antidepressants augment sedation produced by scopolamine by their anticholinergic effects.
2. Respiratory failure: Patients with underlying respiratory disease, like chronic obstructive pulmonary disease or obstructive sleep apnea (with CO_2 retention preoperatively), or who may have received high doses of narcotics, may hypoventilate in the postoperative period, and may be drowsy because of CO_2 retention.
3. Metabolic disorders:
   a. Hypoglycemia: may occur in
      - Neonates (most common in premature babies) and infants
      - Liver failure
      - Patients on insulin or oral hypoglycemic drugs
      - Sepsis

- Malaria
- Alcohol intoxication
   b. Hyperglycemia: may occur in decompensated diabetics, presenting as hyperosmotic hyperglycemic nonketotic coma, or diabetic ketoacidosis
   c. Electrolyte imbalance: hyponatremia, hypernatremia, hypo- or hypercalcemia may all present with delayed emergence
   d. Hypothermia: decreases minimum alveolar concentration of inhalational agents, antagonizes muscle relaxation reversal, and limits drug metabolism. A core temperature of less than 33 °C has a marked anesthetic effect itself and will potentiate the central nervous system depressant effects of anesthetic drugs.[4]
   e. Central anticholinergic syndrome: is a rare entity and is precipitated by drugs including antihistamines, atropine, scopolamine, and antidepressants. It is thought to be due to a decrease in inhibitory anticholinergic activity in the brain, and may manifest as confusion, restlessness, hallucinations, convulsions, and coma, and therefore as delayed awakening from anesthesia. Treatment is with physostigmine 0.04 mg/kg slowly, intravenously.[5]
4. Neurologic disorders: Certain surgical procedures, like carotid endarterectomy, cardiopulmonary bypass, and intracranial procedures, are associated with an increased incidence of postoperative neurological deficits.
   a. Cerebral hypoxia due to any cause may result in delayed awakening.
   Patients with chronic hypertension have an altered cerebral blood flow autoregulation, and any episode of intraoperative hypotension is poorly tolerated and may lead to hypoxia.
   b. Intracerebral hemorrhage, embolism, or thrombosis
   c. Seizures

DIAGNOSIS

If the patient does not wake up from anesthesia, a few rapid tests may aid in diagnosing the underlying issue. These include:

- Patients' vitals, including temperature
- Train of four (TOF) monitoring for residual neuromuscular paralysis
- Arterial blood gas (ABG) analysis with electrolytes
- Blood glucose
- Neurological examination—pupils, cranial nerves, reflexes, response to pain
- Computed tomography (CT) scan, if indicated

MANAGEMENT

Prompt, efficient assessment and treatment of delayed awakening are key to minimizing potential catastrophes. The priority should always be ABC, i.e., airway, breathing, and circulation, which should be reevaluated throughout the course of assessment. Airway obstruction, hypoxia, and hypercarbia should be excluded with the assessment of vital signs, especially the rate and character of spontaneous breathing and oxygen saturation, and physical examination. An ABG analysis aids in diagnosing any respiratory or metabolic derangements.

The patient's medical history and the history of drug intake should be reascertained in cases of delayed emergence to look for any potential associations. It is prudent that if the patient is unable to protect airway reflexes, then it is best to maintain a secure airway (keep them intubated) until fully awake. The anesthetic chart should be looked into and the perioperative management reassessed.

- Confirm that all inhalational and intravenous anesthetic agents are off.
- Check for residual muscular paralysis with TOF if patient is asleep, and reverse accordingly.
  If the patient follows commands, but is still paralysed, it is advisable to sedate the patient and ventilate till adequate recovery from neuromuscular blockade is achieved. An additional dose of reversal agent (neostigmine 2.5 mg/glycopyrrolate 0.5 mg) may be tried. Patients with suxamethonium apnea may need prolonged ventilation.
- Consider:
  - Narcotic reversal: 40 μg IV naloxone; repeat every 2 min up to 0.2 mg
  - Benzodiazepine reversal: 0.2 mg flumazenil every 1 min; max dose = 1 mg
- Measure the patient's temperature and warm if hypothermic.
- Check blood glucose and treat hypo-/hyperglycemia.
- Measure and correct dyselectrolytemia–hyponatremia correction should be performed slowly so as to avoid complications (like central pontine myelinolysis or cardiac failure).
- After all possible drug effects and metabolic causes have been ruled out, consider a thorough neurological examination of the patient to exclude any intracerebral event (ischemic or hemorrhagic stroke). A CT scan may aid diagnosis and guide further course of action.

PREVENTION

With pharmacological advancement and advent of sophisticated monitoring, the incidence of delayed emergence has decreased considerably. Careful titration of drugs to their effects, use of intermediate acting relaxants (like vecuronium and atracurium), use of a nerve stimulator to guide dosing and reversal, and careful evaluation of serum chemistries during the peri and postoperative periods, help prevent delayed awakening from anesthesia. The occurrence of an acute intracerebral event must always be kept in mind while evaluating a patient with an unexplained prolonged emergence.

References

1. Atlee JL. *Complications in Anesthesia*. 2nd ed. Elsevier Health Sciences; 2007:885–887.
2. Radhakrishnan J, Jesudasan S, Jacob R. Delayed awakening or emergence from anaesthesia. *Update Anaesth*. 2001;13:4–6.
3. Morgan Jr GE, Mikhail MS, Murray MJ. *Clinical Anesthesiology*. 4th ed. New York: Lange Medical Books/McGraw Hill; 2005:224–226.
4. Lenhardt R, Marker E, Goll V, et al. Mild intraoperative hypothermia prolongs postoperative recovery. *Anesthesiology*. 1997;87:1318–1323.
5. Brown DV, Heller F, Barkin R. Anticholinergic syndrome after anesthesia: a case report and review. *Am J Ther*. 2004;11:144–153.

Hydrocephalus

Vasudha Singhal[1], Hemanshu Prabhakar[2]

[1]Department of Neuroanaesthesia and Intensive Care, Medanta, The Medicity, Gurgaon, Haryana, India; [2]Department of Neuroanaesthesiology and Critical Care, All India Institute of Medical Sciences, New Delhi, India

DEFINITION

Hydrocephalus (derived from Greek words *hydros* meaning water and *cephalus* meaning head) is defined as the excessive accumulation of cerebrospinal fluid (CSF) in the ventricular system and cisterns of the brain, leading to an increase in intracranial pressure (ICP) and its sequelae. Considering the hydrodynamics of the CSF, Rekate defined hydrocephalus as an active distension of the ventricular system of the brain resulting from inadequate passage of CSF from its point of production within the cerebral ventricles to its point of absorption into the systemic circulation.

VARIANT

Normal pressure hydrocephalus (NPH), affecting mainly the elderly in their sixth or seventh decade of life, is marked by ventricle enlargement without an apparent increase in CSF pressure. NPH exhibits the classic triad of symptoms (popularly known as the Hakim's or Adam's triad)—urinary incontinence, gait disturbance, and dementia (commonly referred to as *wet, wobbly, wacky*). NPH is caused by an increase in ICP due to an abnormal accumulation of CSF in the ventricles of the brain, which can cause the ventricles to enlarge. The ICP gradually falls but still remains slightly elevated compared with baseline measurements. The enlarged ventricles exert pressure on the adjacent cortical tissues, causing the symptoms. NPH may be idiopathic or secondary. Secondary NPH can be due to a subarachnoid hemorrhage, head trauma, tumor, infection in the central nervous system, or a complication of cranial surgery.

Hydrocephalus ex vacuo is a compensatory enlargement of the CSF spaces in response to brain parenchyma loss (as occurs in cerebral atrophy or post trauma) and is not the result of increased CSF pressure.

PATHOPHYSIOLOGY

CSF is produced by the choroid plexuses of the lateral, third, and fourth ventricle. The rate of CSF formation is 0.33 ml/min and with a total volume of about 150 ml, this corresponds to a turnover time of about 5 h. The production of CSF is not pressure regulated, and it continues to be produced even if the reabsorption mechanisms are obstructed. The circulation of CSF is as follows:

Lateral ventricle→interventricular foramen of Monroe→third ventricle→aqueduct of sylvius→fourth ventricle→foramen of Magendie (median aperture)/foramen of Luschka (lateral aperture)→subarachnoid space.

The main sites of absorption of CSF are the arachnoid villi that project into the dural venous sinuses, especially the superior sagittal sinus. As the production of CSF from the choroid plexuses is constant, the rate of absorption of CSF through the arachnoid villi controls the CSF pressure. Hydrocephalus therefore occurs due to one of the following:

1. An abnormal increase in the formation of CSF—as occurs in choroid plexus tumors

2. A blockage of the circulation of the fluid—due to obstruction by a tumor or inflammatory exudates secondary to meningitis, or congenital stenosis of cerebral aqueduct
3. A diminished absorption of the fluid—due to inflammatory exudates, venous thrombosis or pressure on the venous sinuses (vein of Galen malformations, developmental anomalies like craniosynostosis), or obstruction of the internal jugular vein

Depending on the above mechanisms of development of hydrocephalus, Dandy classified hydrocephalus into two types:

- Communicating (or nonobstructive)—due to an abnormal rate of production or absorption of CSF
- Noncommunicating (or obstructive)—due to blockage of CSF circulation

A secondary classification based on the etiology of hydrocephalus may also be helpful:

- Congenital—aqueductal stenosis (most common), Dandy–Walker malformations, porencephaly, spina bifida, Chiari I and II malformations, arachnoid cysts
- Hemorrhagic—subarachnoid hemorrhage, intraventricular hemorrhage
- Inflammatory—syphilis, herpes, meningitis, encephalitis, or mumps
- Neoplastic
- Traumatic
- Degenerative

SIGNS AND SYMPTOMS

The clinical presentation of hydrocephalus differs in infants, children, and adults. In infants, the sutures of the skull are not fused and therefore, disproportionate head size, bulging fontanelle, wide separation of the cranial sutures, prominence of scalp veins, increased limb tone, and "setting sun" of the eyes (attributed to pressure on the midbrain tectum by CSF in the suprapineal recess) are the usual presenting signs. Clinical symptoms include general irritability, poor feeding, shrill high-pitched cry, excessive sleepiness, seizures, vomiting, and delayed developmental milestones.

In older children and adults, the clinical presentation depends on chronicity. Acute dilation of the ventricles presents with signs of increased ICP, such as headache, vomiting, nausea, papilloedema, drowsiness, or coma. Unilateral or bilateral sixth nerve palsy may be present. When hydrocephalus has developed insidiously, cognitive impairment, poor concentration, and behavioral changes are seen. Children may also exhibit the Macewen sign, in which a "cracked pot" sound is noted on percussion of the head.

The presence of bradycardia, hypertension, and irregular breathing pattern should alert the clinician to the presence of increased ICP, and therefore warrants prompt intervention to avoid uncal/cerebellar tonsillar herniation and life-threatening brain stem compression.

DIAGNOSIS

In infants, measurement of the occipitofrontal circumference and plotting this on a centile chart provides a simple and sensitive test for diagnosis of hydrocephalus (head circumference >98th percentile for age). Ultrasound is the imaging modality of choice for monitoring infants with an open fontanelle and imaging the size of ventricles. Also, prenatal diagnosis of hydrocephalus is possible with the use of ultrasound.

Computed tomography and magnetic resonance imaging (MRI) provide the most useful and reliable diagnostic tool in the evaluation of the entire ventricular system and also the underlying etiology of hydrocephalus (Figure 1).

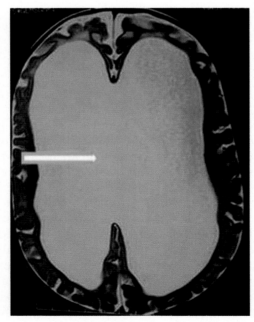

FIGURE 1   A T2-weighted magnetic resonance image of head showing gross dilatation of the lateral ventricles (bold arrow).

- Enlargement of the temporal horns of the lateral ventricles, along with an enlarged third ventricle, favors the diagnosis of hydrocephalus.
- Obliteration of the basal cisterns and effacement of the cortical sulci further support a diagnosis of hydrocephalus with increased ICP.
- Evan's ratio, i.e., the ratio of the largest width of the frontal horns to maximal biparietal diameter, is greater than 30% in hydrocephalus.
- Aqueductal obstruction may be seen as "mickey mouse ventricles" with ballooning of the frontal horns of the lateral ventricles and the third ventricle.
- Upward bowing of the corpus callosum on sagittal MRI suggests acute hydrocephalus.

Other radiological modalities, like skull X-rays, ventriculography, etc. find little scope in modern day practice. Lumbar puncture may be performed to evaluate the CSF in posthemorrhagic and postmeningitic hydrocephalus for protein concentration and to exclude residual infection. Electroencephalography may be obtained in patients with seizures.

PREDISPOSING FACTORS

In neonates, hydrocephalus may occur due to:

1. Intraventricular hemorrhages in premature infants,
2. Infections in the uterus during pregnancy, such as rubella and syphilis,
3. Type II Arnold–Chiari malformation,
4. Aqueduct atresia and stenosis, and
5. Dandy–Walker malformation.

Other factors that can contribute to hydrocephalus among any age group include:

- Lesions or tumors of the brain or spinal cord,
- Central nervous system infections, such as bacterial meningitis or mumps,
- Bleeding in the brain from stroke or head injury,
- Other traumatic injury to the brain.

TREATMENT

Treatment of hydrocephalus is dependent on a number of factors, mainly etiology, severity, age of patient, and response to previous treatments. The patient may be treated conservatively with pharmacotherapy, or surgically using a shunt device or endoscopic third ventriculostomy (ETV).

Medical management: may be tried in patients with hydrocephalus to delay surgical intervention. Acetazolamide (carbonic anhydrase inhibitors) and furosemide have been used to decrease CSF production by the choroid plexus; the effects are, however, not sustained. It may be tried in premature infants with posthemorrhagic hydrocephalus (in the absence of acute hydrocephalus). Pharmacotherapy is only a temporizing measure, and definitive surgical management is needed in the long term.

Surgical management: Bypassing the site of obstruction to CSF flow by diverting the CSF from ventricular cavity to a site where it is readily absorbed is the basic principle underlying the treatment of hydrocephalus. Shunt procedures have, therefore, become the mainstay of treatment in hydrocephalus. ETV is an important alternative in age groups more than one year, for patients with aqueductal stenosis or tumors obstructing flow between the third and fourth ventricle, where there is an adequate CSF reabsorption capacity in the patent subarachnoid space.

The shunt assembly comprises a proximal catheter located in the cerebral ventricles and a distal catheter draining into the selected site of CSF absorption—peritoneal cavity (ventriculoperitoneal shunt), right atrium (ventriculoatrial shunt), or pleural space. A lumboperitoneal shunt is also done in cases of communicating hydrocephalus. The proximal catheter is connected to a one-way resistance valve which controls CSF drainage and is usually placed against the skull, under the skin. The valve designs are based on differential pressures, and may be fixed or programmable. The fixed valves have low, medium, or high pressure alternatives. The operating pressure in programmable valves can be varied by an externally applied magnetic field, so as to prevent overdrainage.

Complications of shunt may be many, and these include:

1. Shunt infection: seen in ~8–10% of all shunt surgeries, especially in the first year of surgery
2. Mechanical complications: like shunt blockage, disconnection, migration, and relative shortening of length
3. Flow-related: CSF overdrainage may lead to subdural hematoma, subdural collections, low-pressure headaches, cranial deformity; and asymmetrical drainage can lead to trapping or isolation of a part of a ventricular system
4. Absorption related: slit ventricular syndrome, ascites, loculations, hydrocele, and perforation of the stomach, large, and small bowel

PROGNOSIS

Prognosis in hydrocephalus depends on the etiology of the disease, age of onset, and the timing of surgical intervention. Review of literature indicates that about half of all children who receive appropriate treatment and follow-up will develop intelligence quotas greater than 85. Patients with congenital hydrocephalus have a better prognostic outcome compared with late onset hydrocephalus due to meningitis. Approximately 50% patients with NPH benefit from shunt installation in the long run.

Further Reading

1. Rekate HL. A contemporary definition and classification of hydrocephalus. *Semin Pediatr Neurol.* March 2009;16(1):9–15.
2. Black PML. Hydrocephalus in adults. In: Youmans JR, ed. *Neurological Surgery.* Philadelphia: WB Saunders Company; 1996:927–944.
3. Hamilton MG. Treatment of hydrocephalus in adults. *Semin Pediatr Neurol.* March 2009;16(1):34–41.
4. Beni-Adani L, Biani N, Ben-Sirah L, Constantini S. The occurrence of obstructive vs absorptive hydrocephalus in newborns and infants: relevance to treatment choices. *Child's Nerv Syst.* December 2006;22(12):1542–1563.
5. Czosnyka M, Whitfield P. Hydrocephalus: a practical guide to CSF dynamics and ventriculoperitoneal shunt. *Adv Clin Neurosci Rehabil.* July/August 2006;6(3):14–17.
6. Factora R, Luciano M. Normal pressure hydrocephalus: diagnosis and new approaches to treatment. *Clin Geriatr Med.* August 2006;22(3):645–657.
7. Kestle JR. Pediatric hydrocephalus: current management. *Neurol Clin.* November 2003;23(4):883–895.
8. Bullivant KJ, Hader W, Hamilton M. A pediatric experience with endoscopic third ventriculostomy for hydrocephalus. *Can J Neurosci Nurs.* March 2009;31(2):16–19.
9. Drake JM. The surgical management of pediatric hydrocephalus. *Neurosurgery.* 2008;62(2):633–642 (February 2008 supplement).
10. Feng H, Huang G, Liao X, et al. Endoscopic third ventriculostomy in the management of obstructive hydrocephalus: an outcome analysis. *J Neurosurg.* April 2004;100(4):626–633.

Normal Perfusion Pressure Breakthrough

Vasudha Singhal[1], Hemanshu Prabhakar[2]

[1]Department of Neuroanaesthesia and Intensive Care, Medanta, The Medicity, Gurgaon, Haryana, India; [2]Department of Neuroanaesthesiology and Critical Care, All India Institute of Medical Sciences, New Delhi, India

DEFINITION

Normal perfusion pressure breakthrough (NPPB) can be defined as the occurrence of multifocal areas of hemorrhage associated with unexplained cerebral edema after the resection of high-flow arteriovenous malformations (AVMs).[1] Various theories have been proposed to explain the hemodynamic basis for this phenomenon.

In 1978, Spetzler and colleagues[2] first introduced the theory of NPPB. They suggested that hypoperfusion of the brain parenchyma surrounding an AVM (caused by an increased blood flow through the low-resistance vascular nidus) could induce local vessels surrounding the AVM nidus to chronically dilate, predisposing them to vasomotor paralysis. Upon restoration of normal perfusion following AVM resection, this impaired autoregulatory capacity may then be unable to compensate for increases in arterial flow and ultimately cause hyperemia, edema, or intracerebral hemorrhage.

However, both the existence and clinical relevance of this theory of NPPB in brain AVMs remain a matter of debate. The incidence of this type of postoperative complication is reported to be lower than 5%.

PATHOPHYSIOLOGY

AVMs are vascular lesions characterized by direct connections between feeding arteries and draining veins without an intervening capillary network. The missing capillary bed creates a low-resistance condition, causing a high flow through the AVM and a hypotensive zone in its immediate vicinity, where the AVM feeders and neighboring normal vessels share the same proximal arterial origin and capillary perfusion pressure is relatively low. This is termed "intracerebral steal," where the increased blood flow through a low-resistance vascular bed diverts flow away from the adjacent brain.[3,4]

Spetzler et al., in their theory of NPPB, proposed that the parenchyma surrounding high-flow AVMs is chronically hypoperfused (due to intracerebral steal) and has an impaired autoregulation mechanism that renders it vulnerable to the restoration of normal perfusion pressure following resection of the AVM. The combination of disturbed autoregulation and normal perfusion pressure results in disruption of local capillary beds, with subsequent hemorrhage and edema.

In NPPB, the capillaries in the adjacent brain parenchyma undergo neovascularization in response to chronic cerebral ischemia through increased capillary density and absent foot processes, making them prone to mechanical weakness, instability, and disruption of the blood–brain barrier, contributing to edema and hemorrhage.[5]

Apart from the NPPB theory, the postoperative hemorrhage and edema following AVM resection have been explained by various other hypotheses. An alternative theory, called the "occlusive hyperemia" theory,[6] proposed a mechanism involving both the arterial feeders and the venous drainage systems, accounting for the postoperative complications. Both the stagnant arterial flow in the former AVM feeders with subsequent worsening of existing hypoperfusion and ischemia, and the venous outflow obstruction in the adjacent parenchyma causing passive hyperemia, engorgement, and further arterial stagnation, contribute to the postoperative hemorrhage and edema significantly. An impairment of the venous drainage system has been noted in up to 75% of the patients with high-flow AVMs.

Such venous overload is seen not only after surgical excision of AVMs but also after embolization of high-flow lesions. Occlusion of the draining venous system in the brain, adjacent to the AVM by a glue embolus, may result in venous outflow obstruction, passive hyperemia, and stagnation in the feeding artery, with subsequent postoperative hemorrhage and edema.[7]

PRESENTATION

Patients with NPPB may present with development of intracranial hemorrhage or with signs of cerebral edema, such as deterioration in GCS, seizures, and fresh neurological deficits, in the immediate postoperative period. Unreversed patients may exhibit delayed awakening or an abnormal pupillary response or focal neurological deficits.

TREATMENT

Postoperative patients presenting with hemorrhage may need to be taken up for urgent evacuation. Intracranial pressure-lowering maneuvers, such as hyperventilation, administration of mannitol, and tight control of blood pressure, need to be adopted for cerebral protection.

As regards perioperative management, NPPB should be diagnosed only after all other correctable causes for malignant brain swelling or bleeding have been excluded.

PREVENTION

Various techniques to reduce the incidence of edema and hemorrhage after AVM obliteration[8,9] include:

- Staged embolization of large AVMs
- Proximal arterial feeder ligation
- Systemic hypotension

In patients with a particularly intense steal phenomenon, arteries are maximally dilated under disautoregulation in the surrounding brain, causing a hyperemic state. At this stage, breakthrough bleeding from the vessels of the impaired surrounding brain (intraoperative NPPB) can be caused by faulty surgical strategies, including (1) occlusion of the drainer in the presence of the residual feeder and (2) inappropriate hemostatic operation for expanded capillaries into which arterial blood flows, i.e., insufficient time or intensity of coagulation. Intraoperative bleeding control should be tackled by managing feeders over 1 mm in diameter with hemoclips, along with adequate capillary coagulation.[10]

Blood pressure control is vital in managing hyperemic complications following complete resection of cerebral AVMs. A direct temporal relationship exists between the cause-and-effect association of hyperperfusion and induced systemic hypotension with resolution of neurological symptoms.[11]

DOES NPPB REALLY EXIST?

NPPB is attributed to cerebral hyperemia due to repressurization of previously hypotensive regions with a loss of autoregulation. More recent investigations, however, contradict many aspects of this theory, casting doubt on the link between impaired vasoreactivity and postoperative complications in the following ways[12]:

- Cerebral hyperemia after an AVM resection is global and is not limited to the ipsilateral side of the AVM.[13] This suggests that mechanisms implicating preoperative focal hypoperfusion due to vascular steal are not the sole cause of postoperative complications.
- There is no relationship between cerebral blood flow changes after resection and the degree of arterial hypotension induced by AVM shunts.[13]
- In hypotensive regions, autoregulatory response is not impaired but is intact and shifted to the left (adaptive autoregulatory displacement),[14] conceptually analogous to the adaptive displacement seen with chronic hypertension and its treatment.
- Cerebrovascular reactivity to carbon dioxide is preserved after AVM resection,[15] suggesting that the vessels in previously hypotensive territories are not paralyzed but have an intact autoregulation.

References

1. Mattei TA. Pathophysiology of normal perfusion pressure breakthrough: more than just abnormal arteries. *Br J Neurosurg*. October 2012;26(5):786–787.
2. Spetzler RF, Wilson CB, Weinstein P, et al. Normal perfusion pressure breakthrough theory. *Clin Neurosurg*. 1978;25:651–672.
3. Taylor CL, Selman WR, Ratcheson RA. Steal affecting the central nervous system. *Neurosurgery*. 2002;50:679–688. discussion 688–89.

4. Symon L. The concept of intracerebral steal. *Int Anesthesiol Clin.* 1969;7:597–615.
5. Sekhon LH, Morgan MK, Spence I. Normal perfusion pressure breakthrough: the role of capillaries. *J Neurosurg.* 1997;86(3):519–524.
6. Al-Rodhan NRF, Sundt Jr TM, Piepgras DG, Nichols DA, Rufenacht D, Stevens LN. Occlusive hyperemia: a theory for the haemodynamic complications following resection of intracerebral arteriovenous malformations. *J Neurosurg.* 1993;78:167–176.
7. Wilson CB, Hieshimia G. A new way to think about an old problem. *J Neurosurg.* 1993;78:165–166.
8. Massoud TF, Hademenos GJ, Young WL, Gao E, Spellman JP. Can induction of systemic hypotension help prevent nidus rupture complicating arteriovenous malformation embolization? Analysis of underlying mechanism achieved using a theoretical model. *Am J Neuroradiol.* 2000;21(7):1255–1267.
9. Zhao JZ, Wang S, Li JS, Sui DL, Zhao YL, Zhang Y. Combination of intraoperative embolisation with surgical resection for treatment of giant cerebral arteriovenous malformations. *J Clin Neurosci.* 2000;7(1):54–59.
10. Kumar S, Kato Y, Sano H, Imizu S, Nagahisa S, Kanno T. Normal perfusion pressure breakthrough in arteriovenous malformation surgery: the concept revisited with a case report. *Neurol India.* January–March, 2004;52(1):111–115.
11. O'Connor TE, Fargen KM, Mocco J. Normal perfusion pressure breakthrough following AVM resection: a case report and review of the literature. *Open J Mod Neurosurg.* 2013;3:66–71.
12. Alexander MA, Connolly ES, Meyers PM. Revisiting normal perfusion pressure breakthrough in light of hemorrhage-induced vasospasm. *World J Radiol.* June 28, 2010;2(6):230–232.
13. Young WL, Kader A, Ornstein E, et al. Cerebral hyperemia after arteriovenous malformation resection is related to "breakthrough" complications but not to feeding artery pressure. Columbia University AVM study project. *Neurosurgery.* 1996;38:1085–1093.
14. Young WL, Pile-Spellman J, Prohovnik I, et al. Columbia University AVM study project: evidence for adaptive autoregulatory displacement in hypotensive cortical territories adjacent to arteriovenous malformations. *Neurosurgery.* 1994;34:601–610.
15. Young WL, Prohovnik I, Ornstein E, et al. The effect of arteriovenous malformation resection on cerebrovascular reactivity to carbon dioxide. *Neurosurgery.* 1990;27:257–267.

Pneumocephalus

Hemanshu Prabhakar, Parmod K. Bithal

Department of Neuroanaesthesiology and Critical Care, All India Institute
of Medical Sciences, New Delhi, India

DEFINITION

Pneumocephalus is defined as an asymptomatic intracranial collection of air, commonly occurring after craniotomy or cranial burr hole. In a retrospective study, the incidence of intracranial air collection varied from 73% in park-bench position, 57% in prone position, and 100% in sitting position.[1] Clinical data on the retrospective review of CT scans indicate that all patients have pneumocephalus in the first 2 days after a supratentorial craniotomy.[2]

VARIANT

Occasionally, high pressure may build up in the air cavity, which results in the development of "tension pneumocephalus," or "inverted pop-up bottle" syndrome. Tension pneumocephalus is, therefore, air in the intracranial compartment that is under pressure and requires immediate evacuation.

CAUSE

The collection of air in the cranial vault is either due to drainage of cerebrospinal fluid, or due to venous blood moving out of the cranium, as in the sitting position, which reduces the brain bulk. Similarly, intraoperative hyperventilation shrinks the brain secondary to hypocapnia. All this creates room for the air to collect, and if not corrected at the end of the procedure, pneumocephalus develops. Some of the common causes for the development of pneumocephalus include the following:

1. Recent craniotomy or craniectomy[3]
2. Prolonged surgery in sitting position
3. Following awake craniotomy
4. Trauma, skull-base fracture, fracture of the skull with laceration of dura
5. Infection, with gas-forming organisms, such as mastoiditis
6. After ventriculostomy
7. Spinal or epidural anesthesia
8. Following surgery on the spine
9. Intravenous catheterization (rarely)
10. Spontaneous pneumocephalus[4]
11. Positive pressure mask ventilation in postoperative patients of transsphenoidal pituitary surgery[5]
12. Use of drugs such as Cabergoline[6]

SIGNS AND SYMPTOMS

Some of the common signs and symptoms are as follows:

1. Deterioration of consciousness with or without lateralizing signs
2. Severe restlessness

3. Generalized convulsions
4. Delayed recovery from anesthesia
5. Arterial hypertension and reflex bradycardia

DIAGNOSIS

The diagnosis of pneumocephalus can be made clinically based on a high index of suspicion. However, a computed tomographic scan can easily diagnose pneumocephalus (Figure 1). The intracranial gas may also be detected by a plain X-ray of the skull. Mt. Fuji sign is very characteristic of pneumocephalus, especially if it is located bilaterally. The sign is characterized by the peaked frontal lobes, which are surrounded and separated by air.

PREDISPOSING FACTORS

Several contributing factors have been implicated in the pathogenesis of pneumocephalus, producing tension effect: nitrous oxide anesthesia, duration of surgery, gross hydrocephalus, a functional ventriculoperitoneal

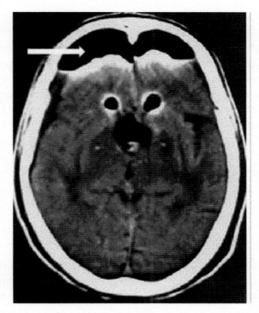

FIGURE 1   A computed tomographic scan showing a large collection of air (bold white arrow).

BOX 1

Factors contributing to development of tension pneumocephalus.

1. Nitrous oxide anesthesia
2. Duration of surgery
3. Gross hydrocephalus
4. Presence of a functional ventriculoperitoneal shunt
5. Intraoperative mannitol or furosemide administration
6. Size of air cavity
7. Surgical position of patient (always observed in sitting position)
8. Head position after surgery

---

shunt, intraoperative mannitol or furosemide administration, size of the air cavity, surgical position of the patient, and position of the head after surgery (Box 1).

TREATMENT

In majority of the cases, pneumocephalus is asymptomatic and requires conservative treatment. In the absence of leaking cerebrospinal fluid, the entrapped air gradually gets absorbed and the pneumocephalus resolves. However, treatment of the primary cause may be essential, especially if pneumocephalus is due to gas-forming organisms. Appropriate antibiotics may be started for control of infection. During the postoperative period, pneumocephalus may be treated by pure oxygen through a face mask that facilitates resorption and prevents desaturation in case of breathing difficulties.

Active intervention is needed in cases of tension pneumocephalus. An emergent frontal twist drill burr hole aspiration of pneumocephalus producing significant symptoms is the treatment of choice. A clinically significant improvement is seen following burr hole evacuation.

PREVENTION

To prevent the development of pneumocephalus, efforts must be directed at minimizing loss of cerebrospinal fluid, maintaining adequate hydration for proper cerebral perfusion, and allowing the brain to regain its normal contour by bringing the end-tidal carbon dioxide to normal levels toward the end of surgery. Subdural injection of saline to displace the residual air may also be useful. Prompt detection of the intracranial hypertension caused by tension pneumocephalus is aided by intracranial pressure monitoring. However, the benefits of intracranial pressure monitoring in the immediate postoperative period must be weighed against the associated risks and complications.

References

1. Toung TJ, McPherson RW, Ahn H, Donham RT, Alano J, Long D. Pneumocephalus: effects of patient position on the incidence and location of aerocele after posterior fossa and upper cervical cord surgery. *Anesth Analg.* 1986;65:65–70.
2. Reasoner DK, Todd MM, Scamman FL, Warner DS. The incidence of pneumocephalus after supratentotial craniotomy. Observations on the disappearance of intracranial air. *Anesthesiology.* 1994;80:1008–1012.
3. Prabhakar H, Bithal PK, Garg A. Tension pneumocephalus after craniotomy in supine position. *J Neurosurg Anesthesiol.* 2003;15:278–281.
4. Nash R, Wilson M, Adams M, Kitchen N. Spontaneous pneumocephalus presenting with alien limb phenomena. *J Laryngol Otol.* 2012;126:733–736.
5. Kopelovich JC, de la Garza GO, Greenlee JD, Graham SM, Udeh CI, O'Brien EK. Pneumocephalus with BiPAP use after transsphenoidal surgery. *J Clin Anesth.* 2012;24:415–418.
6. Machicado JD, Varghese JM, Orlander PR. Cabergoline-induced pneumocephalus in a medically treated macroprolactinoma. *J Clin Endocrinol Metab.* 2012;97:3412–3413.

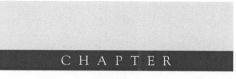

CHAPTER

6

Seizures

Hemanshu Prabhakar, Parmod K. Bithal

Department of Neuroanaesthesiology and Critical Care, All India Institute
of Medical Sciences, New Delhi, India

DEFINITION

Seizure activities are not only difficult to diagnose intraoperative in an anesthetized patient; they are also less recognized clinically, as compared to postoperative seizures in the intensive care unit. Seizure activity may be evident only in cases of incomplete muscle paralysis or use of electrocorticography (ECoG) in the intraoperative period.

Postoperative seizures are, however, a well-recognized entity and defined as seizures with a short onset time, usually occurring in the immediate postoperative period. Nearly 24–38% of all seizures occur during the first 24–72 h postoperative period. Recent data show that the overall incidence of seizures in the postoperative period after surgery for brain tumors is low (8%), even without prophylactic antiepileptic drugs, and the incidence of clinically significant seizure is even lower (3%).[1]

Seizures in the postoperative period put patients at risk of developing cerebral acidosis, brain edema, and raised intracranial pressure.[2]

VARIANTS

Seizures may be focal or generalized. Recognition may be delayed due to the residual anesthetic effect. A rare possibility of nonconvulsive seizures cannot be overlooked. However, this is beyond the scope of this book.

CAUSE

Surgery in the supratentorial compartment carries the risk of seizures. A preexisting history of seizures, an underlying pathology, surgery involving motor cortex, and cortical damage may predispose to seizures in the postoperative period. Intraoperative seizures have been attributed to certain anesthetics. Enflurane is probably the most common proconvulsant anesthetic, although seizure activities have also been reported with use of halothane, isoflurane, and even sevoflurane. Desflurane has shown no proconvulsant activity in humans. Among the intravenous anesthetics, methohexital, ketamine, etomidate, and propofol have shown proconvulsant activities. Seizure-like activities may be observed with use of fentanyl, sufentanil, and alfentanil, but not with morphine and meperidine, at least in humans.[3] Seizures resulting from an overdose toxicity of local anesthetics is also well known.

Postsurgical complications, such as hematoma formation, pneumocephalus, developing infarction, or cortical ischemia, may produce seizures. Posttraumatic or head-injured patients are likely to develop early or delayed seizures.

A common cause of postoperative seizure is alcohol withdrawal, though intraoperative electrolyte imbalance may rarely cause this complication. Febrile convulsions and seizures due to infection are also known.

Although the exact mechanism of development of postoperative seizure remains obscure, free radical formation, disturbed ionic balance, and release of excitatory amino acids have been implicated.[4]

DIAGNOSIS

The diagnosis is clinical and easily recognized in awake postoperative patients. Intraoperative seizure activity can only be monitored under anesthesia with use of ECoG or electroencephalogram.[5]

PREDISPOSING FACTORS

The following are the factors implicated in the development of seizures during the perioperative period:

1. Previous history of seizures
2. Extent of cortical injury
3. Metabolic derangements in the postoperative period, such as hypoxia, hypernatremia (sodium levels more than 160 mEq/L), hyponatremia (sodium levels less than 110 mEq/L), acidosis, and hyperglycemia
4. Surgical retraction
5. Extraaxial lesions, such as aneurysms
6. Inadequate serum levels of antiepileptics
7. Benign tumors
8. Location of tumors, such as supratentorial tumors (those near motor strip area)

COMPLICATIONS

The following are the complications that one should anticipate resulting from seizure activities:

1. Airway obstruction
2. Injury to extremities
3. Structural brain injury
4. Increased risk of cerebral acidosis, cerebral edema, and increased intracranial pressure
5. Hypertension and tachycardia
6. Increased body temperature

TREATMENT

The treatment consists of both symptomatic and specific measures such as the following:

1. Administer 100% oxygen
2. Benzodiazepines such as midazolam

3. Load antiepileptics
4. Tracheal intubation if airway is compromised, and mechanical ventilation of lungs, especially if antiepileptics have resulted in respiratory depression

PREVENTION

Some of the preventive measures suggested for the control of seizures are as follows:

1. Prophylactic antiepileptic therapy of up to 16 weeks
2. Phenytoin 15 mg/kg (about 1 g) over 20 min prior to wound closure followed by 5–6 mg/kg/day (in divided doses) postoperatively
3. Therapeutic serum levels of phenytoin 10 to 20 µg/ml

However, authors of a recently published systematic review found little evidence to suggest that antiepileptic drugs administered prophylactically is effective or not effective in preventing postcraniotomy seizures.[6] In a recent trial on patients with supratentorial meningiomas, authors found that the change in ECoG before and after resection in patients with supratentorial meningioma has a predictive value for early postoperative seizures.[7]

References

1. Manaka S, Ishijima B, Mayanagi Y. Postoperative seizures: epidemiology, pathology and prophylaxis. *Neurol Med Chir Tokyo*. 2003;43:589–600.
2. Wu AS, Trinh VT, Suki D, et al. A prospective randomized trial of perioperative seizure prophylaxis in patients with intraparenchymal brain tumors. *J Neurosurg*. February 8, 2013. [Epub ahead of print].
3. Herrick IA. Seizure activity and anesthetic agents and adjuvants. In: Albin MS, ed. *Text Book of Neuroanesthesia with Neurosurgical and Neuroscience Perspectives*. US: The McGraw-Hill Companies Inc.; 1997:625–642.
4. Layon AJ, Stachniak JB, Day AL. Neurointensive care. In: Cucchiara RF, Black S, Michenfelder JD, eds. *Clinical Neuroanesthesia*. 2nd ed. New York: Churchill-Livingstone Inc; 1998:557–610.
5. Elgueta MF, Vega P, Lema G, Clede L. Should we monitor with bispectral index in all patients at high risk for seizures in the operating room? *Rev Esp Anestesiol Reanim*. September 1, 2012. [Epub ahead of print].
6. Pulman J, Greenhalgh J, Marson AG. Antiepileptic drugs as prophylaxis for post-craniotomy seizures. *Cochrane Database Syst Rev*. 2013;2:CD007286. http://dx.doi.org/10.1002/14651858.CD007286.
7. Fang S, Zhan Y, Xie YF, Shi Q, Dan W. Predictive value of electrocorticography for postoperative epilepsy in patients with supratentorial meningioma. *J Clin Neurosci*. 2013;20:112–116.

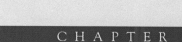

CHAPTER

7

Brain Swelling and Tense Brain

Gyaninder P. Singh, Indu Kapoor

**Department of Neuroanaesthesiology and Critical Care, All India Institute
of Medical Sciences, New Delhi, India**

OUTLINE

Edema refers to abnormal, excessive accumulation of fluid in the cells,
tissues, or body cavities. Brain edema results from excess accumulation of
water in the extracellular and/or intracellular compartments of the brain.
The brain is protected by a closed, rigid cranial cavity that contains brain
tissue, cerebrospinal fluid (CSF), and intravascular blood. Any increase in
either of its components is compensated by reduction or displacement of the

TABLE 1   Classification of Brain Swelling

Vasogenic	Due to shift of fluid from intravascular compartment to extracellular space
Cytotoxic	Due to shift of fluid from extracellular to intracellular compartment
Interstitial	Due to shift of cerebrospinal fluid into the extracellular space
Hyperemic	Due to increase in intravascular volume

other (known as the Monro-Kellie doctrine). If the brain volume increases, the first component to decrease is blood followed by displacement of CSF. The compensation is limited due to the fixed rigid space after the fusion of fontanelles. In adults, due to an unyielding skull, the initial compensatory mechanisms get exhausted early and any further increase in volume of intracranial components leads to a rise in the intracranial pressure (ICP).

Brain swelling, leading to tense brain, may even occur after opening the cranial cavity during a craniotomy. If the tension within the cranial cavity is high, after a craniotomy, the brain may bulge along with the dura mater through the cranial opening. Intraoperatively, brain swelling may occur due to various reasons, causing the brain to become tense. The brain swelling may be classified into four types (see Table 1).[1]

ETIOLOGY

The brain has three anatomical compartments where the excessive fluid can accumulate: the cellular compartment (neurons and supporting cells), the extracellular compartment (interstitial and CSF spaces), and the vascular compartment (arteries, veins, and capillaries). Volume expansion of any one or more of these compartments causes bulk enlargement of brain.

Cellular Compartment

Excessive uptake of fluid by cellular elements of the brain can lead to brain swelling. Derangement of cellular metabolism results in inadequate functioning of energy-dependent Na^+-K^+ pump of the cell membrane, causing cellular retention of Na^+ and water. This process causes the cell to swell (*cytotoxic edema*) (Figure 1(b)). Such swelling occurs during cerebral ischemia. Cytotoxic edema is typically seen after exposure to various intoxicants such as methionine sulfoximine, hydrogen cyanide, lead, hexachlorophene, isoniazid, and so forth; it is also seen in Reye's syndrome.

Extracellular Compartment

Excessive accumulation of fluid in the interstitial space and/or CSF cavities causes the brain to swell. It may occur as a consequence of

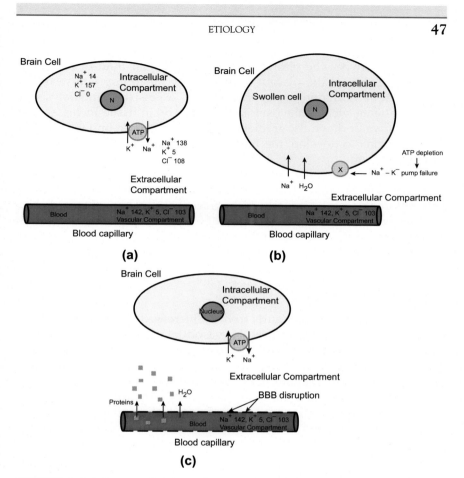

FIGURE 1   Mechanism of brain swelling: (a) normal brain, (b) cytotoxic edema, and (c) vasogenic edema.

disruption of the blood–brain barrier (BBB) with increased permeability of cerebral capillaries (*vasogenic edema* (VE)); osmotic gradient between the plasma and brain extracellular fluid with intact BBB (*osmotic edema*); or due to obstruction of interstitial fluid or CSF outflow (*compressive and hydrocephalic edema*).

VE is the most common type of extracellular edema and is seen in response to head injuries, tumors, infections, inflammations, and cerebrovascular accidents. Disruption of BBB causes intravascular proteins and fluid to penetrate into brain parenchymal extracellular space (Figure 1(c)).[2] The magnitude of edema depends on various factors like severity of BBB dysfunction, size of the lesion, and duration of barrier opening. It increases proportionally with the increase in mean arterial pressure. VE is seen more in the white matter due to lower resistance compared to gray matter which has greater density.

Osmotic edema results when an unfavorable osmotic gradient is established between the plasma and the extracellular fluid of the brain. If the osmolarity of the plasma decreases (e.g., inappropriate secretion of antidiuretic hormone, water intoxication, excessive hemodialysis of uremic patients, etc.) or the osmolarity of the brain tissue increases, the passage of water down the gradient occurs, creating cerebral edema. For osmotic edema to develop, the BBB must be intact to maintain effective osmotic gradient.

Obstruction to the flow of interstitial fluid due to compression by any mass (e.g., a large tumor) may cause the edema of the surrounding tissue (compressive edema). Similarly, in hydrocephalic edema, obstruction to the drainage of CSF leads to collection of CSF proximal to the block, thus causing distention of cavities and retrograde flooding of the extracellular compartment (periventricular edema).

Vascular Compartment

Cerebral engorgement results from an increase in the cerebral blood volume (CBV). It may be caused by vasodilatation or venous outflow obstruction. In the normal brain, the cerebral autoregulation maintains the cerebral blood flow (CBF) according to the physiologic requirement of the brain by regulating the tone and caliber of cerebral arteries and arterioles. However, various pathological conditions (e.g., febrile infections, seizures, malignant hypertension, global ischemia, etc.) may alter metabolic demand and/or disturb arterial tone and caliber. This causes profound arterial dilatation, which may lead to hyperemia and congestion of brain. Obstruction of the cerebral veins or venous dural sinuses also causes congestion of the brain. Venous outflow obstruction can be caused by bacterial meningitis, parasagittal tumors, subdural abscesses, polycythemia, head injury, compression of neck veins, right heart failure, and so forth.

PATHOPHYSIOLOGY OF VE

A cascade of events occurs after injury to the BBB. Filtration of plasma constituents into the brain's extracellular compartment causes reduction in local CBF. It occurs due to volume expansion of the extracellular compartment and an increase in local tissue pressure that compromises the regional microcirculation. This leads to tissue acidosis and formation, and release of toxic substances (bradykinins, glutamate, arachidonic acid, leukotrienes) that further aggravate the edema by increasing the cerebral capillary permeability.[3]

PATHOPHYSIOLOGY OF CYTOTOXIC EDEMA

The molecular cascade initiated by cerebral ischemia results in membrane ionic pump failure. Cellular survival requires Na^+ to be continuously extruded from the intracellular compartment to maintain normal cell volume. Na^+/K^+ ATPase (ionic pump) is energy dependent and requires continuous expenditure of ATP. Cerebral insult leading to ischemia and hypoxia causes depletion of ATP. This is accompanied by an unchecked influx of extracellular ions, mainly Na^+, down their electrochemical gradients.[4] Na^+ influx in turn drives Cl^- inside the cell via chloride channels, and the resultant increase in intracellular osmolarity drives inflow of water (via aquaporin (AQP) channels, among others),[4-6] thereby causing the cells to swell.

Cytotoxic edema occurs in cells of both white and gray matter and astrocytes are more prone for swelling than neurons.[4]

SIGNS AND SYMPTOMS

Signs and symptoms of brain swelling are due to increased ICP. Consistent with the Monro-Kellie doctrine, the consequences of focal or global cerebral edema can be lethal. There may be cerebral ischemia from compromised CBF and increased ICP, causing herniation of brain tissue and resulting in compression of vital brain structures.[7] Elevation of ICP may or may not accompany cerebral edema and yet the cerebral herniation may occur, particularly in patients with focal edema.

Symptoms and signs of brain swelling include headache, dizziness, nausea and vomiting, numbness or weakness, loss of coordination or balance, loss or change of vision, inability to speak, seizures, lethargy, memory loss, irritability, altered behavior, and altered level of consciousness or coma. In infants, the fontanelles may bulge, the head may increase in size, cries may be high-pitched or shrill, and irritability or feeding difficulties may occur. In later stages, abnormalities of vital signs (bradycardia, hypertension) and cardiorespiratory collapse may occur.

CAUSES OF BRAIN SWELLING

Brain swelling can result from numerous causes, including head trauma, infections, brain tumors, stroke, exposure to certain toxins, complications of diabetes (diabetic ketoacidosis), electrolyte imbalance, malignant hypertension, and high altitude sickness.

Intraoperatively, the brain may swell and bulge through the cranial opening due to various reasons. The obstruction to the venous drainage

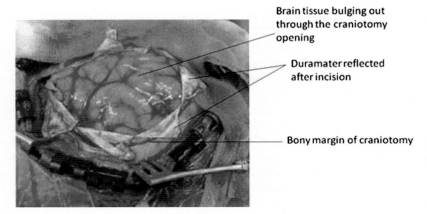

FIGURE 2   The intraoperative tense brain bulging out through the craniotomy opening, after opening the dura mater.

(compression of the neck veins due to excessive flexion or rotation of the neck), rise in intrathoracic pressure (caused by kinking of endotracheal tube, bronchospasm, pulmonary embolus, pneumothorax, venous air embolism causing obstruction to pulmonary outflow, compression of chest or abdomen during prone position), or acute rise in heart rate and blood pressure (due to light plane of anesthesia or inadequate muscle relaxation causing patient movement or bucking over the endotracheal tube, urinary retention,[8] etc.) may all lead to tense brain during the surgery (Figure 2).

DIAGNOSIS

Diagnosis of the brain swelling or edema can be made by clinical signs and symptoms and by radiological findings. An increase in the water content of the brain is seen as a decrease in density, and it appears dark on a computed tomography (CT) scan. On magnetic resonance (MR) imaging, an increase in water molecules is seen as an area of decreased signal (black) on T_1-weighted studies and as an area of increased signal (white) on T_2-weighted studies.

VE primarily involves the white matter of the brain and is thus seen as areas of decreased density on CT and MR (T_1-weighted) that extend along the white matter projections interposed between the normal gray matter (Figure 3(a)). Cytotoxic edema involves both gray and white matter and thus the decreased density on CT and MR (T_1-weighted) can be seen in both the white and gray matter (Figure 3(b)).

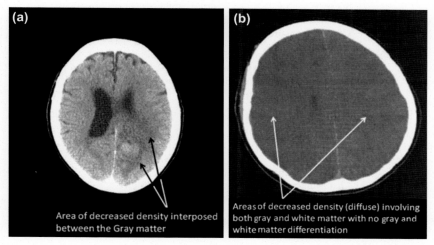

FIGURE 3 Computed tomography scan of brain, showing (a) areas of decreased density interposed between the gray matter (VE) and (b) areas of decreased density involving both gray and white matter (cytotoxic edema) with no gray and white matter differentiation.

TREATMENT

Prompt recognition of these clinical syndromes and institution of targeted therapies is vital to preserve neurologic function, assure a satisfactory clinical outcome, and prevent mortality. Brain edema causes increases in ICP, reduced CBF, inadequate oxygen delivery, energy failure, and further increases of edema. One of the goals of treatment is to interrupt this vicious cycle.[9] Various general and specific measures to prevent and treat cerebral edema are enumerated in Table 2.

General Measures

The principal aim of these measures is to optimize the cerebral perfusion, oxygenation, ionic and osmolar gradients, and venous drainage, while also minimizing cerebral metabolic demands and limiting further increases of edema.

1. *Head elevation and optimizing neck position*: Neutral head position avoids jugular venous compression and impedance of venous outflow from the cranial cavity.[7] Compression around the neck (such as by the tight neck collars or the ribbons used for securing endotracheal tubes) may cause impairment of cerebral venous drainage. Extreme neck flexion or rotation and compression around the neck should thus be avoided. Head elevation to around 30 °C facilitates the cerebrovenous

TABLE 2   Management of Brain Edema

General measures

1. Head elevation and optimizing neck position
2. Ventilation and oxygenation
3. Maintenance of cerebral perfusion pressure
4. Management of hyperglycemia
5. Management of fever
6. Seizure prophylaxis
7. Nutritional support

Specific measures

1. Hyperventilation
2. Osmotherapy (mannitol, hypertonic saline)
3. Loop diuretics (furosemide)
4. Corticosteroids
5. Anti-inflammatory agents
6. Antihypertensive drugs
7. Pharmacological coma
8. Analgesia, sedation, and paralysis
9. Therapeutic hypothermia
10. CSF drainage
11. Operative decompression

drainage and decreases ICP. However, elevation of the head may reduce cerebral perfusion pressure (CPP) and may compromise perfusion to ischemic areas. Thus, both the benefits and risks of head elevation should be carefully considered.

2. *Ventilation and oxygenation*: Both hypoxia and hypercapnia are potent cerebral vasodilators and should be avoided. Patients with low GCS (<9), poor airway reflexes or associated pulmonary insult (e.g. aspiration, contusion, pulmonary edema) should be intubated and ventilation supported. Maintenance of PaO_2 at approximately 100 mm Hg and $PaCO_2$ around 35 mm Hg is recommended.[10] Use of positive end-expiratory pressure during mechanical ventilation (which may be required to maintain adequate oxygenation), may cause increase in central venous pressure and impedance to cerebral venous outflow. This may aggravate cerebral edema and ICP.

3. *Maintenance of CPP*: An adequate amount of isotonic fluids should be used to maintain euvolemia or mild hypervolemia. The goal is to maintain CPP greater than 60 mm Hg with adequate fluid management and use of vasopressor if required. Avoid use of hypotonic fluids and systemic dehydration.

4. *Management of hyperglycemia*: Hyperglycemia can exacerbate brain injury and cerebral edema.[7,11,12] A number of studies have shown that an increased glucose level following injury to the brain is

associated with elevated ICP and increased mortality.[12–16] On the other hand, several studies have demonstrated that tight glycemic control by intensive insulin therapy in head-injured patients leads to increased incidences of hypoglycemia[17–19] and decreased neurological outcome.[20,21] Hence, treatment of hyperglycemia should be based on frequent glucose monitoring and strict precaution to prevent hypoglycemia.[22]

5. *Management of fever*: Deleterious effects of fever on outcome following brain injury have been demonstrated by various authors. Fever causes an increase in oxygen demand and normothermia is strongly recommended in patients with cerebral edema, irrespective of its cause.[7] Acetaminophen in the dose of 325–650 mg orally every 4–6 h or surface cooling methods may be used to control a rise in body temperature.[7]

6. *Seizure prophylaxis*: Anticonsulvants (phenytoin) are used empirically in clinical practice as subclinical seizure activity may cause worsening of edema. However, the benefit of prophylactic use of anticonsvultants in most causes of cerebral edema remains unproven.[7]

7. *Nutritional support*: Prompt institution and maintenance of nutrition is desirable in all patients with brain injury. However, free water intake should be avoided, which may lead to a hypoosmolar state and worsen brain edema.[7] Enteral route of nutrition is preferred unless contraindicated.

Specific Measures

1. *Controlled hyperventilation*: It remains an efficacious therapeutic intervention for control of cerebral edema. Hyperventilation causes a decrease in $PaCO_2$ and a proportional decrease in CBF and CBV. However, aggressive hyperventilation may result in cerebral ischemia.[23] Therefore, the target is to maintain $PaCO_2$ level of approximately 30–35 mm Hg. Vasoconstrictive effect of hyperventilation lasts for 10–20 h beyond which vascular dilatation resulting in an exacerbation of cerebral edema and a rebound rise in ICP may occur. Controlled hyperventilation is used as a rescue for short duration (not beyond 24 h) until more definitive therapies are instituted. Hyperventilation is judiciously reversed over next 6–24 h to avoid cerebral hyperemia and rebound increase in cerebral edema and ICP.[7,24]

2. *Osmotherapy*: Various hyperosmotic agents (urea, glycerol, concentrated human proteins) have been used to ameliorate cerebral edema. However, these are no longer used due to adverse effects, short duration of action, and cost. Mannitol and Hypertonic saline are the major osmotic agent of choice in clinical practice.

Hyperosmolar agents create an osmotic gradient and cause egress of water from the brain tissue into the vasculature. Mannitol (alcohol derivative) is stable in solution and has a long duration of action (4–6h). It is used in a dose of 0.25–1.5mg/kg given intravenously over 30–60min. The maximal effect is observed in 20–40min following administration. Dose may be repeated every 6h and serum osmolality value should not exceed beyond 320mOsm/L. Hypertonic saline in various concentrations (2, 3, 7.5, 10, and 23%) is available. The goal is to increase serum sodium concentration to 145–155mEq/L (serum osmolality around 300–320mOsm/L). Central venous pressure is used to guide the fluid to maintain normovolemia. Adverse effects of mannitol include hypotension, hyperkalemia, renal insufficiency, and pulmonary edema.[7] Hypertonic saline may cause metabolic acidosis, hypokalemia, oliguria, and permanent renal damage. Myelinolysis, during hypertonic saline therapy, typically occurs with rapid correction in serum sodium. According to the Cochrane Database of Systemic Reviews, hypertonic saline significantly reduces the risk of tense brain during craniotomy. A single trial included in this review showed that the duration of intensive care unit and hospital stay are comparable with both mannitol and hypertonic saline.[25]

3. *Loop diuretics*: Furosemide (10–20mg) is the most commonly used drug. Use of this drug along with mannitol produces profound diuresis and may cause volume depletion.[26] However, in another study authors have found that mannitol increases plasma osmolality and reduced water content of the injured and contralateral hemispheres, whereas furosemide has no effect when given alone or in combination with mannitol.[27] Furosemide also has antiepileptic activity regardless of the underlying synaptic and physiologic mechanisms generating the seizure activity.[28]

4. *Steroids*: The main indication for the use of steroids is for the treatment of vasogenic brain edema present along with brain tumors by decreasing tight junction permeability and stabilizing BBB. Dexamethasone (8–32mg) is the preferred agent because of low mineralocorticoid activity.[29,30] Based on the evidence available to date, the treatment with dexamethasone is recommended for symptom relief in adult patients with primary high-grade glioma and cerebral edema.[31] Less consistent response is seen in the treatment of perifocal edema with cerebral abscess, bacterial meningitis, tuberculous infection, and postoperative cerebral edema.[1]

5. *Anti-inflammatory agents*: Nonsteroidal anti-inflammatory drugs (indomethacin, probenecid, ibuprofen) have been found to reduce VE (by reducing vascular permeability) associated with brain tumors.[1]

6. *Antihypertensive drugs*: Formation and spread of VE is directly related to systemic arterial pressure. Thus, any rise in systemic blood pressure should be treated using antihypertensives such as esmolol, labetalol, and enalaprilat. Potent vasodilator (nitroglycerine, nitroprusside) should be avoided as they may exacerbate cerebral edema due to vasodilatation of cerebral vessels.

7. *Analgesia, sedation, and paralysis*: Pain, restlessness, and agitation can all worsen brain edema and increase ICP. Judicious use of analgesics and sedative (morphine, fentanyl, and midazolam) should be used. Paralysis with nondepolarizing agents is used only in refractory cases to control ICP in conjunction with other measures.

8. *CSF drainage*: CSF drainage may be used to resolve the periventricular edema associated with hydrocephalus (interstitial edema).[1]

9. *Pharmacological coma*: This therapy is indicated only for the treatment of cerebral edema associated with refractory increase in ICP. Drugs act by reducing the cerebral metabolic activity, thereby causing coupled reduction in CBF and CBV. This causes lowering of ICP. Barbiturates (pentobarbital or thiopental) are used to produce pharmacological coma. Recommended regimen for pentobarbital is a bolus loading dose of 3–10 mg/kg intravenously followed by continuous intravenous infusion (0.5–3.0 mg/kg/h) titrated to achieve burst suppression on EEG or sustained reduction in ICP. Adverse effects such as systemic hypotension, lowering of CPP, immunosuppression, and hypothermia limit their clinical use. Propofol is another agent used as an alternative to barbiturates. It has the advantage of a short life and an antiseizure property. It decreases cerebral metabolic rate and reduces ICP. Hypotension is the main limiting factor to its use. Higher doses (>5 mg/kg/h infusion) used for a long period (>48 h) may cause propofol infusion syndrome (characterized by cardiac failure, rhabdomyolysis, severe metabolic acidosis, hyperlipidemia, and renal failure), which may be lethal.

10. *Therapeutic hypothermia*: There is clear evidence that hyperthermia is deleterious to brain and normothermia should be achieved. However, the role of therapeutic hypothermia as a measure to reduce cerebral edema is less clear. Few patients with brain edema that results in an increase in ICP benefit from mild therapeutic hypothermia.[32] Therapeutic hypothermia decreases free radical production, inflammation, and ICP. Although a series of pathological and physiological changes as well as potential side effects are observed during hypothermia treatment, it remains a potential therapeutic strategy for brain injuries and needs further study.[33]

11. *Operative decompression*: The removal of a large area of the skull to increase the potential volume of cranial cavity is done to combat massive brain swelling. The decompression may be done by creating an opening in the skull bone (external decompression) with or without resection of brain tissue (internal decompression).

Intraoperative measures to treat a tense and bulging brain include maintaining adequate depth of anesthesia, analgesia, muscle relaxation, and maintaining hemodynamic stability. Extreme neck flexion or rotation, kinking of endotracheal tube, bronchospasm, urinary retention, and other causes should be ruled out. Any acute rise in blood pressure should be treated. Nitrous oxide, if being used, should be stopped and replaced with air. Mannitol or hypertonic saline may be infused, and loop diuretics (furosemide) may be added, titrating the blood pressure. Bolus doses of either thiopentone or propofol may also be given. If the brain still remains tense, consider using intravenous anesthetic agents (propofol infusion) for maintenance of anesthesia instead of inhalational agents. Aspiration of CSF from the ventricles or lumbar puncture if the dura mater is not opened may settle the tense brain.

References

1. Milhorat TH, Pan J. Blood–brain barrier and cerebral edema. In: Cottrell JE, Smith DS, eds. *Anesthesia and Neurosurgery*. 4th ed. St. Louis: Mosby; 2010:115–127.
2. Kuroiwa T, Cahn R, Juhler M, Goping G, Campbell G, Klatzo I. Role of extracellular proteins in the dynamics of vasogenic brain edema. *Acta Neuropathol*. 1985;66:3–11.
3. Baethmann A, Oettinger W, Rothenfusser W, Kempski O, Unterberg A, Geiger R. Brain edema factors: current state with particular references to plasma constituents and glutamate. *Adv Neurol*. 1980;28:175–179.
4. Liang D, Bhatta S, Gerzanich V, Simard JM. Cytotoxic edema: mechanisms of pathological cell swelling. *Neurosurg Focus*. 2009;22:E2.
5. Amiry-Moghaddam M, Ottersen OP. The molecular basis of water transport in the brain. *Nat Rev Neurosci*. 2003;4:991–1001.
6. Badaut J, Lasbennes F, Magistretti PJ, Regli L. Aquaporins in brain: distribution, physiology, and pathophysiology. *J Cereb Blood Flow Metab*. 2002;22:367–378.
7. Raslan A, Bhardwaj A. Medical management of cerebral edema. *Neurosurg Focus*. 2007;22:E12.
8. Bhagat H, Kumar P, Singla N. Urinary retention as the cause of acute brain bulge during pediatric neurosurgery in prone position. *J Neurosurg Anesthesiol*. 2011;23:50–51.
9. Hutchinson P, Timofeev I, Kirkpatrick P. Surgery of brain edema. *Neurosurg Focus*. 2007;22:E14.
10. Rabinstein AA. Treatment of brain edema. *Neurologist*. 2006;12:59–73.
11. Bruno A, Williams LS, Kent TA. How important is hyperglycemia during acute brain infarction? *Neurologist*. 2004;10:195–200.
12. Rovlias A, Kotsou S. The influence of hyperglycemia on neurological outcome in patients with severe head injury. *Neurosurgery*. 2000;46:335–343.
13. Jeremitsky E, Omert LA, Dunham CM, Wilberger J, Rodriguez A. The impact of hyperglycemia on patients with severe brain injury. *J Trauma*. 2005;58:47–50.

14. Lam AM, Winn HR, Cullen BF, Sundling N. Hyperglycemia and neurological outcome in patients with head injury. *J Neurosurg.* 1991;75:545–551.
15. Liu-DeRyke X, Collingridge DS, Orme J, Roller D, Zurasky J, Rhoney DH. Clinical impact of early hyperglycemia during acute phase of traumatic brain injury. *Neurocrit Care.* 2009;11:151–157.
16. Griesdale DE, Tremblay MH, McEwen J, Chittock DR. Glucose control and mortality in patients with severe traumatic brain injury. *Neurocrit Care.* 2009;11:311–316.
17. Bilotta F, Caramia R, Cernak I, et al. Intensive insulin therapy after severe traumatic brain injury: a randomized clinical trial. *Neurocrit Care.* 2008;9:159–166.
18. Bilotta F, Caramia R, Paoloni FP, Delfini R, Rosa G. Safety and efficacy of intensive insulin therapy in critical neurosurgical patients. *Anesthesiology.* 2009;110:611–619.
19. Vespa P, Boonyaputthikul R, McArthur DL, et al. Intensive insulin therapy reduces microdialysis glucose values without altering glucose utilization or improving the lactate/pyruvate ratio after traumatic brain injury. *Crit Care Med.* 2006;34:850–856.
20. Vespa PM, McArthur D, O'Phelan K, et al. Persistently low extracellular glucose correlates with poor outcome 6 months after human traumatic brain injury despite a lack of increased lactate: a microdialysis study. *J Cereb Blood Flow Metab.* 2003;23:865–877.
21. Hill J, Zhao J, Dash PK. High blood glucose does not adversely affect outcome in moderately brain-injured rodents. *J Neurotrauma.* 2010;27:1439–1448.
22. Godoy DA, Napoli MD, Rabinstein AA. Treating hyperglycemia in neurocritical patients: benefits and perils. *Neurocrit Care.* 2010;13:425–438.
23. Stringer WA, Hasso AN, Thompson JR, Hinshaw DB, Jordan KG. Hyperventilation-induced cerebral ischemia in patients with acute brain lesions: demonstration by xenon-enhanced CT. *AJNR Am J Neuroradiol.* 1993;14:475–484.
24. Frank JI. Management of intracranial hypertension. *Med Clin North Am.* 1993;77:61–76.
25. Prabhakar H, Singh GP, Anand V, Kalaivani M. Mannitol versus hypertonic saline for brain relaxation in patients undergoing craniotomy. *Cochrane Database Syst Rev.* 2014;16:7:CD010026.
26. Thenuwara K, Todd MM, Brian Jr JE. Effect of mannitol and furosemide on plasma osmolality and brain water. *Anesthesiology.* 2002;96:416–421.
27. Todd MM, Cutkomp J, Brian JE. Influence of mannitol and furosemide, alone and in combination, on brain water content after fluid percussion injury. *Anesthesiology.* December 2006;105:1176–1181.
28. Hochman DW. The extracellular space and epileptic activity in the adult brain: explaining the antiepileptic effects of furosemide and bumetanide. *Epilepsia.* June 2012;53(suppl 1):18–25.
29. Sinha S, Bastin ME, Wardlaw JM, Armitage PA, Whittle IR. Effects of dexamethasone on peritumoral oedematous brain: a DT-MRI study. *J Neurol Neurosurg Psychiatry.* 2004;75:1632–1635.
30. Papadopoulos MC, Saadoun S, Binder DK, Manlet GT, Krishna S, Verkman AS. Molecular mechanisms of brain tumor edema. *Neuroscience.* 2004;129:1011–1020.
31. Kostaras X, Cusano F, Kline GA, Roa W, Easaw J. Use of dexamethasone in patients with high-grade glioma: a clinical practice guideline. *Curr Oncol.* 2014;21:493–503.
32. Shiozaki T, Sugimoto H, Taneda M, et al. Effect of mild hypothermia on uncontrollable intracranial hypertension after severe head injury. *J Neurosurg.* 1993;79:363–368.
33. Darwazeh R, Yan Y. Mild hypothermia as a treatment for central nervous system injuries: positive or negative effects. *Neural Regener Res.* 2013;8:2677–2686.

COMPLICATIONS RELATED TO SPINAL CORD

Autonomic Disturbances

Vasudha Singhal[1], Richa Aggarwal[2]

[1]Department of Neuroanaesthesia and Intensive Care, Medanta, The Medicity, Gurgaon, Haryana, India; [2]Department of Neuroanaesthesiology and Critical Care, All India Institute of Medical Sciences, New Delhi, India

DEFINITION

Autonomic disturbances are disorders that affect the autonomic neurons of either or both the sympathetic and the parasympathetic nervous systems. Since the autonomic nervous system supplies almost every organ in the body, autonomic diseases influence localized organ function as well as integrated processes that control vital functions in the body such as arterial blood pressure and body temperature. The signs and symptoms present a wide spectrum, ranging from disorders of the cardiovascular system, such as postural hypotension and heart rate disturbances, to dysfunction involving the sudomotor, alimentary, urinary, or sexual systems, and eye and lacrimal glands in the body. Autonomic diseases may present at any age and may be hereditary or acquired. Neuroanesthesiologists may encounter autonomic disturbances most commonly in the setting of trauma patients (spinal cord injury (SCI), traumatic brain injury (TBI)), in diabetics (diabetic neuropathy) and alcoholics, and in patients of Guillain–Barré syndrome and Parkinson's disease.

PATHOPHYSIOLOGY AND CAUSES

Autonomic disturbances may arise due to a dysfunction of the central or peripheral nervous system pathways. The autonomic nervous system has a craniosacral parasympathetic and a thoracolumbar sympathetic pathway.

Sympathetic outputs arise in brain and brain stem centers, descend into the spinal cord, and synapse with neurons in the intermediolateral cell mass in the thoracic and upper lumbar segments. Axons originating in the spinal cord synapse with cells in paravertebral ganglia, which, in turn, provide sympathetic output to remote target organs. Preganglionic sympathetic synapses use acetylcholine as the major neurotransmitter, while the postganglionic synapses use noradrenaline.

Parasympathetic outflow originates from the cranial and sacral segments, and these axons synapse in ganglia are located near their target organs. Acetylcholine is the major neurotransmitter in both pre- and postganglionic synapses.[1]

Disruption at any level in the transmission pathway may cause autonomic disturbances.

Causes for autonomic neuropathy may be hereditary or acquired. The common causes are best classified on an etiological basis:

1. Aging
2. Trauma: TBI, SCI
3. Systemic diseases:
   a. Diabetic neuropathy: the prevalence of autonomic impairment in diabetes is estimated to be ~54% in type 1 and ~73% in type 2 diabetic patients[2]
   b. Hepatic disease
   c. Uremic neuropathy
   d. Amyloidosis
   e. Subacute combined degeneration

4. Infections: HIV, leprosy, and Chagas' disease
5. Drugs and toxins: botulism, cancer chemotherapeutic drugs like vincristine and cisplatin, amiodarone, pyridoxine overdose
6. Immune mediated: Guillain–Barré syndrome, rheumatoid arthritis, systemic lupus erythematosus, systemic sclerosis, Eaton–Lambert syndrome, anti-N-methyl-D-aspartate (NMDA) receptor encephalitis, etc.
7. Hereditary: Anderson–Fabry disease, MEN type 2B
8. Idiopathic

Dysautonomia frequently occurs in patients with severe TBI. A younger age and diffuse axonal injury could be risk factors for facilitating the development of dysautonomia.[3] Almost 10% of patients with severe TBI have dysautonomic crises during their intensive care unit (ICU) stay. Dysautonomic crises determined a worse short-term neurologic recovery, a greater morbidity, and a longer ICU stay.[4]

Autonomic dysreflexia (AD), seen in spinal cord injuries above T6 level, is a potentially dangerous clinical syndrome resulting in acute, uncontrolled hypertension, typically triggered by bladder or bowel distension.

AD is a clinical emergency. The patients usually give a history of headache, blurring of vision, spots in the visual field, nasal congestion, and a sense of anxiety or malaise.

There is significant rise in systolic and diastolic blood pressure (BP). An increase in systolic blood pressure of more than 20–30 mm Hg is considered a dysreflexic episode.[5] This sudden increase in BP is associated with bradycardia. Clinically, the patient may have profuse sweating and flushing of the skin above the level of lesion. AD occurs more often in chronic stages of SCI but can occur early. It is more severe in complete tetraplegia than in incomplete lesions.[6]

SIGNS AND SYMPTOMS

Postural hypotension is the most commonly recognized symptom of autonomic neuropathy. Any symptom affecting a single organ or system should be carefully evaluated for the possibility of an underlying disease.

The clinical features[7] may be classified on the basis of system involvement.

Cardiovascular System

Postural hypotension, supine hypertension, lability of BP, bradycardia, tachycardia—all may be manifestations of an autonomic disease.

Orthostatic hypotension is defined as a fall in BP of 20 mm Hg systolic or 10 mm Hg diastolic on sitting, standing, or during a 60° head-up tilt. The patient complains of dizziness, visual disturbances, and cognitive deficits due to decreased perfusion pressure of organs above the heart level, most notably the brain. If BP falls precipitously, syncope may occur. Nonspecific symptoms such as weakness, tiredness, and fatigue may be seen.

Hypertension may be seen as a part of AD in high spinal cord injuries precipitated by bladder or bowel distension, and may cause a throbbing headache, palpitations, sweating, and flushing over the face and neck. In tetanus, hypertension may be precipitated by muscle spasms or tracheal suction in ventilated patients. Intermittent hypertension may occur in the Guillain–Barré syndrome, porphyria, posterior fossa tumors, and pheochromocytoma, often without a clear precipitating cause. In tetanus and Guillain-Barré syndrome, hypertension is usually accompanied with tachycardia due to an increased sympathetic discharge. Sustained hypertension caused by increased sympathetic activity may occur in subarachnoid hemorrhage.

Bradycardia may be seen with hypertension in cerebral tumors and spinal cord injuries. In high spinal cord injuries, the lack of sympathetic activity and the unopposed vagal tone precipitates bradycardia. In neurally mediated syncope, severe bradycardia is seen with hypotension. In diabetes mellitus, the presence of cardiac vagal neuropathy may increase the likelihood of a cardiopulmonary arrest during anesthesia.

Sudomotor System

Anhidrosis or hypohidrosis (reduced or no sweating) is seen in autonomic failure. At times, hyperhidrosis (increased sweating) in segmental areas may occur as a compensatory response to diminished sudomotor activity elsewhere. In SCIs, the level of lesion is conspicuous by a band of hyperhidrosis above and anhidrosis below the particular level. Hyperhidrosis in the face and neck may be seen in AD in high spinal cord lesions, and in parkinsonism. Localized sweating over face and neck caused by food (gustatory sweating) may be seen in diabetes and after parotid surgery.

Hypothermia may be seen in hypothalamic disorders and in the elderly. In high spinal lesions, poikilothermia is evident due to lack of shivering in thermogenesis and during the acute phase of neurogenic shock.

Alimentary System

Reduced salivation, altered taste, dry mouth (xerostomia) leading to dental decay, and dysphagia may occur in autonomic diseases. Gastroparesis in diabetics may cause abdominal distension, bloating, and vomiting of undigested food. Constipation or diarrhea may occur. Diarrhea is commonly seen in patients with diabetes mellitus, especially at night, due to incomplete digestion, altered bowel flora, and abnormal motility.

Kidneys and Urinary Tract

Nocturia is common in primary autonomic failure. There may be urinary frequency, urgency, incontinence, or retention. In SCI, the loss of sacral parasympathetic function causes an atonic bladder with urinary retention. Such patients are also prone to urinary calculi, especially when immobility increases calcium excretion.

Sexual Function

In males, decreased parasympathetic activity may result in erectile dysfunction, while diminished sympathetic activity leads to ejaculatory dysfunction. Priapism, caused by abnormal spinal reflexes, may occur in patients with spinal cord lesions. In females, vaginal dryness and difficulty in achieving an orgasm may be seen.

Eye and Lacrimal Glands

Loss of sympathetic innervation in Horner's syndrome may cause ptosis and miosis. Night vision may be impaired. Dilated pupils, with blurred vision and reduced tolerance to sunlight, may be seen in parasympathetic failure. Cycloplegia may also increase intraocular pressure and contribute to glaucoma.

Impaired lacrimation may be seen in primary autonomic failure and Sjogren's syndrome. Crocodile tears syndrome may cause excessive and inappropriate lacrimation.

Respiratory System

Stridor may result from the weakness of the cricoarytenoid muscles. Abnormal responses following activation of reflexes from the respiratory tract, such as during tracheal suction, may cause profound cardiovascular disturbances; in tetanus, severe hypertension and tachycardia may occur, while in high cervical cord transection, bradycardia and cardiac arrest may occur. In diabetics, reduced bronchoconstrictor reflexes have been detected, contributing to reduced responses to hypoxia.

Unexplained weight loss and absence of warning signs of hypoglycemia are also characteristics in patients with autonomic disturbances.

DIAGNOSIS

The patient's clinical history directs the evaluation of autonomic diseases.

- An acute onset of autonomic symptoms, along with mild weakness or numbness, should prompt the evaluation for Guillain–Barré syndrome. A cerebrospinal fluid picture of albuminocytologic dissociation may be confirmatory, but may appear late during the course of the disease.
- A chronic onset should trigger evaluation for other neurological disorders, like Parkinson's disease.
- A detailed family history is important to rule out any familial or genetic causes.
- Drug or toxin exposure should be suspected.
- The patients' medication should be thoroughly reviewed:
  - Increased sympathetic activity is seen with amphetamines, cocaine, tricyclic antidepressants, monoamine oxidase inhibitors, and beta-adrenergic agonists.
  - Decreased sympathetic activity may be seen with centrally active agents, such as clonidine, methyldopa, reserpine, and barbiturates, and peripherally acting agents (e.g., alpha- or beta-adrenergic antagonists).
  - Increased parasympathetic activity may be seen with anticholinesterase inhibitors like pyridostigmine.
  - Decreased parasympathetic activity may be seen with antidepressants, phenothiazines, anticholinergic agents, and botulinum toxicity.

Tests for systemic diseases causing secondary autonomic failure should be done.

- Glycosylated hemoglobin is indicative of diabetes mellitus.
- HIV testing should be done in patients with suspected HIV.
- Autoimmune screening helps to evaluate for collagen vascular disorders.

Cardiovascular evaluation includes the following:

- Standing and supine BP and pulse measurements
- Electrocardiogram (ECG) to measure beat-to-beat variation of resting-rate interval with respiration and during Valsalva maneuver
- Head-up tilt testing

Other more sophisticated laboratory tests for evaluation of autonomic dysfunction[8] include, but are not limited to, plasma norepinephrine (supine and standing), genetic testing for inherited neuropathies, amyloid investigations, nerve conduction studies, cystometry, doppler studies, positron emission tomography for cardiac sympathetic dysfunction, thermoregulatory sweat testing, quantitative sudomotor axon reflex test (to test thermoregulatory pathways), penile plethysmography, and so forth.

PREDISPOSING FACTORS

Diabetes is the most important predisposing factor for autonomic neuropathy in clinical practice. Diabetic patients who are overweight, elderly, hypertensive, and with high blood cholesterol have an additional risk.

Alcoholics are also prone to develop autonomic disturbances.

Other medical conditions such as lupus, HIV, cancer, Parkinson's disease, and botulism increase the risk of dysautonomia.

TREATMENT

Management of patients with autonomic disturbances begins with initial diagnosis and incorporates patient education about the condition and its implications. This may range from measures to prevent orthostatic hypotension to improvements in self-care and hygiene in diabetes mellitus. Patients should be monitored for drug efficacy and side effects. Management strategies revolve around the following:

- Treatment of underlying cause
- Orthostatic hypotension:
  - Head-up tilt of the bed at night
  - Performing positional changes, like standing up, slowly and gradually
  - Volume replacement (increased fluid intake)
  - Salt supplementation
  - Medication (such as fluorohydrocortisone, midrodine)
  - Wearing compressive stockings
- Gastrointestinal dysfunction:
  - Gastroparesis in patients with diabetic autonomic neuropathy is improved by rigorous control of blood glucose concentrations.
  - Advise patients to eat small meals and eat often.
  - Lowering the fat content of the diet.
  - Prokinetic agents for gastroparesis like metoclopramide, domperidone, and erythromycin can be used. A jejunostomy tube may rarely be required.
  - Bowel hypomotility can be helped with:
    - Increased dietary fiber and increased fluid intake.
    - Use of stool softeners and/or an osmotic laxative.
    - Gluten-free diet and restriction of lactose should be tried.
    - Colestyramine, clonidine, somatostatin analogs, pancreatic enzyme supplements, and even antibiotics (such as metronidazole) have been tried.[9]

- Genital autonomic neuropathy:
  - Using a drug like sildenafil (selective PDE5 inhibitor) to induce erection.
  - Using a vacuum pump to force blood into the penis to induce an erection.
  - Vaginal lubricants and estrogen creams to combat dryness.
- Autonomic dysfunction of the urinary tract:
  - Timed voiding schedules and bladder contractions increased by a Valsalva maneuver.
  - Clean intermittent self-catheterization.
  - Desmopressin may be used for symptoms of nocturia.
  - Cholinergic agonists in bladder hypotonia (for example, bethanechol; has a limited role).
- Hyperhidrosis:
  - Anticholinergic agents (for example, trihexyphenidyl and propantheline) may be helpful but doses required may limit use (anticholinergic side effects).
  - Intracutaneous injection of botulinum toxin type A is often beneficial.
  - Sympathectomy is rarely required.
  - There is no effective treatment for hypohidrosis.
- Immunoglobulins are used to improve clinical and immunologic aspects of the disease; these may decrease autoantibody production and increase solubilization and removal of immune complexes.
- Treatment of AD after SCI: Initial management involves placing the patient in an upright posture and loosening of any clothing or constrictive devices. Upright posture leads to pooling of blood in abdominal and lower extremity vessels causing reduction in arterial pressure. The cause for AD should be searched for, which in 85% of cases is related to bladder or bowel distension. If there is no indwelling catheter, catheterize the patient. If the catheter is already in place, check for obstruction and blockage. If BP remains high after emptying bladder, check the rectum for stool impaction.

  Monitor BP every 2–5 min until the patient stabilizes. Antihypertensive drugs should be used if systolic BP remains 150 mm Hg or higher. Antihypertensives with a rapid onset and short duration of action should be used. The most commonly used agents are nifedipine, nitrates, and captopril. However, only nifedipine is supported by controlled trials (level 2). Nifedipine is given using the "bite and swallow" method in a dose of 10 mg and not sublingually. It causes a modest fall in systolic and diastolic BP, though sometimes drop in BP can be dramatic. Nitrates are often used but contraindicated if patient has taken sildenafil in the last 24 h. Captopril is given sublingually in a dose of 25 mg.[10]

If left untreated, AD can cause seizures, retinal hemorrhage, pulmonary edema, renal insufficiency, myocardial infarction, cerebral hemorrhage, and even death, from sustained, severe peripheral hypertension.

The patient should be monitored for at least 2 h after resolution of AD, as it may recur. The patients should follow preventive measures to mitigate further episodes of AD such as intermittent catheterization, care of indwelling catheters, a regular bowel program, and routine skin care for prevention of pressure ulcers.

PREVENTION

Addressing conditions that might cause secondary neuropathy might help prevent its development. Regulating blood sugar levels by eating a low sugar and high fiber diet to keep diabetes under control is the primary way of prevention. Lifestyle changes like quitting smoking and alcohol, exercising regularly, creating healthy eating habits, losing weight, and controlling BP can all help to minimize symptoms of autonomic neuropathy in diabetics.

References

1. Mathias CJ. Disorders of the autonomic nervous system. In: *Neurology in Clinical Practice*. Boston, MA: Butterworth-Heinemann; 1996:1953–1981.
2. Low PA, Benrud-Larson LM, Sletten DM, et al. Autonomic symptoms and diabetic neuropathy: a population-based study. *Diabetes Care*. December 2004;27(12): 2942–2947.
3. Lv LQ, Hou LJ, Yu MK, et al. Risk factors related to dysautonomia after severe traumatic brain injury. *J Trauma*. September 2011;71(3):538–542.
4. Fernández-Ortega JF, Prieto-Palomino MA, Muñoz-López A, Lebron-Gallardo M, Cabrera-Ortiz H, Quesada-García G. Prognostic influence and computed tomography findings in dysautonomic crises after traumatic brain injury. *J Trauma*. November 2006; 61(5):1129–1133.
5. Mathias CJ, Bannister R. Autonomic disturbances in spinal cord lesions. In: Mathias CJ, ed. *Autonomic Failure: A Textbook of Clinical Disorders of the Autonomic Nervous System*. Oxford: Oxford University Press; 2002:839–881.
6. Curt A, Nitsche B, Rodic B, Schurch B, Dietz V. Assessment of autonomic dysreflexia in patients with spinal cord injury. *J Neurol Neurosurg Psychiatry*. 1997;62:473–477.
7. Mathias CJ. Autonomic diseases: clinical features and laboratory evaluation. *J Neurol Neurosurg Psychiatry*. 2003;74(suppl III):iii31–iii41.
8. Low PA. Laboratory evaluation of autonomic function. *Suppl Clin Neurophysiol*. 2004;57:358–368.
9. Freeman R. Autonomic peripheral neuropathy. *Lancet*. April 2–8, 2005;365(9466): 1259–1270.
10. Krassioukov A, Warburton DE, Teasell R, Eng JJ. The SCIRE research team. A systematic review of the management of autonomic dysreflexia following spinal cord injury. *Arch Phys Med Rehabil*. 2009;90(4):682–695.

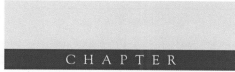

CHAPTER

9

Pneumorrhachis

Gyaninder P. Singh, Indu Kapoor

Department of Neuroanaesthesiology and Critical Care, All India Institute
of Medical Sciences, New Delhi, India

DEFINITION

Pneumorrhachis is the presence of air within the spinal canal (either in the intra- or extradural space). It is a rare phenomenon and is often asymptomatic. This condition was first reported in 1977 by Gordon et al.[1] who used the term "pneumomyelogram" to describe air around the dura mater spinalis and has since been described by various terms in the literature (such as intraspinal pneumocele, spinal pneumatosis, spinal emphysema, aerorachia, pneumosaccus, air myelogram, etc.). The term "pneumorrhachis" was coined by Newbold et al. in 1987 to describe air in the spinal canal.[2] Depending on the location of air, pneumorrahachis may be extradural (epidural) or intradural (subarachnoid), the former being more common.

ETIOLOGY

Pneumorrhachis may be primary (intraspinal origin) or secondary to occurrence of air in other parts of the body. Pneumorrhachis is almost always associated with air in other body compartments and cavities. It is particularly seen in conjunction with pneumocephalus, pneumothorax, pneumomediastinum, pneumopericardium, pneumoperitonium, and subcutaneous emphysema.[3-5] Distribution of air in the spinal canal may be confined to isolated cervical, thoracic, lumbar, or sacral region or may be widely spread to more than one area[6] or even the entire spine.[5] Localization and distribution of air depends on site, rate, and volume of air entry, capacity of intraspinal space, and patient positioning.[3]

Pneumorrhachis may be classified into following three types, depending upon the cause:

1. *Nontraumatic*: caused by conditions that produce high intrathoracic pressures such as violent cough due to bronchial asthma[4,7] or acute bronchitis, airway obstruction due to aspiration of foreign body,[8] after cardiopulmonary resuscitation, inhalational drug abuse such as Ecstasy[9] or marijuana,[10] persistent forceful vomiting, invasive tumor progression, postradiation changes,[11] paraparesis,[12] and leukemia.[13]
2. *Traumatic*: caused by trauma to head,[3,14] neck,[15] thorax,[16,17] abdomen, pelvis,[18] or spine.[19]
3. *Iatrogenic*: caused by surgery (over head, neck, thorax, abdomen, or spine),[20-22] anesthesiological procedure (spinal or epidural anesthesia),[23] or diagnostic interventions involving lumbar puncture.

SIGNS AND SYMPTOMS

Pneumorrhachis is usually asymptomatic but may sometimes present with symptoms either of itself or its underlying pathology. As the accumulated air occupies intraspinal (and sometimes even intracranial) space, it may cause syndromes of intracranial and intraspinal hypertension or hypotension as a result of increase or decrease of intracranial and intraspinal pressures, respectively.[3] Pneumorrhachis may be associated with pain[24] and/or neurological deficits.[5,21,25] The entrapped intraspinal air may act as space occupying lesion and exert pressure on the spinal cord and nerve roots.

DIAGNOSIS

Since pneumorrhachis is mostly asymptomatic and clinically nonspecific, the diagnosis of pneumorrhachis is primarily radiological. Plain radiograph of the spine may be useful to detect larger volumes of air and for early

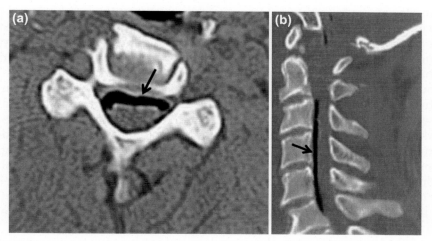

FIGURE 1   CT scan of the spine: (a) axial and (b) sagittal image. The black arrow shows collection of air (pneumorrhachis) in the anterior part of the spinal canal.

detection of the possible associated injuries. The air is seen as linear lucency along the spinal canal on lateral chest radiograph; the diagnostic imaging of choice is a spinal computerized tomography (CT) scan (Figure 1). Nevertheless, it may be difficult to differentiate intradural pneumorrhachis from extradural on a CT scan. Magnetic resonance imaging (MRI) is more sensitive and may be used for differential diagnosis. Since pneumorrhachis is frequently associated with air distribution in other parts of the body, a total-body CT scan or MRI may be necessary to identify the etiolology.

DIFFERENTIAL DIAGNOSIS

Differentiation of intraspinal air from free intraspinal gas is essential. The intraspinal gas may be formed from degenerative,[26] malignant,[27] inflammatory,[28] or infectious disease by gas-forming organism.[29] The composition of intraspinal gas is different from that of intraspinal air accumulation, though both have the same low density and cannot be clearly differentiated on a CT examination.

TREATMENT

Pneumorrhachis per se is a rare entity and often asymptomatic. The air gradually gets reabsorbed spontaneously into the circulation over a period of days, and thus the patients of pneumorrhachis are usually managed conservatively. However, pneumorrhachis may be associated with decreased intraspinal and intracranial pressure due to leak of cerebrospinal fluid (CSF). A significant and persistent CSF leak may need surgical repair because of the high risk of meningitis. On the other hand, increased intraspinal pressure due to entrapped air under pressure may lead to tension pneumorrhachis requiring decompression by percutaneous insertion of Tuohy needle and air aspiration. Since a wide range of etiologies is associated with the occurrence of pneumorrhachis, a meticulous evaluation is important to identify the cause and treat appropriately. Any underlying pathological conditions causing pneumorrhachis, such as fistulas between intrathoracic and intraspinal space may require surgical intervention. If a patient with pneumorrhachis requires general anesthesia for any surgical procedure, use of nitrous oxide should be avoided as it diffuses into the air-filled space and causes expansion.

Other treatment approaches include use of intravenous steroids (dexamethasone), administration of high concentration of inspired oxygen to promote reabsorption of air, and hyperbaric oxygen therapy. However, there are reported cases where pneumorrhachis is managed conservatively without any complications.[30]

CONCLUSION

Pneumorrhachis in itself is a rare and often self-limiting condition. It is almost exceptionally associated with collection of air in other body cavities or compartments. Pneumorrhachis is primarily a radiological diagnosis, and a spinal CT is the diagnostic tool of choice. There is a multitude of etiologies associated with pneumorrhachis and thus thorough evaluation is essential to recognize the cause and for adequate management of the underlying pathology. Pneumorrhachis associated with trauma is believed to be a marker of severe injury and is thought to be associated with an increased morbidity and mortality. The management of patients should be individualized and often require inter- and multidisciplinary approaches.

References

1. Gordon IJ, Hardman DR. The traumatic pneumomyelogram. A previously undescribed entity. *Neuroradiology*. 1977;13:107–108.
2. Newbold RG, Wiener MD, Vogler 3rd JB, Martinez S. Traumatic pneumorrhachis. *AJR*. 1987;148:615–616.
3. Oertel MF, Korinth MC, Reines MHT, Krings T, Terbeck S, Gilsbach JM. Pathogenesis, diagnosis and management of pneumorrhachis. *Eur Spine J*. 2006;15:S636–S643.

4. Manden PK, Siddiqui AH. Pneumorrhachis, pneumomediastinum, pneumopericardium and subcutaneous emphysema as complications of bronchial asthma. *Ann Thorac Med.* 2009;4:143–145.
5. Wosko J, Dabrowski W, Zadora P, Fijalkowska A, Grzycka-Kowalczyk L. Pneumocephalus and pneumorrhachis after chest wall injury. *Anestezjol Intensywna Ter.* 2011; 43:40–44.
6. Chibbaro S, Selem M, Tacconi L. Cervicothoracolumbar pneumorachis. Case report and review of the literature. *Surg Neurol.* 2005;64:80–82.
7. Tsuji H, Takazakura E, Terada Y, Makino H, Yasuda A, Oiko Y. CT demonstration of spinal epidural emphysema complicating bronchial asthma and violent coughing. *J Comput Assist Tomogr.* 1989;13:38–39.
8. Tambe P, Kasat LS, Tambe AP. Epidural emphysema associated with subcutaneous emphysema following foreign body in the airway. *Pediatr Surg Int.* 2005;21:721–722.
9. Bernaerts A, Verniest T, Vanhoenacker F, Van den Brande P, Petre C, De Schepper AM. Pneumomediastinum and epidural pneumatosis after inhalation of "Ecstasy". *Eur Radiol.* 2003;13:642–643.
10. Hazouard E, Koninck JC, Attucci S, Fauchier-Rolland F, Brunereau L, Diot P. Pneumorachis and pneumomediastinum caused by repeated Muller's maneuvers: complications of marijuana smoking. *Ann Emerg Med.* 2001;38:694–697.
11. Wippold FJ, Schnapf D, Bennett LL, Friedman AC. Esophago-subarachnoidal fistula: an unusual complication of esophageal carcinoma. *J Comput Assist Tomogr.* 1982;6:147–149.
12. Kim KY, Kang JH, Lee MH, Han Y, Choi DW. Atypical traumatic pneumorrhachis accompanied by paraparesis. *Ann Rehabil Med.* 2014;38:410–414.
13. Showkat HI, Jan A, Sarmast AH, Bhat GM, Jan BM, Bashir Y. Pneumomediastinum, pneumorachis, subcutaneous emphysema: an unusual complication of leukemia in a child. *World J Clin Cases.* 2013;1:224–226.
14. Coskun S, Sahin M, Cobanoglu M, Kilicaslan I. Entire pneumorrhachis due to isolated head trauma. *Am J Emerg Med.* 2009;27:902.e3–902.e6.
15. Alkan A, Baysal T, Saras K, Sigirci A, Kutlu R. Early MRI findings in stab wound of the cervical spine two case reports. *Neuroradiology.* 2002;44:64–66.
16. Hwang WC, Kim HC. CT demonstration of spinal epidural air after chest trauma. *Eur Radiol.* 2002;10:396–397.
17. Adams MT, Nadalo L, Dunn EL. Air in the spinal canal following blunt thoracic trauma. *J Trauma.* 2003;55:386.
18. Chimon JL, Cantos EL. CT recognition of spinal epidural air after pelvic trauma. *J Comput Assist Tomogr.* 1990;14:795–796.
19. Oertel MF, Korinth MC, Reinges MH, Gilsbach JM. Pneumorrhachis of the entire spinal canal. *J Neurol Neurosurg Psychiatry.* 2005;76:1036.
20. Ristagno RL, Hiratzka LF, Rost Jr RC. An unusual case of pneumorrhachis following resection of lung carcinoma. *Chest.* 2002;121:1712–1714.
21. Prabhakar H, Bithal PK, Ghosh I, Dash HH. Pneumorrhachis presenting as quadriplegia following surgery in the prone position. *Br J Anaesth.* 2006;97:901–903.
22. Uemura K, Behr R, Roosen K. Symptomatic intraspinal air entrapment. *Br J Neurosurg.* 2000;14:154–156.
23. Hirsch M, Katz Y, Sasson A. Spinal cord compression by unusual epidural air accumulation after continuous epidural analgesia. *Am J Roentgenol.* 1989;153:887–888.
24. Overdiek N, Grisales DA, Gravenstein D, Bosek V, Nishman R, Modell JH. Subdural air collection: a likely source of radicular pain after lumbar epidural. *J Clin Anesth.* 2001;13:392–397.
25. Krishnam, Mallick A. Air in the epidural space leading to a neurological deficit. *Anaesthesia.* 2003;58:292–293.

26. Ford LT, Gilula LA, Murphy WA, Gado M. Analysis of gas in vacuum lumbar disc. *Am J Roentgenol*. 1977;128:1056–1057.
27. Kennedy C, Phillips R, Kendall B. Epidural gas: an unusual complication of metastatic oesophageal carcinoma. *Neuroradiology*. 1990;32:67–69.
28. Burke V, Mall JC. Epidural gas: an unusual complication of Crohn disease. *Am J Neuroradiol*. 1984;5:105–106.
29. Thompson GR, Crawford GE. Pneumorachis caused by metastatic gas gangrene. *Diagn Microbiol Infect Dis*. 2009;63:108–110.
30. Jung H, Lee SC, Lee DH, Kim GJ. Spontaneous pneumomediastinum with concurrent pneumorrhachis. *Korean J Thorac Cardiovasc Surg*. 2014;47:569–571.

10

Postoperative Paraplegia and Quadriplegia

Ankur Luthra[1], Hemanshu Prabhakar[2]

[1]Department of Neuroanaesthesia and Intensive Care, Medanta, The Medicity, Gurgaon, Haryana, India; [2]Department of Neuroanaesthesiology and Critical Care, All India Institute of Medical Sciences, New Delhi, India

Postoperative paraplegia refers to new onset neurological deficit which occurs as a result of damage/insult to the spinal cord below T1 whereas quadriplegia/tetraplegia with or without respiratory dysfunction will occur when the insult is above the first thoracic vertebra. Usually it affects the cervical spinal nerves resulting in complete paralysis of both arms and legs. In addition to the arms and legs being paralyzed, the chest and abdominal muscles will be affected resulting in weakened breathing (paradoxical respiration) and the inability to properly cough and clear the secretions from the chest.

Anterior cord syndrome is when the damage is in the front of the spinal cord, so a patient can have loss of motor power, decreased sensations to pain, temperature and touch below their level of injury. Pressure and joint sensations can be preserved. It is possible for some patients with this injury to later recover some movement if motor recovery is evident days after the initial injury.

Posterior cord syndrome is when the damage is in the posterior aspect of the spinal cord. This type of injury may leave a patient with good muscular power, and temperature and pain sensations; however, they may have problems in coordinating movement of their limbs.

ETIOPATHOGENESIS

Paraplegia is one of the major mortifying complications. Occasional case reports of midcervical quadriplegia in the postoperative period after posterior fossa procedures performed in the sitting position have been reported in the literature. Hitselberger and House mentioned five unreported cases of midcervical quadriplegia after cerebellopontine angle neuroma resection performed in the sitting position.[1] Acute focal pressure on the spinal cord, along with the flexion of the neck, was the postulated mechanism. Matjasko and colleagues reported a case of quadriparesis due to sitting position in a patient with severe cervical stenosis.[2]

Wilder highlighted the fact that acute flexion of the neck in a patient under general anesthesia in the sitting position may cause stretching of the cord at the level of fifth cervical vertebra[3] due to which regional cord perfusion is compromised, especially if intraoperative hypotension occurs.

According to a previous report, quadriplegia can also be a major complication of lumbar spinal surgery. Several possible mechanisms have been held responsible for cervical spinal cord damage.[4]

First, neuromuscular blocking drugs cause a decrease in the tone in the cervical musculature during general anesthesia so that already present spondylitic bars may cause compression of the spinal cord. Haisa and Kondo[5] demonstrated slight intervertebral disk bulge which occurred during surgery because of acute neck flexion that led to compression and cord stretching, leading to myelomalacia.

Second, blood flow may be impaired in the upper spinal cord as a result of prone position with hyperflexion. Wilder[3] suggested that flexion of the cervical spine during general anesthesia may produce enough spinal cord stretching to alter the autoregulation by mechanically affecting the spinal cord vessels.

When the neck position is changed from neutral position to full flexion, the entire cervical cord is elongated by 10% of its initial length as compared to the neutral position.[6] Hence the longitudinal arteries are stretched and constricted with this elongation.

Anatomically, the cervical spinal cord receives its major share of blood from the longitudinal trunks (anterior and posterior spinal arteries), supplied by radicular branches of vertebral arteries.[7,8] Turnbull et al.[9] demonstrated that the cervical cord receives zero to eight radicular arteries.

Because of the very critical sources of blood supply to the spinal cord, any pathology that interferes with the arterial supply can cause ischemia, infarction, or both. The vertical extensity of spinal cord infarction depends upon the limit of vascular occlusion and collateralization.

Though spinal arteries are least susceptible to atherosclerosis, but multiple aortic atheromas may occasionally be the cause of infarction or ischemia. Various other possible sources of infarction are emboli originating from disk substance, [10]infection, [11]or stasis of blood because of extreme neck rotation or hyperflexion in the prone position.[12]

The vertebral body in its anterior most and lateral extents receive nutritional vessels termed anterior central arteries, sourcing from the anterior branches of paired vertebral arteries at the same or adjacent level.[7,8] In contrast to the bony territory of the spinal cord, the radicular arteries which are the major sources of blood to the cervical spinal cord originate eccentrically and unilaterally form the paired vertebral arteries, passing through the root sheath of dura mater along with the nerve roots to the cervical cord with increasing obliquity from the cranial to caudal end, and contribute to blood supplying the longitudinal arterial trunk of the spinal cord.[7,8] Therefore, the levels of cord ischemia are not the same as the levels of the vertebral column.

Few case reports also describe the use of oxidized cellulose (Surgicel) as a hemostat in spine surgeries which may swell up and cause spinal cord compression resulting in paraplegia. Oxidized cellulose is used commonly in many surgical fields as a hemostat. However, its tendency to swell up once placed causes increase in the compression risk of the cord in closed or bone walled spaces.

SIGNS AND SYMPTOMS

Complete cessation of motor activity and loss of sensation either immediately postoperatively or can be delayed up to as long as 48 h postsurgery may be considered as an ongoing complication of spine surgery. This may be associated with urinary or bowel incontinence and areflexia in the involved myotomes.

Inactivity due to paraplegia and quadriplegia can cause multiple problems:

- Pressure sores
- Spastic limbs
- Pneumonia
- Urinary tract infection
- Osteoporosis
- Chronic pain

Paraplegic and quadriplegic patients may also become depressed because of:

- Social isolation
- Lack of emotional support
- Increased dependence on others

DIAGNOSIS AND SPINAL CORD MONITORING

During surgery, when the spine is subjected to corrective forces, while the spinal canal is invaded surgically, or when a bony resection is to be performed, the cord is always at risk of injury. The incidence of paraplegia after scoliosis surgery in the absence of spinal cord monitoring has been reported to be between 3.7% and 6.9%[13] but can be reduced to 0.5% by intraoperative monitoring (IOM).[14] The American Academy of Neurology published guidelines on IOM stating that "extensive evidence favours the use of monitoring as a safe and efficacious tool in clinical situations where there is a significant risk to the nervous system, provided we appreciate its limitations." It is now considered mandatory to do spinal cord monitoring for these procedures.

IOM ideally detects abnormalities in the function of spinal cord early in order that the surgeon is alarmed and can take appropriate steps to correct them before irreversible damage occurs. The time, between a change in the electrophysiological recordings after overdistraction, and the onset of irreversible damage, however, is in the order of only 5–6 min in animal studies.[15]

A motor deficit is functionally more damaging to the patient than a sensory deficit. It is important to consider while evaluating the advantages of these methods of monitoring, few of which will assess motor tracts, and few will assess the sensory tracts of the cord.

As the anesthetic technique can have multitude effects on the ability to monitor spinal cord function accurately, the knowledge of intraoperative spinal cord monitoring is essential to the anesthetist. There are four main methods of IOM: the Stagnara wake-up test, ankle clonus test, somato-sensory-evoked potentials (SSEPs), and motor-evoked potentials (MEPs).

Ankle Clonus Test

This was the first test to be used historically. Clonus is repetitive rhythmic movement elicited by the stretch reflex. The clonus test is usually done at emergence, either at the conclusion of surgery or during a wake-up test. All muscle paralysis has to be antagonized. There is only a limited and brief period between anesthesia and wakefulness when it is possible to elicit clonus. The foot is dorsiflexed sharply at the ankle joint. Spinal cord injury is described by complete absence of repeated movements at the ankle joint.

In the neurologically intact awake patients, cortical centers have a descending inhibitory influence on the reflex, and clonus is thus not elicited. In healthy individuals during general anesthesia, cortical centers are abolished and there is a loss of descending inhibition via the spinal pathways on the ankle reflex. Clonus may, hence, be appreciated on ankle stretch, especially during awakening from general anesthesia. If the spinal cord is damaged whatsoever, the cord undergoes a period of brief spinal shock, and there is complete loss of reflex activity accompanied by flaccid paralysis. During recovery from general anesthesia in these patients, the ankle clonus reflex will definitely not be present.

This test is easy to apply and has a high level of sensitivity (100%) and specificity (99.7%).[16] However, the test can only be done intermittently, and the absence of clonus could be not only due to spinal cord damage, but also to an excessive depth of anesthesia. Further, the presence of clonus does not exclude cord damage; other regions of the cord may be damaged leaving the ankle stretch reflex intact.

Stagnara Wake-Up Test

This test was first described in 1973. Preoperatively, this test is to be explained to the patient; it includes the patient performing a specified motor action, usually in the lower limbs, to verbal command during the surgery. This test assesses the functional integrity of the motor pathways (lower and upper motor neurons) involved in doing this motor task. The test however does not evaluate the integrity of the peripheral nervous system.

The surgeon must give the anesthesiologist adequate warning for the need to do a wake-up test as muscle relaxant effect has to be reversed and the plane of anesthesia lightened. As the patient regains consciousness, they are asked first to perform an action involving muscle groups above the level of cord damage, usually involving the upper limbs (for example, to grip the anesthesiologist's fingers). When a positive response is elicited, the patient is asked to move their legs, and the response to this command is noted. If the patient is able to move his legs, anesthesia is then deepened and surgery continued. If the patient is not able to move their legs, adequate corrective measures are applied immediately.

A wake-up test should be easy and rapid to institute as far as possible which requires an anesthetic technique that is reliable, but has to be quickly reversed as many times as the surgeon demands. Awakening should be smooth to decrease the risk of tracheal extubation. Further, the patient should not feel any pain during the test and have no subsequent recall of intraoperative events.

This test has a number of disadvantages. First, it requires the patient to be fully cooperative. Second, there is a risk to the patient that he may move or fall from the operating table and become accidentally extubated, often in the prone position. Third, it requires considerable skill from the anesthesiologist. Fourth, it does not allow continuous monitoring of motor pathways. The appearance of a change in these recordings and permanent injury to the nervous system can occur more than 20 min after the final corrective force is applied to the spine.[15] It is, therefore, possible that a wake-up test could be normal after the final corrective maneuver has been applied but before the occurrence of the causative neurological deficit.

The value of the Stagnara wake-up test in spinal cord monitoring should hence be confined to situations in which electrophysiological monitoring techniques are unavailable, fail, or produce equivocal results.

Somatosensory-Evoked Potentials

SSEPs are elicited by electrically stimulating a mixed nerve (usually the posterior tibial, peroneal, or sural nerves), and the response is recorded from the electrodes at distant sites cephalad to the level at which surgery is being done. The stimulus is applied to the peripheral nerve on the right and the left limb alternatively as a square wave for 0.1–0.3 ms, and at a frequency of 3–7 Hz. The intensity varies depending upon the electrodes and quality of skin contact, but is in the frequency range of 25–40 mA. Recording electrodes are placed in the cervical region over the spinous processes or over the somatosensory cortex on the scalp, or are placed during surgery in the epidural space. Adequate baseline data is obtained after skin incision which allows a stable plane of general anesthesia to be established during baseline recordings because anesthetic agents affect SSEPs. During surgery, the responses are recorded in a sequential manner. The functional integrity of the sensory pathways is then determined by comparing the change of amplitude and the latency change of the responses obtained during surgery to baseline values. An amplitude reduction of the response by 50% and an increase in the latency by 10% are considered by most authors as significant.[14,17] The amplitude response is considered as the primary criterion.

The pathways involved in the recorded SSEPs starts from a peripheral nerve, the dorsomedial tracts of the cord and, depending on the placement of electrode, the cerebral cortex. The physiological role of these tracts is to carry sensations of proprioception and light touch. It must be clearly stated that responses are not obtained from motor tracts, or from the anterolateral sensory tracts of the spinal cord (which are carrying pain and temperature sensations). Two important aspects are highlighted thereby. First, because of the closer proximity of the dorsomedial sensory tracts to the motor tracts in the cord, it is presumed that when using SSEPs, any damage to the motor tracts will be alarmed by a change in SSEPs. But this cannot be guaranteed. Second, the supply of the corticospinal motor tracts is different from that of the dorsomedial sensory tracts so hypoperfusion in the region of the anterior spinal artery may cause ischemia in the anterolateral tracts, not affecting the dorsomedial tracts. It is, therefore, quite possible to have normal recordings from SSEPs throughout surgery, but to have a paraplegic patient postoperatively.[18-20] Furthermore, in patients with preexisting neurological disorders, reliable data can only be recorded in 75–85% of patients.[21]

Effectiveness of SSEP Monitoring

A large retrospective multicentric study of over 51,000 procedures stated that SSEP monitoring was found to have a sensitivity of 92% and specificity of 98.9%. The false negative rate was 0.127% (normal SSEPs throughout the case but a neurological deficit postoperatively). The false positive rate was 1.51% (SSEP had changed, but no new neurological deficit postoperatively), or one in 67 procedures. Other studies have found a higher false positive rate (14.7%), [22]and that SSEP monitoring has a lower specificity, 85.33%, but a sensitivity of 100%, probably explained by the smaller number of cases.

Motor-Evoked Potentials

As a result of the various problems using SSEPs as a monitoring tool during spinal surgery, and reports of postoperative paraplegia despite apparently normal intraoperative SSEPs, efforts have been made to monitor motor tracts of the spinal cord as a more sensitive indicator of motor function.

MEP monitoring was used clinically over 10 years ago.[23] Monitoring techniques are divided according to the site of stimulation (motor cortex or spinal cord); method of stimulation (electrical potential or magnetic field); and the site of recording (spinal cord or peripheral mixed nerve and muscle). Each variation of this technique has its own advantages and disadvantages. The principle is the same throughout; stimulation by whatever means cephalad to the site of surgery causes prodromal stimulation of motor tracts in the spinal cord, and of peripheral nerve and muscles caudal to the site of surgery. Disturbance of motor pathway function by surgery leads to a reduction in amplitude and an increase in latency of the recorded responses.

The motor cortex is stimulated by electrical or magnetic means. Magnetic equipment is bulky and difficult to work with but is not affected by the quality of contact of electrodes. Recorded responses are classified into myogenic or neurogenic. Myogenic responses arise from the summated electromyography (EMG) activity of a muscle, such as tibialis anterior, in response to stimulation. Neurogenic recordings result from the summated electrical activity of a peripheral nerve or the spinal cord. The advantage of recording EMG response is its large amplitude. The main problem is its varying morphology. While recording EMG responses, the depth of neuromuscular relaxation is of utmost importance because if it is too deep, responses are not obtained and if only residual block is present, then there is a risk of injury to the patient, due to the violent movements that might occur in response to stimulation. Myorelaxants should be administered by continuous infusion, and depth of muscular block monitored. The first twitch of the train of four response should be maintained at 10–20% of baseline.[24] However, neurogenic responses, can be recorded under completely myorelaxed state to avoid patient injury, and are thus more reliable in terms of latency, amplitude, and morphology.

Effectiveness of MEP Monitoring

MEP monitoring is less reliable in patients who have a preexisting neurological deficit.[24] Furthermore, there are reports of preserved neurogenic MEPs associated with postoperative motor deficit[25], which suggests the sensitivity of MEPs is less than 100%.

SSEP monitoring has become an accepted standard of patient care during spinal surgery. Because it is less affected by the technical difficulties associated with MEP monitoring, it is widely being used. However, MEP monitoring is becoming an accepted standard and the two methods should be regarded as complementary, with the use of a wake-up test reserved for situations where such monitoring is not possible or responses are significantly attenuated during surgery.

PREDISPOSING FACTORS, PREVENTION, AND TREATMENT

Few of the predisposing factors include:

1. Age more than 60 years
2. Severe atherosclerotic disease
3. Aortic aneurysms/dissections in severe hypertensive individuals
4. Prolonged aortic cross-clamping
5. Extensive scoliotic deformity
6. Degenerative disk disease
7. Cervical spondylosis

8. Midcervical quadriplegia in sitting position due to extreme flexion
9. Intraoperative hypotension
10. Severe anemia and massive blood loss
11. Epidural hematoma in patients with coagulopathy

Prevention essentially includes careful positioning of the patient with special emphasis on neck flexion (at least a two finger-breadth space should be allowed between the chin and sternum) during sitting position, intraoperative SSEP/MEP monitoring, and avoiding hypotensive anesthesia and major blood loss are some of the key factors in preventing postoperative paraplegia and quadriplegia.

TREATMENT

1. Consider early surgical decompression of the spinal cord in the setting of a deteriorating cord injury that may improve neurologic recovery, although one can never be sure that it will. Consider early spinal stabilization wherever indicated.
2. Methylprednisolone sodium succinate is not recommended anymore for acute spinal cord injury, because there is no class I or II evidence to support its benefit. Rather, there is a higher incidence of infection, sepsis, diabetic complications, prolonged intensive care unit length of stay, and death with steroid use (level 1 recommendations).
   In the National Acute Spinal Cord Injury Study (NASCIS) II study, 1992, Bracken et al. recommended administration of methylprednisolone (30 mg/kg in 30 min then 5.4 mg/kg/h during first 23 h). This would allow reduction of spinal cord edema and inflammation and inhibit the extension of the secondary lesion. The authors did show a statistically significant beneficial effect on motor function, provided that the drug was administered in the first 8 h following trauma. However, the complication rate and the mortality were identical. Its administration in the prehospital course in US is currently recommended and largely spread in the initial management of spine trauma with deficient neurological signs.
   The NASCIS III study, whose results were published in 1997, compared methylprednisolone (30 mg/kg followed by 5.4 mg/kg/h) for 24 h to same dose methylprednisolone for 48 h and following administration of tirilazad mesylate 2.5 mg/kg every 6 h for 48 h. Patients receiving this drug for 48 h had better functional recovery (but higher infectious complication rate, such as pneumonia) than those treated for 24 h only when the process was initiated between 3 and 8 h after the trauma. For those patients who presented before 3 h, all the three protocols were identical. Rates of mortality were similar. There was no placebo.

3. Secondary injury prevention includes adequate skin care and pressure sore development. Repositioning at regular intervals to provide pressure relief or turn at least every 2 h while maintaining spinal precautions should be followed. The area under the patient should be kept clean and dry and temperature elevation is to be avoided. Routinely, assess nutritional status on admission and regularly thereafter. Keep monitoring the skin for excoriation under pressure garments and splints.

4. Prevention and treatment of venous thromboembolism: Apply mechanical compression devices as early as possible after injury if lower limb injury does not preclude it. Begin Low molecular weight heparin (enoxaparin 40 mg subcutaneous once a day) or UFH (Unfractionated) (5000 U subcutaneous BD twice a day) plus intermittent pneumatic compression, in patients once homeostasis is achieved and there is no further evidence of bleeding. Intracranial bleeding, spinal hematoma, or hemothorax are potential contraindications to the administration of these prophylactic agents, but they may be resumed once bleeding has stabilized. Consider placing an inferior vena cava filter in those patients who have an active episode of bleeding anticipated to persist for more than 48–72 h and begin prophylactic anticoagulants as soon as feasible.

5. Initiate stress ulcer prophylaxis. Start early enteral nutrition.

6. Consider tracheostomy for quadriplegic patients who show prolonged ventilator dependence. Prevention of ventilator-associated pneumonia and early weaning may be facilitated by early tracheostomy.

References

1. Hitselberger WE, House WF. A warning regarding the sitting position for acoustic tumour surgery. *Arch Otolaryngol.* 1980;106:69.
2. Matjasko J, Petrozza P, Cohen M, Steinberg P. Anaesthesia and surgery in the seated position. Analysis of 554 cases. *Neurosurgery.* 1985;17:695–702.
3. Wilder BL. Hypothesis: the etiology of mid cervical quadriplegia after operation with the patient in sitting position. *Neurosurgery.* 1982;11:530–531.
4. Turker RJ, Slack C, Regan Q. Thoracic paraplegia after lumbar spinal surgery. *J Spinal Disord.* 1995;8(3):195–200.
5. Haisa T, Kondo T. Midcervical flexion myelopathy after posterior fossa surgery in the sitting position: case report. *Neurosurgery.* 1996;38(4):819–821.
6. Dominguez J, Rivas JJ, Lobato RD, Diaz V, Larru E. Irreversible tetraplegia after tracheal resection. *Ann Thorac Surg.* 1996;62(1):278–280.
7. Ozgen S, Pait TG, Caglar YS. The V2 segment of the vertebral artery and its branches. *J Neurosurg Spine.* 2004;1(3):299–305.
8. Yuh WT, Marsh III EE, Wang AK, et al. MR imaging of spinal cord and vertebral body infarction. *AJNR Am J Neuroradiol.* 1992;13(1):145–154.
9. Turnbull IM, Brieg A, Hassler O. Blood supply of cervical spinal cord in man: a microangiographic cadaver study. *J Neurosurg.* 1966;24(6):951–965.

10. Kestle JR, Resch L, Tator CH, Kucharczyk W. Intervertebral disc embolization resulting in spinal cord infarction: case report. *J Neurosurg*. 1989;71(6):938–941.
11. Zouaoui A, Hidden G. The cervical vertebral venous plexus and anastomoses with the cranial venous sinuses. *Bull Assoc Anat (Nancy)*. 1987;71(212):7–13.
12. Yuan Q, Dougherty L, Margulies SS. In vivo human cervical spinal cord deformation and displacement in flexion. *Spine*. 1998;23(15):1677–1683.
13. Epstein NE, Danto J, Nardi D. Evaluation of intraoperative somatosensory-evoked potential monitoring during 100 cervical operations. *Spine*. 1993;18:737–747.
14. Nuwer MR, Dawson EG, Carlson LG, et al. Somatosensory evoked potential monitoring reduces neurological deficits after scoliosis surgery: results of a large multicenter study. *Electroenceph Clin Neurophysiol*. 1995;96:6–11.
15. Owen JH, Naito M, Bridwell KH, Oakley DM. Relationship between duration of spinal cord ischaemia and postoperative neurologic deficits in animals. *Spine*. 1990;15:846–851.
16. Hoppenfeld S, Gross A, Andrews C, Lonner B. The ankle clonus test for assessment of the integrity of the spinal cord during operations for scoliosis. *J Bone Joint Surg Am*. 1997;79:208–212.
17. Dawson EG, Sherman JE, Kanim LEA, Nuwer MR. Spinal cord monitoring. Results of the scoliosis research society and the European spinal deformity society survey. *Spine*. 1991;16(Suppl.):361–364.
18. Ben-David B, Haller G, Taylor P. Anterior spinal fusion complicated by paraplegia. A case report of a false-negative somatosensory-evoked potential. *Spine*. 1987;12:536–539.
19. Ginsburg HH, Shetter AG, Raudzens PA. Postoperative paraplegia with preserved intra-operative somatosensory evoked potentials. *J Neurosurg*. 1985;63:296–300.
20. Pelosi L, Jardine A, Webb JK. Neurological complications of anterior spinal surgery for kyphosis with normal somatosensory evoked potentials. *J Neurol Neurosurg Psychiatry*. 1999;66:662–664.
21. Owen JH. The application of intraoperative monitoring during surgery for spinal deformity. *Spine*. 1999;24:2649–2662.
22. Papastefanou SL, Henderson LM, Smith NJ, et al. Surface electrode somatosensory-evoked potentials in spinal surgery. *Spine*. 2000;25:2467–2472.
23. Edmonds HJ, Paloheimo MP, Backman MH, et al. Transcranial magnetic motor evoked potentials (tcMMEP) for functional monitoring of motor pathways during scoliosis surgery. *Spine*. 1989;14:683–686.
24. Herdmann J, Lumenta CB, Huse KOW. Magnetic stimulation for monitoring of motor pathways in spinal procedures. *Spine*. 1993;18:551–559.
25. Minahan RE, Sepkuty JP, Lesser RP, et al. Anterior spinal cord injury with preserved neurogenic 'motor' evoked potentials. *Clin Neurophysiol*. 2001;112:1442–1450.

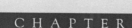

CHAPTER

11

Spinal Shock

Vasudha Singhal[1], Richa Aggarwal[2]

[1]Department of Neuroanaesthesia and Intensive Care, Medanta, The Medicity, Gurgaon, Haryana, India; [2]Department of Neuroanaesthesiology and Critical Care, All India Institute of Medical Sciences, New Delhi, India

DEFINITION

Spinal shock occurs following an acute spinal cord injury and involves a reversible loss of all neurological function, including reflexes and rectal tone, below a particular level. It is defined as a state of transient physiologic (rather than anatomic) reflex depression of cord function below the level of injury, with associated loss of all sensorimotor functions. It is not a "shock" in the sense of a circulatory collapse, but a state of depressed spinal reflexes caudal to cord injury.

Spinal shock was first described by Whytt in 1750 as a loss of sensation accompanied by motor paralysis with initial loss but gradual recovery of reflexes, following a spinal cord injury (SCI)—most often a complete transection.[1]

Reflexes generally return in a specific pattern after spinal shock, with cutaneous or polysynaptic reflexes returning before deep tendon reflexes. Ko et al.[2] described a specific pattern of reflex return with the delayed plantar reflex (DPR) returning first, followed by the bulbocavernosus and cremasteric reflexes, and finally the ankle and knee jerk reflexes. The bulbocavernosus reflex usually returns 1–3 days after the injury. It is elicited by squeezing the penile glans or the clitoris (or tugging on the foley catheter) and feeling for an involuntary contraction of the anus.

The DPR is a pathological response elicited by an unusually strong stimulation of the sole of the foot and is characterized by a slow and protracted plantar flexion of the great toe and/or other toes and slow return to the neutral position. Presence of this reflex has a prognostic significance in spinal shock.[3] The presence of a DPR immediately following injury has a poor prognostic correlation with recovery of ambulation.

VARIANT

Spinal shock is often confused with neurogenic shock. Neurogenic shock describes the hemodynamic changes resulting from a sudden loss of autonomic tone due to spinal cord injury. It is commonly seen when the level of the injury is above T6. Spinal shock, on the other hand, refers to loss of all sensation below the level of injury and is not circulatory in nature. Both may, however, coexist in a patient.

Neurogenic shock is a type of distributive shock, consisting of the hemodynamic triad of hypotension, bradycardia, and peripheral vasodilatation, attributed to severe central nervous system damage (head trauma, cervical cord trauma, or high thoracic cord injuries), resulting in loss of sympathetic stimulation to the blood vessels and unopposed vagal activity. Patients may be poikilothermic and may not be able to regulate their body temperature due to profound vasodilatation and heat loss. There is systemic hypotension due to a decrease in sympathetic fiber-mediated arterial and venous vascular resistance, along with venous pooling and loss of preload, with or without bradycardia. The bradycardia is often exacerbated by suctioning, defecation, turning, and hypoxia. The hypotension places patients at increased risk of secondary spinal cord ischemia due to impairment of autoregulation. Fluid resuscitation and vasopressors remain the mainstay of treatment. Norepinephrine is started initially but in refractory cases epinephrine and vasopressin infusions may be required. Bradycardia usually responds to atropine and glycopyrrolate but in severe cases dopamine infusion is required.

Important to note here is that shock associated with a spinal cord injury must always be considered hemorrhagic until proven otherwise.[4] This differentiation is very necessary as the management to both forms of shock vary—while hypovolemic shock requires aggressive fluid resuscitation to treat hypotension and a thorough evaluation to exclude any ongoing blood loss, the choice of therapy in neurogenic shock is vasopressors to overcome low blood pressure, as the patients may be refractory to fluid resuscitation. Also, hemorrhagic shock is associated with tachycardia, but the loss of thoracic sympathetic innervation (T1–T5) may inhibit tachycardia and vasoconstriction as signs of hypovolemia, in patients where both conditions coexist. Moreover, neurogenic shock can persist for 1–6 weeks after the injury.

CAUSE

The mechanism of injury that causes spinal shock is usually traumatic in origin, due to transection, distraction, compression, bruising, hemorrhage, or ischemia of the cord or by injury to blood vessels supplying it. There occurs a sudden loss of conduction in the spinal cord as a result of the migration of potassium ions from the intracellular to extracellular spaces. This is associated with a transient loss of somatic and automatic reflex activity below the level of spinal cord segment damage.

The pathophysiology of spinal shock is best explained by the four-phase model of spinal shock proposed by Ditunno et al.[4] in 2004:

Phase I: Areflexia/hyporeflexia—occurs from 0 to 1 day post injury. All deep tendon reflexes caudal to the cord injury are absent, and muscles are flaccid and paralyzed. This occurs due to the loss of background excitation of spinal motor neurons and interneurons from the supraspinal axons.
Phase II: Initial reflexes return—lasts 1–3 days after injury. It is marked by the return of polysynaptic cutaneous reflexes like bulbocavernosus, due to denervation supersensitivity to neurotransmitters in partially denervated spinal neurons.
Phase III: Initial hyperreflexia—occurs between 4 days and 1 month post injury. The deep tendon reflexes reappear during this period, resulting from axon supported synapse growth.
Phase IV: Final hyperreflexia—occurring between 1 and 12 months post injury. This occurs from soma-supported synapse growth. Cutaneous reflexes, deep tendon reflexes, and the Babinski sign become hyperactive and respond to minimal stimuli. The time of detrusor or bladder recovery is usually 4–6 weeks. Vasovagal hypotension and bradyarrhythmias resolve in 3–6 weeks.

Autonomic dysreflexia may emerge in phase III or IV of spinal shock recovery. It usually occurs due to a distended viscus, like the bowel or bladder, acting as a stimulus causing massive sympathetic outflow below the zone of injury, which is upregulated by supraspinal input. It often manifests with episodic hypertension, flushing, diaphoresis, and tachycardia.[5]

SIGNS AND SYMPTOMS

Spinal shock is characterized by flaccid, areflexic paralysis of skeletal and smooth muscles. There is a complete loss of autonomic function below the level of the lesion, resulting in loss of urinary bladder tone and paralytic ileus. Sweating and piloerection are diminished or absent. Since vasomotor tone is lost, dependent lower extremities may become edematous and patients may be particularly vulnerable to deep venous thrombosis and pulmonary embolism. Temperature regulation is affected. Genital reflexes are lost. Sensation below the level of the lesion may be completely absent. Autonomic dysfunction is worse with higher levels of injury. In injuries above the T6 level, the sympathetic outflow is diminished with a persistent parasympathetic output by the vagus nerve, resulting in bradycardia and hypotension. Paralysis of the intercostals and abdominal musculature impairs both expansion of the lungs and diaphragmatic stabilization, dramatically compromising vital capacity, deep breathing, and cough strength. Patients usually require mechanical ventilation during acute hospitalization. High cervical lesions have the highest incidence of ventilation complications, like nosocomial pneumonias, and are most difficult to wean off mechanical ventilation.

As spinal shock resolves, patients with upper motor neuron lesions gradually develop spasticity, which predisposes them to pain, contractures and pressure ulcers. Osteoporosis and heterotopic ossification are common long term complications in patients with spinal cord injuries. Pressure ulcers due to soft tissue necrosis caused by constant unrelieved pressure and excessive frictional or shearing forces, are the commonest hurdles in patient rehabilitation.

TREATMENT[6]

- Airway, Breathing, Circulation:
  - Patients presenting with spinal shock almost always need intubation and mechanical ventilation.
  - Initial resuscitation with intravenous fluids to maintain optimal tissue perfusion and to resolve shock is the first treatment priority.
  - Initial base deficit or lactate level can be used to determine the severity of shock and the need for ongoing fluid resuscitation or the need for vasopressors.

- All potential causes of hemodynamic instability, including hemorrhage, pneumothorax, myocardial injury, pericardial tamponade, sepsis related to abdominal injury, and other traumatic and medical etiologies need to be ruled out.
- In the setting of neurogenic shock, it is essential to first ensure that intravascular volume is restored, then vasopressors (dopamine, norepinephrine, phenylephrine) may be used to treat hypotension.[7]
- High cervical injury patients may frequently require cardiovascular interventions, such as the use of vasopressors, atropine, aminophylline, or pacemakers for symptomatic bradycardia.[8]
- An ideal vasopressor in the setting of bradycardia should have both α- and β-adrenergic actions, such as dopamine, norepinephrine, or epinephrine, to counter the loss of sympathetic tone and provide chronotropic support to the heart.
- Temperature monitoring is essential during the acute management phase, as patients with SCI above T6 may experience hypothermia as well as reduced ability to dissipate body heat.
- Consider placing a nasogastric tube for abdominal decompression.
- Maintaining skin integrity and preventing pressure sores during the acute hospitalization phase following SCI is critical to optimizing patient outcomes and minimizing complications.
  - Place the patient on a pressure reduction mattress.
  - Reposition to provide pressure relief or turn at least every 2h while maintaining spinal precautions.
  - Keep the area under the patient clean and dry and avoid temperature elevation.
  - Assess nutritional status on admission and regularly thereafter.
  - Inspect the skin under pressure garments and splints.
- Prevention and treatment of venous thromboembolism:
  - Apply mechanical compression devices early after injury.
  - Begin low molecular weight heparin, or unfractionated heparin plus intermittent pneumatic compression, in all patients.
- Patients with acute SCI are at high risk for respiratory complications. Respiratory complications (including ventilatory failure, atelectasis, pneumonia, and pleural effusions) are most common with C1–C4 level injuries (84% incidence).[9]
  - Perform a tracheotomy early in the hospitalization of patients who are likely to remain ventilator-dependent or to wean slowly from mechanical ventilation over an extended period of time.
  - Treat retained secretions due to expiratory muscle weakness with manually assisted coughing ("quad coughing"), pulmonary hygiene, mechanical insufflation–exsufflation, or similar expiratory aids in addition to suctioning.
- Place an indwelling urinary catheter as part of the initial patient assessment.

II. COMPLICATIONS RELATED TO SPINAL CORD

- Priapism is usually self-limited in acute SCI and does not require treatment.
- Initiate gastrointestinal stress ulcer prophylaxis.
  - Evaluate swallowing function prior to oral feeding in any acute SCI patient.
  - Dysphagia occurs in at least 15% of patients with recent cervical SCI and may result in aspiration pneumonia.[10]
  - Bowel distention and inadequate evacuation can lead to nausea and vomiting, high gastric residuals, anorexia, poor lung expansion, and inadequate venous return. Therefore, attention to bowel evacuation early after injury can prevent complications and reduce acute care length of stay.
  - Early enteral nutrition should be initiated within 24–48 h of spinal shock.

PROGNOSIS

Functional recovery in patients with spinal shock remains poor. Life expectancy for such patients has increased in recent years with better rehabilitation services. Pneumonia, pulmonary embolism, septicemia, and suicides remain the leading causes of death in patients with complete spinal cord injury.

References

1. Sherrington CS. *The Integrative Action of the Nervous System*. London: Constable & Company Ltd; 1906.
2. Ko HY, Ditunno Jr JF, Graziani V, et al. The pattern of reflex recovery during spinal shock. *Spinal Cord*. 1999;37:402–409.
3. Weinstein DE, Ko HY, Graziani V, Ditunno Jr JF. Prognostic significance of the delayed plantar reflex following spinal cord injury. *J Spinal Cord Med*. April 1997;20(2):207–211.
4. Atkinson PP, Atkinson JL. Spinal shock. *Mayo Clin Proc*. 1996;71:384–389.
5. Ditunno JF, Little JW, Tessler A, et al. Spinal shock revisited: a four-phase model. *Spinal Cord*. 2004;42:383–395.
6. Early acute management in adults with spinal cord injury. *J Spinal Cord Med*. 2008;31(4):408.
7. Stevens RD, Bhardwaj A, Kirsch JR, Mirski MA. Critical care and perioperative management in traumatic spinal cord injury. *Neurosurg Anesthesiol*. July 2003;15(3):215–229.
8. Bilello JF, Davis JW, Cunningham MA, Groom TF, Lemaster D, Sue LP. Cervical spinal cord injury and the need for cardiovascular intervention. *Arch Surg*. October 2003;138(10):1127–1129.
9. Jackson AB, Groomes TE. Incidence of respiratory complications following spinal cord injury. *Arch Phys Med Rehabil*. March 1994;75(3):270–275.
10. Kirshblum S, Johnston MV, Brown J, O'Connor KC, Jarosz P. Predictors of dysphagia after spinal cord injury. *Arch Phys Med Rehabil*. September 1999;80(9):111–115.

Further Reading

1. Silver JR. Early autonomic dysreflexia. *Spinal Cord*. 2000;38:229–233.

COMPLICATIONS RELATED TO CARDIO-VASCULAR SYSTEM

Aneurysm/Arteriovenous Malformation Rupture

Hemanshu Prabhakar, Indu Kapoor

Department of Neuroanaesthesiology and Critical Care, All India Institute of Medical Sciences, New Delhi, India

DEFINITION

Rupture of the intracranial aneurysm or an arteriovenous malformation during surgical clipping or coil embolization is one of the most devastating complications in neurosurgery. It is defined as a fresh or new leak in the existing vascular pathology occurring during the intraoperative course. The complication may occur any time from induction of

© 2016 Elsevier Inc. All rights reserved.

anesthesia to application of the negative pressure vacuum drain at the end of surgery.[1,2] The majority of aneurysms rupture during dissection and clip application. The complication is more catastrophic in neuroradiologic suites as the patients are heparinized. Intraoperative rupture may occur at a rate of 7–35%[3] and may be due to various causes mentioned below. In the Analysis of Treatment by Endovascular approach to Nonruptured Aneurysms (ATENA) study, the rate varies from 2.4% to 3.9% in aneurysm more than 3 mm and less than or equal to 3 mm, respectively.[4] However, in the Clinical and Anatomic Results in the Treatment of Ruptured Intracranial Aneurysms (CLARITY) study, the frequency of aneurysm rupture is higher in patients with middle cerebral artery aneurysm, patients under 65 years of age, and hypertensive patients.[5]

PATHOPHYSIOLOGY

The rupture of aneurysm during induction of anesthesia and tracheal intubation occurs as a result of wide fluctuations in the mean arterial pressure. It is an important goal to minimize the transmural pressure at the time of induction of anesthesia without affecting the cerebral perfusion pressure. Transmural pressure is the difference of the mean arterial pressure and the intracranial pressure. Sudden fluctuation in the mean arterial pressure disturbs this equation and results in disruption or rupture of the aneurysm (Figure 1). Factors affecting the mean arterial pressure or the intracranial pressure may alter the transmural gradient, thereby, increasing the susceptibility of aneurysmal rupture.

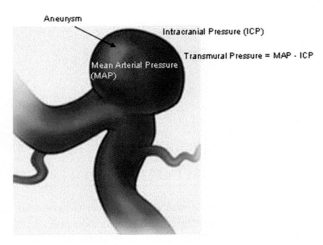

FIGURE 1   Schematic diagram showing the determinants of the transmural pressure.

CAUSE

The risk of rupture of aneurysm is related to size, large arteries, location, transmural pressure gradient, technical causes such as temporary arterial occlusion, experience of the surgeon, and days since ictus. Posterior inferior cerebellar arteries and the anterior and posterior communicating arteries are more likely to rupture.[6] In a neuroradiological suite, the cause may be coil protrusion and microcatheter perforation[7] and aneurysm in middle cerebral artery. Injecting the contrast may increase the intraluminal pressure causing rupture.

SIGNS AND SYMPTOMS

The features of aneurysmal rupture vary depending on the time of rupture. A sudden increase in blood pressure associated with or without bradycardia during or immediately after induction of general anesthesia is suggestive of ruptured aneurysm. This also results in increased intracranial pressure. The brain may swell, making exposure and dissection of aneurysm difficult. However, in most of the cases the aneurysm ruptures during dissection or application of temporary clip, it can be easily appreciated by sudden gush of blood from the pathological vessel.

DIAGNOSIS

Sudden hemodynamic fluctuations should raise suspicion of ruptured aneurysm. The diagnosis may also be made with use of transcranial Doppler ultrasound.

Intraoperative rupture at the time of dissection or clipping can be visually confirmed by sudden gush of arterial blood from the operative site.

PREDISPOSING FACTORS

According to the authors of one study, patients undergoing coiling, independent predictors of intraoperative aneurysm rupture were Asian race, black race, chronic obstructive pulmonary disease, and lower initial Hunt and Hess Grade. Hyperlipidemia and lower initial Hunt and Hess Grade were both independent predictors of intraoperative aneurysm rupture among those undergoing clipping.[8]

TREATMENT

The most important step in the event of intraoperative ruptured aneurysm is a good communication between the anesthetist and the surgeon or the interventional radiologist.

Should a rupture occur during induction of anesthesia and prior to surgery, decision to proceed with the surgery should be carefully considered as the raised intracranial pressure greatly impairs surgical dissection and exposure of the aneurysm. However, the experience and skill of the surgeon may be a reason to proceed with the surgery and immediate clipping of the ruptured aneurysm. All during the event, it is essential that the vitals of the patients be carefully monitored and maintained. It has therefore been suggested, that the patient's blood pressure be reduced by 20–25% below the baseline values at the time of induction. To attenuate the hemodynamic response to tracheal intubation, prophylactic measures may be taken as suggested in the literature. Use of narcotics, lidocaine, and a bolus of intravenous anesthetic agent may be helpful in this regard. It is important to avoid hyperventilation all during this period as sudden reduction in arterial carbon dioxide levels may reduce intracranial pressure. This increases the transmural pressure and may lead to rupture of the aneurysm.

If the aneurysm ruptures during dissection or clipping, it is important to take measures to reduce the brain bulk and maintain intravascular volume status, maintaining systemic and cerebral hemodynamics targeting adequate cerebral perfusion pressure, controlling intracranial pressure, and reducing the transmural pressure. The mean arterial pressure may be reduced to the lower limit of cerebral autoregulation (50–60 mmHg) as this facilitates surgical clipping. Agents such as thiopentone sodium, propofol, or etomidate may be used to lower the blood pressure. Etomidate is especially helpful in hemodynamically unstable patients. These agents also provide some cerebral protection when temporary clips are applied to the main vessel. Ipsilateral carotid compressions for short duration have also been suggested. Once clipped, the arterial pressures may be raised to preoperative values. If large amount of blood has been lost, it is prudent to transfuse colloids, whole blood, and blood products to maintain intravascular volume status.

Managing this complication in radiological suite is more challenging and difficult. Lowering the blood pressure is generally helpful as it reduces the amount of subarachnoid bleed. As these patients are heparinized, immediate reversal of heparin should be carried out using protamine sulfate. Protamine sulfate should be administered in the dose of 1 mg for each 100 units of heparin given. In extreme situations, transfusion of platelet concentrates may also be required. Measures to reduce the intracranial pressure by hyperventilation (up to end-tidal carbon dioxide of 30 mmHg), mannitol, or placing an external ventricular drain may be needed. Antiepileptic prophylaxis with phenytoin or levetiracetam should be started as these patients become prone to seizures.

PREVENTION

Both the anesthetist and the surgeon play an important role in preventing this catastrophic event. Avoiding extreme fluctuations of blood pressure at the time of induction of anesthesia is essential. Strict measures should be taken to avoid coughing at the time of tracheal intubation. Hyperventilation should be avoided during initial stage till the dura is opened so as to avoid intracranial hypotension. It has also been suggested that mannitol should be administered after the dural opening.

References

1. Pong RP, Lam AM. Anesthetic management of cerebral aneurysm surgery. In: Cottrell JE, Young WL, eds. *Neuroanesthesia*. 5th ed. Mosby Elsevier; 2010:218–246.
2. Prabhakar H, Bithal PK, Chouhan RS, Dash HH. Rupture of intracranial aneurysm after partial clipping due to aspiration drainage system. *Middle East J Anesthesiol*. 2008;19:1185–1190.
3. Wong JM, Ziewacz JE, Ho AL, et al. Patterns in neurosurgical adverse events: open cerebrovascular neurosurgery. *Neurosurg Focus*. 2012;33:E15.
4. Pierot L, Barbe C, Spelle L, ATENA investigators. Endovascular treatment of very small unruptured aneurysms: rate of procedural complications, clinical outcome, and anatomical results. *Stroke*. 2010;41:2855–2859.
5. Pierot L, Cognard C, Anxionnat R, Ricolfi F, CLARITY Investigators. Ruptured intracranial aneurysms: factors affecting the rate and outcome of endovascular treatment complications in a series of 782 patients (CLARITY study). *Radiology*. 2010;256:916–923.
6. Leipzig TJ, Morgan J, Horner TG, Payner T, Redelman K, Johnson CS. Analysis of intraoperative rupture in the surgical treatment of 1694 saccular aneurysms. *Neurosurgery*. 2005;56:455–468.
7. Luo CB, Teng MMH, Chang FC, Lin CJ, Guo WY, Chang CY. Intraprocedure aneurysm rupture in embolization: clinical outcome with imaging correlation. *J Chin Med Assoc*. 2012;75:281–285.
8. Elijovich L, Higashida RT, Lawton MT, Duckwiler G, Giannotta S, Johnston C, Cerebral Aneurysm Rerupture After Treatment (CARAT) Investigators. Predictors and outcomes of intraprocedural rupture in patients treated for ruptured intracranial aneurysms: the CARAT study. *Stroke*. 2008;39:1501–1506.

CHAPTER

13

Vasospasm

Charu Mahajan[1], Nidhi Gupta[2]

[1]Department of Neuroanaesthesiology and Critical Care, All India Institute
of Medical Sciences, New Delhi, India; [2]Department of Neuroanaesthesia,
Indraprastha Apollo Hospital, New Delhi, India

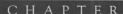

OUTLINE

Cerebral vasospasm implies narrowing of blood vessels resulting in decreased cerebral blood flow to distal tissues resulting in ischemia. It has been variously defined[1] in the literature by different authors:

1. *Clinical vasospasm* defined as neurological deterioration deemed secondary to vasospasm after other causes are eliminated. It is seen in 20–40% of patients.
2. *Delayed cerebral ischemia* (DCI) defined as clinically symptomatic vasospasm or infarction on computed tomography (CT) attributable to vasospasm.
3. *Angiographic vasospasm* defined as moderate-to-severe arterial narrowing on digital subtraction angiography not attributable to atherosclerosis, catheter-induced spasm, or vessel hypoplasia. About

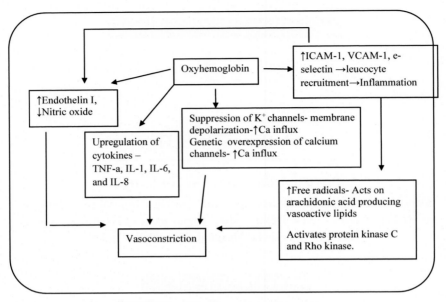

FIGURE 1   Etiopathogenesis of vasospasm.

70% of patients may have angiographic narrowing but clinically may not be evident in all.

4. *Transcranial Doppler (TCD) spasm*, defined as any mean flow velocity >120 cm/s.

PATHOPHYSIOLOGY

It occurs mostly between 3 and 21 days post hemorrhage. The arteries have thin adventitia through which blood breakdown products reach tunica media and cause vasoconstriction (Figure 1) .

The various possible mechanisms involved are:

- Neuronal apoptosis
- Scavenging or decreased production of nitric oxide (NO)
- Increased endothelin 1 levels
- Direct oxidative stress on smooth muscle cells
- Free radical production and lipid peroxidation of cell membranes
- Modification of potassium and calcium channels
- Rho kinase induced proliferation and growth of vascular smooth muscle cells

- Ischemia producing cortical spreading depolarization[2]
- Overexpression of genes

CLINICAL PRESENTATION

Altered consciousness, disorientation, occurrence of new focal neurological deficit corresponding to the artery involved, usually seen 3–14 days after subarachnoid hemorrhage (SAH). We have to exclude other causes of neurological deterioration like hydrocephalus, rebleeding, electrolyte disorders, seizures, and hypoxia.

DIAGNOSIS

The various modalities for diagnosis of vasospasm are:

Digital subtraction angiography is the gold standard for diagnosing cerebral vasospasm. It also has a therapeutic role as it allows intra-arterial administration of vasodilators or balloon angioplasty. The disadvantages are it is an invasive procedure with risk of vessel injury, is expensive, and repeated frequent studies are not possible.

CT angiography is a minimally invasive and less expensive alternative for angiography.

Magnetic resonance angiography (MRA) is a noninvasive technique that requires neither contrast nor radiation exposure. Time of flight–MRA sequence is specific for diagnosis of vasospasm. It is, however, expensive and requires patient cooperation during long study period.

TCD can measure an increase in cerebral blood flow velocity present in cerebral vasospasm. Normal middle cerebral artery (MCA) blood flow velocity is <120 cm/s, velocity from 120 to 200 cm/s indicates mild vasospasm and >200 cm/s is taken as severe vasospasm. Also an increase by 50 cm/s in 24 h indicates the presence of vasospasm. Lindegaard index helps in differentiation of vasospasm and hyperemia; it is a ratio of flow velocities in ipsilateral MCA to extracranial internal carotid artery. Normal ratio is <3, 3–6 indicates mild vasospasm, and >6 denotes severe vasospasm.

Cerebral blood flow (CBF) studies. The various CBF studies performed like single-photon emission computed tomography, positron emission tomography, xenon-enhanced CT, and diffusion and perfusion weighted magnetic resonance imaging studies can also detect ischemia secondary to vasospasm. Cerebral microdialysis and electroencephalography are the other lesser utilized modalities for diagnosis of vasospasm.

MANAGEMENT

Triple-H therapy	• Aims to raise CBF by increasing intravascular volume, vascular resistance, and decreasing viscosity. • Several studies have found no reduction in delayed ischemic neurological deficit or improvement in outcome. • The various complications of triple-H therapy are pulmonary edema, myocardial ischemia, congestive cardiac failure, electrolyte imbalance, dilutional coagulopathy, and rupture of unsecured aneurysm. • In 2010, a systematic review aimed to compare the three components and concluded hypertension is more effective in increasing cerebral blood flow.[3] • The American Heart Association/American Society of Anesthesiologists guidelines[4] recommend maintenance of euvolemia and normal circulating blood volume for prevention of DCI (class I; level of evidence B). • In patients who develop DCI, hypertension can be induced provided cardiac status permits it (class I, level of evidence B).[4]
Calcium channel blockers (CCBs)	• CCBs block calcium influx into the cell through L-type voltage gated calcium channels thereby reducing vasospasm. • Nimodipine has little vasodilatory action on vasospastic vessels but improves outcome by its neuroprotective action.[5] • Oral nimodipine 60 mg, 4 times a day should be administered to all patients for 21 days from the day of hemorrhage (class I, level of evidence I).[4] • Nicardipine prolonged-release implants placed in cisterns or in ventricles have shown positive results in preventing and relieving vasospasm.[6,7] • In several studies, fasudil hydrochloride, a potent antagonist of rho-kinase, has been used by intravenous and intra-arterial route for treating vasospasm. • A meta-analysis shows significant reduction in angiographic vasospasm and vasospasm-related infarcts with intravenous fasudil administration. Requires further large randomized controlled trials for validation.[8] • Side effects like convulsions, intracerebral hemorrhage and raised alkaline phosphatase, aspartate aminotransferase, alanine transaminase have been reported after fasudil administration. • Verapamil has been tried by intra-arterial route; inconsistent results.[9]
Endothelin receptor antagonist	• Clazosentan, an endothelin A receptor antagonist reduced the incidence of angiographic vasospasm in a dose-dependent manner but was associated with increased rates of pulmonary complications, hypotension, and anemia (CONSCIOUS-1 trial).[10] • In a subsequent trial (CONSCIOUS-2), clazosentan failed to improve outcome in patients treated with surgical clipping.[11] • CONSCIOUS-3 trial was undertaken to assess whether clazosentan reduced vasospasm-related morbidity and all-cause mortality in aneurysmal subarachnoid hemorrhage (SAH) patients treated by endovascular coiling. It was stopped prematurely following completion of CONSCIOUS-2 and no improvement in clinical outcome was found.[12]

Magnesium	• It is a calcium antagonist, N-methyl-D-aspartate receptor antagonist, decreases glutamate release, and has neuroprotective effects. • The Magnesium in Aneurysmal Subarachnoid Hemorrhage (MASH) trial, showed nonsignificant reductions in delayed cerebral as well as 3-month poor clinical outcomes.[13] • Subsequently, intravenous magnesium sulfate for the Aneurysmal Subarachnoid Hemorrhage trial and the MASH-2 trial demonstrated almost similar outcome in both groups.[14,15]
Statins	• These are 3-hydroxy-3-methylglutaryl-CoA reductase inhibitors which increase nitric oxide synthetase levels causing smooth muscle relaxation and vasodilation. • Earlier studies showed conflicting results. • Simvastatin in the Aneurysmal Subarachnoid Hemorrhage (STASH)-2 trial showed no benefit of statins in ameliorating vasospasm.[16]
Erythropoietin (EPO)	EPO has been found to have neuroprotective, antiapoptotic, antioxidative, and neurotrophic properties. A phase II randomized controlled trial showed decrease in incidence of severe vasospasm and delayed ischemic deficit in patients having aneurysmal SAH who received EPO.[17]
Phosphodiesterase inhibitors	Milrinone is a phosphodiesterase III inhibitor with ionotropic and vasodilator effects. Has been used by both intravenous and intra-arterial routes. However, hypotension may ensue after its administration. Papaverine inhibits cAMP and cGMP phosphodiesterases in smooth muscles causing vasodilatation. May be administered via intra-arterial or intracisternal route. The various side effects reported are hypotension, raised intracranial pressure, transient neurological deficits (mydriasis, brain stem depression), seizures, and thrombocytopenia.[18] The vasodilatory effect is short-lived and may require repeat administration.
Sildenafil citrate, NO donors	Experimental data only.
Angioplasty	• Usually done for refractory vasospasm. • Balloon angioplasty mechanically dilates the proximal parts of large spastic intracranial vessels. • Various complications described are thrombosis at an angioplasty site, vessel rupture, hemorrhagic infarction, and rebleeding from an unprotected aneurysm following vessel dilatation. • Pharmacological angioplasty treats even distal, small, and difficult to reach vessels. • Various intra-arterial agents used are CCBs, papaverine, and milrinone. • Cerebral angioplasty and/or selective intra-arterial vasodilator therapy is reasonable in patients with symptomatic cerebral vasospasm, particularly those who are not rapidly responding to hypertensive therapy (class IIa; level of evidence B).[5]

CONCLUSION

The morbidity and mortality associated even in treated SAH patients, makes it one of the most researched areas ranging from molecular to clinical studies. The multifactorial etiology makes it imperative to devise a treatment modality which targets several steps at a time.

References

1. Frontera JA, Fernandez A, Schmidt JM, et al. Defining vasospasm after subarachnoid hemorrhage: what is the most clinically relevant definition? *Stroke*. 2009;40:1963–1968.
2. Dreier JP, Woitzik J, Fabricius M, et al. Delayed ischaemic neurological deficits after subarachnoid haemorrhage are associated with clusters of spreading depolarizations. *Brain*. 2006;129(Pt 12):3224–3227.
3. Dankbaar JW, Slooter AJC, Rinkel GJ, Schaaf IC. Effect of different components of triple-H therapy on cerebral perfusion in patients with aneurysmal subarachnoid haemorrhage: a systematic review. *Crit Care*. 2010;14:R23.
4. Connolly ES, Rabinstein AA, Carhuapoma JR, et al. Guidelines for the management of aneurysmal subarachnoid hemorrhage: a guideline for healthcare professionals from the American Heart Association/American Stroke Association. *Stroke*. 2012;43(6):1711–1737.
5. Pickard JD, Murray GD, Illingworth R, et al. Effect of oral nimodipine on cerebral infarction and outcome after subarachnoid haemorrhage: British aneurysm nimodipine trial. *BMJ*. March 11, 1989;298(6674):636–642.
6. Barth M, Thome C, Schmiedek P, Weiss C, Kasuya H, Vajkoczy P. Characterization of functional outcome and quality of life following subarachnoid hemorrhage in patients treated with and without nicardipine prolonged-release implants: clinical article. *J Neurosurg*. 2009;110(5):955–960.
7. Schneider UC, Dreher S, Hoffmann KT, Schmiedek P, Kasuya H, Vajkoczy P. The use of nicardipine prolonged release implants (NPRI) in microsurgical clipping after aneurysmal subarachnoid haemorrhage: comparison with endovascular treatment. *Acta Neurochir*. 2011;153(11):2119–2212.
8. Liu GJ, Wang ZJ, Wang YF, et al. Systematic assessment and meta-analysis of the efficacy and safety of fasudil in the treatment of cerebral vasospasm in patients with subarachnoid hemorrhage. *Eur J Clin Pharmacol*. 2012;68(2):131–139.
9. Kimball MM, Velat GJ, Hoh BL. Participants in the international multi-disciplinary consensus conference on the critical care management of subarachnoid hemorrhage. Critical care guidelines on the endovascular management of cerebral vasospasm. *Neurocrit Care*. 2011;15(2):336–341.
10. Macdonald RL, Kassell NF, Mayer S, et al. Clazosentan to overcome neurological ischemia and infarction occurring after subarachnoid hemorrhage (CONSCIOUS-1): randomized, double-blind, placebo-controlled phase 2 dose-finding trial. *Stroke*. 2008;39:3015–3021.
11. Macdonald RL, Higashida RT, Keller E, et al. Clazosentan, an endothelin receptor antagonist, in patients with aneurysmal subarachnoid haemorrhage undergoing surgical clipping: a randomised, double-blind, placebo-controlled phase 3 trial (CONSCIOUS-2). *Lancet Neurol*. 2011;10:618–625.
12. MacDonald RL, Higashida RT, Keller E, et al. Randomized trial of clazosentan in patients with aneurysmal subarachnoid hemorrhage undergoing endovascular coiling. *Stroke*. 2012;43(6):1463–1469.
13. van den Bergh WM, Algra A, van Kooten F, et al. MASH study group. Magnesium sulfate in aneurysmal subarachnoid hemorrhage: a randomized controlled trial. *Stroke*. 2005;36(5):1011–1015.

14. Wong GKC, Chan MTV, Boet R, Poon WS, Gin T. Intravenous magnesium sulfate after aneurysmal subarachnoid hemorrhage: a prospective randomized pilot study. *J Neurosurg Anesthesiol.* 2006;1(2):142–148.
15. Dorhout Mees SM, Algra A, Vandertop WP, et al. Magnesium for aneurysmal subarachnoid haemorrhage (MASH-2): a randomized placebo-controlled trial. *Lancet.* 2012;380(9836):44–49.
16. Kirkpatrick PJ, Turner CL, Smith C, Hutchinson PJ, Murray GD, for the STASH Collaborators. Simvastatin in aneurysmal subarachnoid haemorrhage (STASH): a multicentre randomised phase 3 trial. *Lancet Neurol.* 2014;13:666–675.
17. Tseng MY, Hutchinson PJ, Richards HK, et al. Acute systemic erythropoietin therapy to reduce delayed ischemic deficits following aneurysmal subarachnoid hemorrhage: a Phase II randomized, double-blind, placebo-controlled trial: clinical article. *J Neurosurg.* 2009;111(1):171–180.
18. Liu JK, Couldwell WT. Intraarterial papaverine infusions for the treatment of cerebral vasospasm induced by aneurysmal subarachnoid hemorrhage. *Neurocrit care.* 2005;2:124–132.

CHAPTER

14

Electrocardiogram Abnormalities

Richa Aggarwal, Hemanshu Prabhakar

Department of Neuroanaesthesiology and Critical Care, All India Institute of Medical Sciences, New Delhi, India

DEFINITION

The close association between the brain and the heart makes the heart vulnerable during any neurologic insult. This may be reflected in the electrocardiogram (ECG) and could vary between sinus tachycardia to asystole (flat ECG). The abnormalities could be a change in the rhythm or the morphology of the ECG.

VARIANTS

Morphologic ECG changes noted in neurologically compromised patients may be isolated P, Q, U, and T wave changes, QRS complex changes, and the ST-T segment changes.

However, rhythm changes observed in the ECG may range from all possible benign dysrhythmias, such as sinus bradycardia or tachycardia, to potentially fatal dysrhythmias, such as ventricular tachycardia, ventricular fibrillation, and asystole.[1]

CAUSES

Various neurologic causes have been attributed to bringing about changes in the ECG. The conditions may be as follows:

1. Subarachnoid hemorrhage (SAH)
2. Traumatic brain injury (TBI), both in adults and pediatrics[2]
3. Brain tumors
4. Stroke
5. Spinal cord injury (SCI)
6. Electroconvulsive therapy (ECT)
7. Electrolyte abnormalities: potassium, calcium
8. During hemodynamic instability
9. Raised intracranial pressure (ICP)
10. Meningitis
11. Venous air embolism
12. During hyperventilation
13. Pharmacological causes such as the use of papaverine or hydrogen peroxide
14. Technical causes such as during magnetic resonance imaging (MRI) or faulty ECG electrodes
15. Therapeutic hypothermia
16. Epilepsy

It has been suggested through experimental studies that the insula in the brain has a cardiac chronotropic organization. This may be involved in the genesis of arrhythmias seen in epilepsy or after cerebral hemorrhage or stroke.[3]

SIGNS AND SYMPTOMS

In a majority of cases, patients remain asymptomatic, especially during their preoperative period. However, during the intraoperative period, care has to be taken and vigilance maintained. Hemodynamic instability may be observed in some cases. Some anesthetics, such as halothane, produce myocardial depression and may be dangerous. Under the influence of anesthetic agents, there remains a possibility that potentially fatal dysrhythmias may precipitate.

DIAGNOSIS

ECG is a routine preoperative investigation. Intraoperative monitoring of ECG is also a routine procedure. Therefore, changes in the rhythm or morphology of the ECG are easily noticeable and can be diagnosed on monitoring. Some of the characteristic ECG changes observed in clinical conditions are mentioned below.

Patients with SAH show ECG changes in 40–100% cases; more are observed in poor-grade patients.[1] The changes include T wave inversion, ST segment depression, prolongation of QT interval, and appearance of U and Q waves. Rhythmic disturbances may include sinus bradycardia or tachycardia, atrioventricular dissociation, and serious ones such as the ventricular tachycardia and fibrillation.

Severe head injury may produce T wave inversion,[4] ST segment depression,[2] and prolonged QT interval. Both adults and pediatrics are susceptible to these changes.

Brain tumors may be associated with ECG changes,[5] which are more often observed in those involving the limbic system compared to the tumors of extralimbic location. The most frequent change noted is the prolonged QTc interval.

The ST segment changes, T inversion, and fibrillations may be observed in patients suffering from stroke.[6] Raised intracranial pressure results in prominent U waves, ST-T changes, and notched T wave along with shortening and prolongation of QT intervals.[7]

SCIs may produce ECG changes such as sinus pause, shifting sinus pacemaker, nodal escape beats atrial fibrillations, ventricular premature contractions, ventricular tachycardia, and ST-T changes.

Some of the common ECG changes observed following TBI are prolonged QTc intervals, ST-T changes, increased P wave amplitude, heart blocks, supraventricular tachycardia, and sinus tachycardia.

ECT is known to produce nonspecific changes in ST-T waves.[8]

The common ECG changes noted during raised ICP are sinus bradycardia, QT prolongation, ST segment changes, and T or U wave abnormalities. The presence of J wave has also been reported.[9] ECG changes mimicking myocardial infarction have been reported during meningitis.[10]

Following venous air embolism and secondary to desaturation, ECG changes may be observed in some situations. The changes involve the ST-T segment and are usually reversible. Bradycardia has been reported with use of drugs such as papaverine[11] and hydrogen peroxide.[12]

Faulty placement of electrodes may show abnormalities in the ECG, which need to be carefully judged. Therapeutic hypothermia used in a neurosurgical setup, especially as a cerebroprotective strategy, may result in changes in the ECG morphology.[13] Sinus bradycardia, presence of J wave, prolonged QT interval, T wave changes, heart blocks, junctional rhythm, and atrial fibrillations may be seen. Similarly, during seizures, ECG changes appear in the form of sinus tachycardia and shortening or prolongation of the QTc interval.[14]

TREATMENT

In most of the cases, these ECG changes are transient and do not require treatment or active management. The changes revert to a normal rhythm on correction of the inciting factor. However, in situations where patients become hemodynamically unstable, treating these ECG changes may become mandatory. An arterial blood gas analysis is helpful in identifying electrolyte abnormalities.

Treat hypertension, hypotension, tachycardia, and bradycardia. Hypotension secondary to blood loss may be treated with crystalloids, colloids, and blood and blood products, if required. The electrolytes need to be corrected to normal values; details are discussed in other sections of the book.

ECG changes due to SCIs may be corrected using atropine, propranolol, or even bilateral vagal nerve resection. With increasing duration of time after an injury, the ECG changes usually disappear.

PREVENTION

Whereas naturally occurring pathological conditions may not be preventable, some of the conditions that may be easily controlled in order to avoid occurrence of ECG changes include:

1. Correct electrolyte abnormalities.
2. Avoid hemodynamic fluctuations.
3. Avoid hyperventilation or use cautiously.
4. Avoid factors that may increase ICP.
5. Minimize the use of drugs such as papaverine and hydrogen peroxide.

References

1. Pong RP, Lam AM. Anesthetic management of cerebral aneurysm surgery. In: Cottrell JE, Young WL, eds. *Neuroanesthesia*. 5th ed. Mosby Elsevier; 2010:218–246.
2. Dash M, Bithal PK, Prabhakar H, Chouhan RS, Mohanty B. ECG changes in pediatric patients with severe head injury. *J Neurosurg Anesthesiol*. 2003;15:270–273.

3. Oppenheimer SM, Cechetto DF, Hachinski VC. Cerebrogenic cardiac arrhythmias. *Arch Neurol.* 1990;47:513–519.
4. La Rocca R, Materia V, Pasquini A, La Rosa FC, Marte F, Patanè S. T-wave inversion after a severe head injury without ischemic heart disease. *Int J Cardiol.* 2011;151:e43–44.
5. Koepp M, Kern A, Schmidt D. Electrocardiographic changes in patients with brain tumors. *Arch Neurol.* 1995;52:152–155.
6. Kumar AP, Babu E, Subrahmanyam D. Cerebrogenic tachyarrhythmia in acute stroke. *J Neurosci Rural Pract.* 2012;3:204–206.
7. Jachuck J, Ramani PS, Clark F, Kalbag RM. Electrocardiographic abnormalities associated with raised intracranial pressure. *Br Med J.* 1975;1:242–244.
8. Messina AG, Paranicas M, Katz B, Markowitz J, Yao FS, Devereux RB. Effect of electroconvulsive therapy on the electrocardiogram and echocardiogram. *Anesth Analg.* 1992;75:511–514.
9. Milewska A, Guzik P, Rudzka M, et al. J-wave formation in patients with acute intracranial hypertension. *J Electrocardiol.* 2009;42:420–423.
10. Brander L, Weinberger D, Henzen C. Heart and brain: a case of focal myocytolysis in severe pneumococcal meningoencephalitis with review of the contemporary literature. *Anaesth Intensive Care.* 2003;31:202–207.
11. Rath GP, Mukta, Prabhakar H, Dash HH, Suri A. Haemodynamic changes following intracisternal papaverine instillation during intracranial aneurysmal surgery. *Br J Anaesth.* 2006;97:848–850.
12. Prabhakar H, Bithal PK, Pandia MP, Gupta M, Rath GP. Bradycardia due to hydrogen peroxide irrigation during craniotomy for craniopharyngioma. *J Clin Neurosc.* 2007;14:488–490.
13. de Souza D, Riera AR, Bombig MT, et al. Electrocardiographic changes by accidental hypothermia in an urban and a tropical region. *J Electrocardiol.* 2007;40:47–52.
14. Moseley BD, Wirrell EC, Nickels K, Johnson JN, Ackerman MJ, Britton J. Electrocardiographic and oximetric changes during partial complex and generalized seizures. *Epilepsy Res.* 2011;95:237–245.

Hemodynamic Instability

Charu Mahajan, Hemanshu Prabhakar

Department of Neuroanaesthesiology and Critical Care, All India Institute
of Medical Sciences, New Delhi, India

O U T L I N E

The utmost objective of anesthetic management of neurosurgical patients is the maintenance of adequate cerebral perfusion pressure (CPP) that prevents any secondary injury to the brain and spinal cord. Hemodynamic instability is often encountered intraoperatively or postoperatively and encompasses both hypotension and hypertension along with changes in heart rate. Specifically related to the brain, hypotension may decrease cerebral blood flow (CBF) causing ischemia, while hypertension may raise CBF, thereby increasing intracranial pressure (ICP) and edema and may even cause hemorrhaging. An interplay of systemic, neurogenic, and cardiogenic factors make blood pressure (BP) labile.

PREVENTION

Careful intraoperative positioning, monitoring of vitals, maintenance of adequate central venous pressure, and hematocrit are mainstays for the prevention of intraoperative hemodynamic variability. Arterial BP monitoring

TABLE 1   Reasons for Hemodynamic Instability in Neurosurgical Patients

Hypertension	Hypotension
Systemic • Essential hypertension • Laryngoscopy and intubation • Incision • Pin fixation • Light level of anesthesia • Pain • Hypercarbia • Bladder distension • Autonomic neuropathy (e.g. Guillain–Barré syndrome) **Neurosurgical** • Raised ICP: Tumor, ICH, SAH, AIS, TBI • Brain stem handling • Emergence • Induced hypertension for vasospasm • Postcarotid endarterectomy • Autonomic dysreflexia (SCI above T6)	**Systemic** • Preexisting cardiomyopathy • Arrhythmias • Cardiac failure • MI • Hypovolemia due to decreased intake, diuretics, Diabetes insipidus, cerebral salt wasting syndrome, hemorrhage from systemic injuries, surgical blood loss • Anesthesia drugs • Anaphylaxis • Sepsis • Tension Pneumothorax • Cardiac tamponade • Adrenal insufficiency • Autonomic neuropathy **Neurosurgical** • Neurogenic stunned myocardium • Spinal shock • Carotid body stimulation • TCR • Brain stem handling • Hypothalamic lesions • Pituitary failure
Bradycardia	**Tachycardia**
• As part of the Cushing reflex (bradycardia, hypotension, and respiratory disturbances) • Brain stem handling during surgery • As part of TCR • Vagal stimulation • Acute spinal shock • Autonomic dysreflexia • Cardiac conduction disturbances • Drugs (calcium channel blockers, β-blockers, digitalis, etc.) • Hypothyroidism • Hypothermia • Hypoxia	• Hypovolemia • Sudden blood loss • Pain • Fever • Hypercarbia • Lighter plane of anesthesia • Brain stem handling • Cardiac causes • Drugs (anticholinergics, adrenaline, dopamine, etc.) • Hyperthyroidism

ICH, Intracranial Hemorrhage; SAH, Subarachnoid hemorrhage; AIS, Acute ischemic stroke; TBI, Traumatic brain injury; SCI, Spinal cord injury.

III. COMPLICATIONS RELATED TO CARDIO-VASCULAR SYSTEM

with transducer zeroed at the level of external auditory meatus gives an accurate beat-to-beat measurement. Noninvasive cardiac output monitors can be used in patients with preexisting heart disease.

HEMODYNAMIC INSTABILITY IN SPECIFIC SITUATIONS

Craniotomy for Tumor Excision

Brain stem handling during tumor excision is common, and it manifests as hypertension or hypotension, bradycardia or tachycardia (Table 2). Surgeons should be immediately informed so that surgical stimulus can be promptly withdrawn. It is not advisable to pharmacologically treat it because it may mask further brain stem handling. Massive blood loss may result in hypovolemic hypotension and require fluids, blood, and resuscitation. Trigeminocardiac reflex (TCR) may result in bradycardia and hypotension due to stimulation of any sensory branch of a trigeminal nerve along its intracranial or extracranial course.[1] It usually resolves on its own if stimulation is stopped, but in severe cases, a vagolytic may have to be administered. However, it should also be remembered that TCR may also manifest as a pressor response.[2] At the end of craniotomy closure, negative pressure applied via a vacuum device connected to a drain placed in the extradural space has been reported to cause a sudden decrease in ICP, resulting in bradycardia.[3]

Carotid Endarterectomy

Incidences of hypertension and hypotension after carotid endarterectomy is 9% and 12%, respectively.[5] Preoperative hypertension is a significant risk factor for the development of postoperative hypertension, which in turn increases the incidence of neurological deficit and operative mortality.[5,6] Even 21% of preoperative normotensive patients have raised pressure in the postoperative period.[6] Postoperative hypertension may lead to hematoma formation in the neck at the surgical site, cerebral hyperperfusion syndrome, or even myocardial infarction (MI). Hyperperfusion syndrome is characterized by headache, seizures, focal neurologic signs,

TABLE 2   Hemodynamic Response During Stimulation of Structures[4]

Structures	Response
Trigeminal nerve stimulation	Hypotension and bradycardia or hypertension and tachycardia
Vagus nerve stimulation	Hypotension and/or bradycardia
Brain stem handling	Hypotension/hypertension, bradycardia/tachycardia

brain edema, and intracerebral hemorrhage. Carotid body denervation at the time of surgery is a reason for BP variability during and after surgery. While dissecting the common carotid artery, precaution has to be taken not to damage the vagus nerve and carotid sinus.[7] Cross-clamping of the carotid artery intraoperatively decreases CBF, leading to activation of baroreceptors and compensatory increases in arterial pressure. With the application of a shunt or removal of a clamp, normal pressures are restored. Bradycardia and hypotension may occur intraoperatively during stretching of carotid sinus. Carotid sheath infiltration with local anesthetic blunts the hemodynamic alterations occurring due to handling of carotid artery. Postoperatively, hypotension is less commonly encountered and may be due to carotid body hypersensitivity or the effects of overtreatment with antihypertensives. This usually responds to fluids or low-dose vasopressor. However, if it fails to respond, MI has to be ruled out.

Subarachnoid Hemorrhage

Sudden hemorrhage from an aneurysm raises ICP, which causes ischemia of the hypothalamus. This results in intense sympathetic stimulation, which increases arterial pressure to maintain CPP. But this catecholamine surge also produces myocardial injury, which may present as spectra of chest pain, dyspnea, hypoxemia, left ventricular systolic dysfunction, cardiogenic shock with pulmonary edema, and elevated cardiac markers. Such patients may need additional cardiac output monitoring for management of hypotension. In the postoperative period, therapeutic hypertension may be instituted for treating vasospasm if cardiac status allows it. This requires fluids and drugs like dopamine, dobutamine, phenylephrine, or noradrenaline.

Minimally Invasive Procedures

Endoscopic procedures run a high risk of bradycardia and hypertension because of raised ICP caused by continuous inflow of irrigation fluid through neuroendoscope. Stimulation of the floor of the third ventricle or distortion of posterior hypothalamus may also result in bradycardia.[8] Stimulation of subthalamic nucleus is known to cause an increase in heart rate and blood pressure and should be borne in mind during deep brain stimulation.[9]

TREATMENT OF HYPERTENSION

The cause of hypertension should be searched for and adequately treated. The Cushing reflex is a protective mechanism in which BP tries to rise above ICP to maintain CPP. Thus, lowering ICP should be the first

TABLE 3   Antihypertensive Agents

Sympatholytics	
β-adrenergic blockers: Metoprolol, Esmolol, Mixed α- and β-adrenergic antagonist labetalol	No known adverse effect on ICP; caution during Cushing reflex: may accentuate bradycardia.
α-adrenergic antagonist: phentolamine	↓CBF if CPP significantly decreases.
Clonidine	↓CBF by direct α_2 mediated action on cerebral vessels.[10]
Angiotensin-converting enzyme inhibitors: Captopril, Enalapril, Lisinopril, Ramipril	Cause leftward shift of autoregulation curve with shortened plateau phase.[11]
Angiotensin receptor blockade Losartan	Preserves CBF; has a role in hypertensive patients with history of stroke.
Calcium channel blockers Diltiazem, Nicardipine, Nifedipine, Verapamil, Felodipine	Cause cerebral vasodilation and may ↑ICP.[11]
Vasodilators: hydralazine, NTG, SNP	Cerebral vasodilation→↑CBV and ↑ICP with ↓MAP and CPP.
Diuretics: Thiazides, loop diuretics, potassium-sparing diuretics.	May be added along with other drugs. If patient is already on osmotic diuretics, may be avoided.

step in such cases. Intraoperative, adequate depth of anesthesia and analgesia should be ensured. Inform the surgeon of any sudden change in arterial pressure.

Emergence hypertension can be prevented by extubating the trachea in deeper levels or by pharmacological means. As this phenomenon is transient, short-acting β-blockers effectively control BP without compromising the patient's state for extubation (Table 1).

In cases where all reasons of hypertension are ruled out and control of BP is mandatory, pharmacological treatment is required. The various agents used for treating hypertension and their effects on cerebral hemodynamics are discussed (Table 3). Calcium channel blockers, nitroglycerine, sodium nitroprusside, and hydralazine may all cross the blood–brain barrier and may increase CBF, ICP, and impair autoregulation.

TREATMENT OF HYPOTENSION

- Find and treat the cause.
- The surgical field should be continuously assessed for blood loss. Resuscitation has to be done with fluids and blood when required.

III. COMPLICATIONS RELATED TO CARDIO-VASCULAR SYSTEM

- Pharmacological treatment: Phenylephrine is a pure vasoconstrictor and may even cause reflex bradycardia. It is commonly used for the maintenance of BP in patients with traumatic brain injury (TBI), postsurgical patients, and for inducing hypertension in subarachnoid hemorrhage patients with vasospasm. Dopamine, epinephrine, and norepinephrine belong to the vasoconstrictor-inotrope group. Norepinephrine increases BP by peripheral vasoconstriction, and unlike epinephrine and dopamine, it does not increase heart rate. However, if the blood–brain barrier is defective, then its β-mimetic activity may increase the cerebral metabolism and blood flow. Dobutamine and milrinone are the inotropes with vasodilatory action helpful in low-cardiac output states. Presently, in literature there are no recommendations for using a particular vasopressor. Though, some have found norepinephrine more efficient for maintaining cerebral perfusion pressure, the evidence is not strong enough[12].

MANAGEMENT OF BRADYCARDIA AND TACHYCARDIA

The reasons for bradycardia and tachycardia should be sought and treated. Any traction or stimulation of the brain structures may produce this change. The surgeon should be asked to promptly withdraw the stimulus. This is often transient and should resolve immediately on its own.

Bradycardia in asymptomatic patients does not require treatment. However, if associated with hypotension and other symptoms of compromised perfusion, it should be immediately treated. Isoprenaline and atropine are often used for this purpose. In refractory cases, transcutaneous pacing may have to be done. Tachycardia with hypertension may be treated with short-acting β-blockers. Cardiac causes of tachycardia have to be treated accordingly.

References

1. Arasho B, Sandu N, Spiriev T, Prabhakar H, Schaller B. Management of the trigeminocardiac reflex: facts and own experience. *Neurol India*. 2009;57:375–380.
2. Meng Q, Zhang W, Yang Y, et al. Cardiovascular responses during percutaneous radiofrequency thermocoagulation therapy in primary trigeminal neuralgia. *J Neurosurg Anesthesiol*. 2008;20:131–135.
3. Wasnick JD, Lien CA, Rubin LA, Fraser RA. Unexplained bradycardia during craniotomy closure. The role of intracranial hypotension. *Anesth Analg*. 1993;76:432–433.
4. Black S, Cucchiara RF. Tumor surgery. In: Cucchiara RF, Black S, Michenfelder JD, eds. *Clinical Neuroanesthesia*. New York: Churcill Livingstone; 1998:343.
5. Wong JH, Findlay JM, Suarez Almazor ME. Hemodynamic instability after carotid endarterectomy: risk factors and associations with operative complications. *Neurosurgery*. 1997;41:35–41.

6. Towne JB, Bernhard VM. The relationship of postoperative hypertension to complications following carotid endarterectomy. *Surgery*. 1980;88:575–580.
7. Biller J, Feinberg WM, Castaldo JE, et al. Guidelines for carotid endarterectomy: a statement for healthcare professionals from a special writing group of the stroke council, American Heart Association. *Circulation*. 1998;97(5):501–509.
8. El-Dawlatty AA, Murshid WR, Elshimy A, Maqboul MA, Samarkandi A, Takrouri MS. The incidence of bradycardia during endoscopic third ventriculostomy. *Anesth Analg*. 2000;91:1142–1144.
9. Kaufmann H, Bhattacharya KF, Voustianiouk A, Gracies JM. Stimulation of the subthalmic nucleus increases heart rate in patients with Parkinson disease. *Neurology*. 2002;59:1657–1658.
10. Coughlan MG, Lee JG, Bosnjak ZJ, Schmeling WT, Kampine JP, Warltier DC. Direct coronary and cerebral vascular responses to dexmedetomidine. Significance of endogenous nitric oxide synthesis. *Anesthesiology*. 1992;77:998–1006.
11. Tietjen CS, Hurn PD, Ulatowski JA, Kirsch JR. Treatment modalities for hypertensive patients with intracranial pathology: options and risks. *Crit Care Med*. 1996;24:311–322.
12. Steiner LA, Johnston AJ, Czosnyka M, et al. Direct comparison of cerebrovascular effects of norepinephrine and dopamine in head injured patients. *Crit Care Med*. 2004;32:1049–1054.

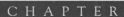

C H A P T E R

16

Vascular Injuries

Charu Mahajan, Hemanshu Prabhakar

Department of Neuroanaesthesiology and Critical Care, All India Institute
of Medical Sciences, New Delhi, India

The inadvertent rupture of a vessel is not an uncommon complication during neurosurgical procedures. Other than major blood loss and its resultant complications, it carries a high risk of ischemia and permanent neurological deficits. This requires prompt management to minimize the morbidity and mortality associated with it.

Vascular injuries may be classified based on the following:

1. Location: intracranial or spinal
2. Type: arterial, venous, or capillary

INTRACRANIAL

A large vessel injury may result in cortical ischemia, while damage to perforating vessels results in deep-brain ischemia. Torrential bleeding from a major artery may lead to rapid blood loss and hemodynamic instability and needs immediate control. The sphenopalatine artery, internal carotid artery (ICA), cavernous portion of ICA, and cavernous venous sinus are the structures vulnerable to damage during transsphenoidal approach for pituitary tumors. Bleeding through a major vessel during an endoscopic surgery obscures the vision and is impossible to take control of. The majority of vascular injuries may be avoided if the surgeon adheres to a strict midline course. Important vessels traverse the base of the skull, and any surgery in this area carries significant risk of vessel damage. Intraoperative aneurysm rupture is not an uncommon entity and requires urgent control by means of a clip.

Venous injury can occur due to the inadvertent opening of a sinus or damage to a cortical vein. Retractor injury is also an important cause of cortical vein injury. Prolonged application of the retractor blade can cause the vessel to stretch and needs to be released intermittently.

During neurointerventional procedures, vascular injury can be seen as contrast leakage on an angiogram. An awake patient may complain of sudden headache, and neurological deterioration may require urgent intubation. A minor leak may be closed endovascularly by stent placement. The onset of Cushing reflex entails a rapid intracranial pressure (ICP) lowering regime and an urgent craniotomy for the evacuation of hematoma.

SPINAL

Anterior cervical diskectomy and fusion is a safe procedure, but rare reports of vertebral artery injury are present in the literature. During cervical corpectomy and craniovertebral junction surgeries, a vertebral artery or the ICA may be damaged. It has been seen that 60–90% of patients with vertebral artery injury underwent anterior cervical corpectomy.[1] This procedure carries a high risk of vessel injury, more so at higher cervical vertebrae. The vessel injury has been reported to occur at the time of drilling, screw placement, or by the instruments themselves. The incidence of major vascular injury during lumbar spinal surgery ranges from 1 to 5 per 10,000 or even higher.[2] About 30% of these comprise of arterial injury.[3] The aorta bifurcates at the level of L4–L5 intervertebral disc into the right and left common iliac arteries. Thus, the major vessels like the aorta, common iliac artery, inferior vena cava, common iliac veins, or the internal iliac vein may get injured during thoracic and lumbar spinal surgeries. A malpositioned thoracic pedicle screw may cause aortic injury and can be rapidly fatal. The left common iliac artery lies just anterior to L4–L5 intervertebral disc and is the most commonly injured vessel in the literature.[4] The Adamkiewicz artery usually arises on the left side between T9–T12 but can originate anywhere between T5–L2. It supplies lumbar and sacral cord, and if damaged, it can result in anterior cord syndrome.

PREDISPOSING FACTORS

During intracranial surgery, vessels trapped inside a tumor or surgical field in close proximity to major vessels or venous sinuses increase the chances of vessel damage. The highest risk of aneurysm rupture is during its dissection. Level L4–L5 is closely related to the common iliac vessel and is the most common site for vascular injury during spine surgery.[5]

Factors predisposing to vessel injury during spinal surgery are defect or degeneration of the fibrous annulus or the anterior longitudinal ligament, adhesion of prevertebral structures to the anterior longitudinal ligament, and in complex operative settings such as redo surgeries, aggressive exploration, and complex patient positioning.[4,6]

CLINICAL COURSE

This can be divided into acute, subacute, and chronic. The acute effects of major vessel injury are mainly due to sudden blood loss resulting in tachycardia, hypotension, and shock. The surgical field may be flooded with blood, and vessel injury may be easily diagnosed. But at times, bleeding may not be apparent in cases of posterior lumbar spine surgery or if blood collects in the retroperitoneal space. Having a high index of suspicion for a patient with sudden, unexplained hypotension may be life saving. If the patient survives, the subacute effects are as a consequence of massive blood transfusion and its complications. The patient may develop new neurological deficits depending on the vessel involved. The watershed areas of the spinal cord are prone to ischemia, and depending on the vessel affected, the patient may develop anterior, posterior, or central cord syndrome. The sequelae of an arterial injury are formation of pseudoaneurysm or an arteriovenous fistula even months or years later. Delayed effects of a cortical vein bleed are edema, normal pressure hydrocephalus, and cortical vein thrombosis.

PREVENTION

Preoperative radiographic visualization of the vessel course helps in learning about any anomalous positions of a major vessel. Surgery in close vicinity to vascular structures has to be performed cautiously to avoid any injury. Surgical skill is also a determining factor of vascular injury. Adequate visualization of the surgical field and dissection planes, avoiding blind instrumentation, and avoiding contact injury from instruments like ultrasonic aspirators, drills, and screws is essential for prevention of any vascular injury.[7] In case of cervical corpectomy, midline landmarks should be carefully followed and excessive lateral placement of screws has to be avoided to prevent injuring vertebral artery. The ICA or even thyroid arteries may be damaged by the retractors during anterior cervical spine approach. Despite all the precautions, accidental injury may occur anytime.

MANAGEMENT

Management will depend upon the size of the vessel, whether the vessel is arterial or venous, and its location.

Local Management

Once bleeding occurs from a vessel, compression is applied at the point of bleeding and packing is done with cottonoids and local hemostats. Low-flow arterial bleeding from small perforating vessels can be controlled by cauterization. Electrocautery carries a risk of thrombosis and thermal damage to the vessel itself and even to the adjacent neural structures. It can be used for a small vessel or capillary bleed, but it is ineffective for a major vessel or sinus bleed. A major arterial bleed may have to be controlled by hemostatic clips or even angiographic embolization. Similarly, for an aneurysm rupture, proximal clip application may be done to clear the surgical field for subsequent permanent clip application. Care has to be taken not to coagulate contiguous cortical veins and avoid placing a retractor in the area of the coagulated vein. Topical application of various local hemostats controls capillary, venous, and even small arterial bleed. These are absorbable gelatin sponges with thrombin, fibrillated collagen, oxidized cellulose, fibrin sealants, and a gelatin–thrombin matrix. Crushed muscle tissue contains thromboplastin and can be applied for local hemostasis. For a sinus injury, hemostatic biomaterial agents and dural patch are required for its repair. For an aortic or inferior vena cava injury, an urgent laparotomy has to be performed for direct repair of the vessel.

Systemic Management

The main aim of systemic management is to provide hemodynamic stability by transfusion of adequate crystalloids, colloids, and blood and its components. Transient-controlled hypotension may assist the surgeon in visualizing the point of vessel injury and taking prompt control. However, it should not be allowed for longer periods.

Endovascular Management

Over the past decade, there has been an upsurge in endovascular repair of vascular complications during surgery. Repair of arterial injuries can be undertaken endovascularly, especially in patients who are stable. An arterial injury may subsequently present as a pseudoaneurysm and require endovascular placement of a stent or coil occlusion. Venous thrombolysis may be done endovascularly for major sinus thrombosis.

CONCLUSION

Iatrogenic vascular injuries may be less commonly encountered in daily practice, but they carry a high risk of morbidity and mortality. A high index of suspicion and prompt management are critical for good outcomes.

References

1. Inamasu J, H Guiot B. Vascular injury and complication in neurosurgical spine surgery. A review article. *Acta Neurochir Wien*. 2006;148:375–387.
2. Papadoulas S, Konstantinou D, Kourea HP, et al. Vascular injury complicating lumbar disc surgery. A systematic review. *Eur J Vasc Endovasc Surg*. 2002;24:189–195.
3. Skippage P, Raja J, McFarland R, et al. Endovascular repair of iliac artery injury complicating lumbar disc surgery. *Eur Spine J*. 2008;17(suppl 2):S228–S231.
4. Szolar DH, Preidler KW, Steiner H, et al. Vascular complications in lumbar disk surgery: report of four cases. *Neuroradiology*. 1996;38:521–525.
5. Sadhasivan S, Kayner AM. Iatrogenic arteriovenous fistula during lumbar microdiscectomy. *Anesth Analg*. 2004;99:1815–1817.
6. Prabhakar H, Bithal PK, Dash M, Chaturvedi A. Rupture of aorta and inferior vena cava during lumbar disc surgery. *Acta Neurochir Wien*. 2005;147:327–329.
7. Kassam A, Snyderman CH, Carrau RL, Gardner P, Mintz A. Endoneurosurgical hemostasis techniques: lessons learned from 400 cases. article E7 *Neurosurg Focus*. 2005;19(1).

COMPLICATIONS
RELATED TO
COAGULATION

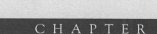

CHAPTER

17

Coagulopathy

Charu Mahajan, Hemanshu Prabhakar

Department of Neuroanaesthesiology and Critical Care, All India Institute
of Medical Sciences, New Delhi, India

DEFINITION

Coagulopathy is defined as a condition in which the blood's ability to clot is impaired. Sometimes the term is used to represent both hypocoagulability and hypercoagulability. In this chapter we will be limiting our discussion primarily to hypocoagulability.

CAUSES

The normal coagulation cascade at a localized site seals any breach in vascular continuity and limits blood loss. Failure of this process to advance places the patient at risk of bleeding. The main concern is bleeding in a closed compartment, such as intracranial or intraspinal, which may result in hazardous consequences. The major causes of coagulopathy in a neurosurgical patient are listed in Table 1. Patients with a history of venous thromboembolism, stroke, coronary artery stents, prosthetic heart valves, and intracardiac thrombus are usually on anticoagulant therapy and antiplatelet drugs. They may present for some elective neurosurgical procedure or for emergency surgery secondary to development of an intracranial hemorrhage requiring urgent reversal of coagulopathy. The decision regarding cessation of drug therapy has to be taken in consultation with cardiologist, hematologist, and neurosurgeon. Patient and his family should be explained clearly about the risk of development of thromboembolism with cessation of drugs or occurrence of bleeding in case they are continued (Table 2).

TABLE 1 List of Various Causes of Coagulopathy

Congenital

Hemophilia
Von Villebrands disease
Factor V, factor VIII, protein C, antithrombin III deficiency
Afibrinogenemia

Acquired

Massive blood loss
Dilution of coagulation factors and platelets by fluid resuscitation and blood transfusion
Disseminated intravascular coagulopathy
Sepsis
Drugs
- antiplatelet agents—aspirin and other NSAIDS
  Clopidogrel, ticlopidine
  Glycoprotein IIb/IIa receptor antagonist (tirofiban, eptifibatide)
- anticoagulants (warfarin, heparin, enoxaparin, dalteparin)
- fibrinolytics (streptokinase, urokinase, alteplase, reteplase)
Severe liver disease
Vitamin K deficiency
Thrombocytopenic purpura
Hypothermia
Citrate toxicity

NSAIDS, Nonsteroidal antiinflammatory drugs.

TABLE 2   Work Up for Diagnosis of Coagulopathy

Complete Medical History (Present and Past)
Past surgical history
History of trauma
Drug history
Family history
Physical examination
Laboratory tests[3] for
* enzymatic coagulation
  Prothrombin time/international normalized ratio, Activated Partial
  thromboplastin time, thrombin time, thrombin–antithrombin III complex,
  prothrombin cleavage fragments, thromboelastography, rotational
  thromboelastometry.
* fibrinolyis
  d-dimer, fibrinogen degradation product, plasminogen activator
  inhibitor-1,
  throboelastography, rotational thromboelastometry.
* platelets
  Platelet count, bleeding time, platelet function analyzer, rapid platelet
  function assay.
  Whole-blood impedence aggregometry, thromboelastography, rotational
  thromboelastometry.

BRAIN TUMORS

Brain tumors are known to cause coagulation abnormalities resulting in either hypercoagulability or less commonly hypocoagulability. Patients with benign tumors were found to have reduced coagulant property while those with malignant tumors had increased fibrinolytic activity.[1] This hemostatic abnormality is due to hyperfibrinolysis either primary or secondary to disseminated intravascular coagulopathy (DIC).[2] Tissue plasminogen activator released from tumor cells or from brain parenchyma during surgery may lead to development of DIC. This consumptive coagulopathy thus results in hyperfibrinolysis raising the risk of bleeding.

TRAUMATIC BRAIN INJURY

After head injury, release of tissue thromboplastin from brain may result in hypercoagulability and ischemic lesions.[3] Subsequently, coagulation factor consumption results in DIC and bleeding diathesis[3] (Figure 1). Other reasons attributing to coagulopathy may include hypoperfusion, massive blood loss, dilutional thrombocytopenia, hypothermia, and acidosis. Combined trauma and hypoperfusion causes activation of protein C-mediated coagulopathy while chronic protein C depletion causes predisposition to infection and thromboembolic events.[3]

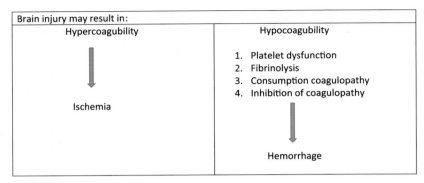

FIGURE 1   Mechanism of development of coagulopathy after brain injury.[3]

ACUTE ISCHEMIC STROKE

Patients with acute ischemic stroke often also have coronary artery disease and are on antiplatelet drugs. Before being taken for surgery these patients have to be assessed for risk of coagulopathy and thromboembolism. Further, patients with acute ischemic stroke may develop thrombolytic-related intracerebral hemorrhage (ICH) and may present in operation room for evacuation of hematoma. In this scenario, reversal of coagulopathy is desirable for prevention of enlargement of hematoma.

INTRACRANIAL HEMORRHAGE

An important cause of hemorrhagic stroke in elderly population is drug-induced coagulopathy. This requires immediate reversal of coagulopathy to limit extent of intracranial bleed and for any surgical intervention if required.

The commonly used tests are platelet count, prothrombin time/international normalized ratio, activated partial thromboplastin time, and blood transfusion. The others may not be available in usual practice. Thromboelastography or rotational thromboelastometry can measure complete hemostatic function including enzymatic function, fibrinolysis, and platelet action.[3] The real-time information enables to achieve goal-directed therapy with transfusion of the particular component of blood that is deficient.

MANAGEMENT

Patients should be thoroughly evaluated in preoperative period by history, physical examination, and appropriate coagulation tests when required. Neurosurgical procedures (neurosurgery, spinal surgery) belong to the high risk group for bleeding and their thrombotic risk stratification can be done based on their evaluation.[5,6]

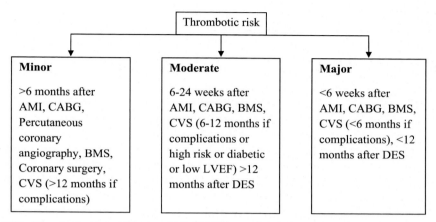

Minor	Moderate	Major
>6 months after AMI, CABG, Percutaneous coronary angiography, BMS, Coronary surgery, CVS (>12 months if complications)	6-24 weeks after AMI, CABG, BMS, CVS (6-12 months if complications or high risk or diabetic or low LVEF) >12 months after DES	<6 weeks after AMI, CABG, BMS, CVS (<6 months if complications), <12 months after DES

Table: Thrombotic risk stratification. AMI, ACUTE myocardial infarction; CABG, coronary artery bypass grafting; BMS, bare metal stent; CVS, cerebrovascular stroke; DES, drug eluting stent.

Warfarin is an oral anticoagulant which interferes with vitamin K metabolism thus affecting factors II, VII, IX, X, and protein C and S. Patients with mechanical heart valves, chronic atrial fibrillation, and venous thromboembolism are usually on warfarin. For surgical procedure, it is stopped 4–5 days prior to allow INR to decrease below 1.5. An emergency surgery or an intracranial bleed requires urgent reversal of warfarin anticoagulation. This can be carried out by administration of prothrombin complex concentrate (PCC) or fresh frozen plasma (FFP), containing vitamin K-dependent factors (II,VII, IX, X). PCC is the product of choice and has several advantages over FFP.[7] It is given in dose of 25–50 U/kg and about 90% of patients achieve normal INR within 15 min of administration.[5] A second dose may be repeated if INR fails to reach target value. A limiting factor for PCC use is its availability and it also carries risk of thrombosis. FFP is universally available and can be administered in dose of 15–20 mL/kg. The main disadvantage is high volume load produced by its transfusion and low concentration of factor IX which hinders the INR correction when its value is above 5. Vitamin K should be coadministered along with PCC or FFP. It can be given by oral, intravenous, intramuscular, and subcutaneous route. It is given in dose of 5 mg intravenously and takes 24 h for lowering of INR.[8]

Recombinant factor VIIa (rFVIIa) is used as a hemostatic agent both for surgical prophylaxis and treatment of bleeding episodes in patients having hemophilia A or B and factor VII deficiency.[9] It has also been used for anticoagulation reversal, in ICH/trauma patients and for achieving perioperative hemostasis. In patients with warfarin induced ICH, rFVIIa reversed its action earlier than PCC and FFP.[10] However, it also runs a small risk of thrombotic complications.

In patients with intracranial bleed due to traumatic brain injury (TBI), antifibrinolytics, aprotinin, tranexamic acid, aminocaproic acid, or rFVIIa are often used as hemostatic agents to reduce the occurrence or size of intracranial bleed. Several randomized controlled trials support these agents but Cochrane systematic review performed to compare these drugs found no reliable evidence to support the effectiveness of these drugs in reducing mortality or disability in patients with TBI.[11]

The narrow therapeutic ranged unfractionated heparin (UFH) has made way for low molecular weight heparin (LMWH) which needs no monitoring. However, in cases with high bleeding risk UFH may be preferable as it has short duration of action and its effect can be readily reversed with protamine (1 mg protamine for 100 U heparin).[5] LMWH has to be stopped at least 24 h before surgery.[12] UFH has to be discontinued at least 6 h before surgery.[5,12] Patients with intracranial bleed (anticoagulants have to be stopped immediately) with high thrombotic risk may be planned for temporary inferior vena cava filter after discussion with hematologist and intervention radiologist.[5]

Dual antiplatelet therapy should be continued for 4–6 weeks in patients with bare metal stents and for 6–12 months after drug eluting stents. Any elective procedure should be deferred during this period (<6 weeks for BMS and <6 months for drug eluting stent) and only life saving surgeries should be undertaken.[6] For patient with moderate to mild hemorrhagic risk and high thrombotic risk, low dose aspirin can be continued till surgery. However, neurosurgical interventions are at high risk of bleeding and thus antiplatelet agent (APA) is generally stopped prior to surgery (aspirin, 7 days; clopidogrel, 10 days; ticlopidine, 12 days).[6] In these patients who have high thrombotic risk, bridging therapy with heparin may be considered. APAs cause platelet dysfunction and before taking up a patient for urgent neurosurgical surgery, their action has to be reversed by platelet transfusion. Prophylactic transfusion of platelets is associated with infectious and immunological complications and is not warranted. Usual dose for reversal is one unit platelet per 5–10 kg prior to surgery. Desmopressin enhances hemostasis by raising levels of factor VIII and Von Willebrandt factor and increases platelet adhesiveness. It has been used effectively in surgical patients to reverse the effect of antiplatelet drugs and to decrease risk of perioperative bleeding. It is given in dose of 0.3 μg/kg body weight. Further studies are warranted in TBI and ICH patients.[13]

Fibrinolytics and thrombolytics require urgent infusion of cryoprecipitate which is a good source of fibrinogen.

TABLE 3   Prevention of Coagulopathy

Embolization of feeding vessel in case of highly vascular tumors before taking up for surgery
Careful positioning to avoid venous bleeding (abdomen should be free in prone position)
Transfusion of FFP, cryoprecipitate, and platelets when required
Maintenance of body temperature
Antifibrinolytics administration
Vitamin K
Calcium
Correction of lactate levels

PREVENTION

Patients with congenital coagulation disorders should be adequately prepared prior to surgery in consultation with a hematologist.

Patients having massive blood loss when resuscitated with fluids and packed red cells may develop dilutional coagulopathy. Primary prevention of blood loss during surgery should be the first step to be targeted (Table 3). In cases of hemorrhage and blood loss, whole blood has to be replaced. But limitation in its availability makes it necessary to be replaced by packed red blood cells (pRBCs) along with its components. The higher ratio of platelets/FFP/pRBC administration 1:1:2 or even 1:1:1 is being popularized but still needs further studies to be validated. Early administration of tranexamic acid in bleeding trauma patients reduces the risk of death.[4] Further, CRASH-3 trial results will elucidate its role in isolated traumatic brain injury.

CONCLUSION

In clinical practice, we often come across patients with an altered coagulation profile due to various causes. Decision regarding its management depends upon urgency of procedure, the risk of bleeding associated with surgery, and thrombotic risk associated with the patient's underlying condition.

References

1. Sawaya RE, Ligon BL. Thromboembolic complications associated with brain tumors. *J Neuro-Oncol*. 1994;22:173–181.
2. Goh KY, Tsoi WC, Feng CS, Wickham N, Poon WS. Haemostatic changes during surgery for primary brain tumours. *J Neurol Neurosurg Psychiatry*. September 1997;63(3):334–338.

3. Laroche M, Kutcher ME, Huang MC, Cohen MJ, Manley GT. Coagulopathy after traumatic brain injury. *Neurosurgery.* 2012;70(6):1334–1345.
4. Roberts I, Shakur H, Coats T, et al. The CRASH-2 trial: a randomized controlled trial and economic evaluation of th effects of tranexamic acid on death, vascular occlusive events and transfusion requirement in bleeding trauma patients. *Health Technol Assess.* 2013;17(10):1–79.
5. Thachil J, Gatt A, Martlew V. Management of surgical patients receiving anticoagulation and antiplatelet agents. *Br J Surg.* 2008;95:1437–1448.
6. Liau JV, Lopez-Forte C, Sapena L, Ferrandis R. Perioperative management of antiplatelet agents in noncardiac surgery. *Eur J Anesthesiol.* 2009;26(3):181–187.
7. Makris M, Greaves M, Phillips WS, Kitchen S, Rosendaal FR, Preston EF. Emergency oral anticoagulant reversal: the relative efficacy of infusions of fresh frozen plasma and clotting factor concentrate on correction of the coagulopathy. *Thromb Haemostasis.* 1997;77:477–480.
8. Powner DJ, Hartwell EA, Hoots WK. Counteracting the effects of anticoagulants and antiplatelet agents during neurosurgical emergencies. *Neurosurgery.* 2005;57:823–831.
9. Hawryluk GW, Cusimano MD. The role of recombinant activated factor VII in neurosurgery: hope or hype? *J Neurosurg.* 2006;105(6):859–868.
10. Woo CH, Patel N, Conell C, et al. Rapid warfarin reversal in the setting of intracranial hemorrhage:a comparison of plasma, recombinant activated factor VII and prothrombin complex concentrate. *World Neurosurg.* 2014;81(1):110–115.
11. Perel P, Roberts I, Shakur H, Thinkhamrop B, Phuenpathom N, Yutthakasemsunt S. Hemostatic drugs for traumatic brain injury. *Cochrane Database Syst Rev.* January 20, 2010;(1):CD007877.
12. Douketis JD, Spyropoulos AC, Spencer FA, et al. Perioperative management of antithrombotic therapy and prevention of thrombosis, 9th ed: American College of Chest Physicians evidence-based clinical practice guidelines. *Chest.* 2012;141(suppl 2): e326S–e350S.
13. Beynon C, Hertle DN, Unterberg AW, Sakowitz OW. Clinical review: traumatic brain injury in patients receiving antiplatelet medication. *Crit Care.* 2012;16:228.

Postoperative Hematoma

Charu Mahajan, Hemanshu Prabhakar
Department of Neuroanaesthesiology and Critical Care, All India Institute
of Medical Sciences, New Delhi, India

DEFINITION

Development of a postoperative hematoma is a common complication after intracranial surgery; the gravity depends on the amount of collected blood. Some amount of blood may be frequently seen on subsequent scan in almost 10.8–50% of operated patients.[1] For practical purpose, we define postoperative hematoma as intracranial collection of blood following craniotomy which is clinically symptomatic and requires evacuation. On this basis, the incidence varies from 0.8 to 6.9%.[1]

SITE

The site of hematoma may be at primary surgical site or at a remote area away from the operative field. It can be subdural, epidural, or intra-parenchymal. Acute brain decompression may cause rupture of a bridging vein causing subdural hematoma away from the site of surgery.[2] In cases where dura is stripped from skull, bleeding from middle meningeal artery may lead to formation of an epidural hematoma.

Risk factors/predisposing factors:

- Uncontrolled hypertension
- Bleeding disorders
- Drug therapy—aspirin, clopidogrel, heparin, low molecular weight heparin.
- Vascular disease
- Hypothermia

Causes

- Coagulopathies and hematological abnormalities
- Drug-causing coagulation disorders
- Intraoperative hypertension
- Massive blood loss/dilutional coagulopathy
- Excessive brain dehydration and cerebrospinal fluid drainage[1]
- Retraction injury[3]
- Residual tumor
- Inadequate surgical hemostasis
- Normal pressure perfusion breakthrough

SIGNS AND SYMPTOMS

The cranial vault is closed and rigid, so the presence of hematoma may lead to raised intracranial pressure (ICP) and appearance of its features. An awake patient, who has recovered completely from anesthesia after craniotomy but deteriorates subsequently, indicates development of an intracranial hematoma. Altered consciousness, reduction in Glasgow coma scale, impaired papillary reactions, and/or appearance of new focal neurological deficits related to the site of bleeding may occur. In patients who are sedated and being ventilated, ICP monitoring may provide an early indication of postoperative intracranial hemorrhage. Early changes in respiratory pattern, arrhythmias, and appearance of Cushing reflex are suggestive of posterior fossa hematoma.

DIAGNOSIS

Intraoperative computed tomography (CT) scan or magnetic resonance imaging can help in the early detection of intracranial hematoma, though most of them form in the postoperative period. The first 6 h are most crucial and should be closely observed, though delayed hematomas are also known to occur.[4] Neurological examination is of utmost importance for diagnosis. Intracranial pressure monitoring and transcranial Doppler may also help in giving an early warning of raised ICP. Though it is not specific but it has been suggested as a warning tool in patients at high risk of postoperative bleeding.[1] An urgent CT scan is required to be done immediately for confirmation of hematoma.

TREATMENT

If the hematoma is causing mass effect and clinical symptoms, it has to be evacuated as soon as possible. Patient should be urgently shifted to operating room for its surgical evacuation.

PREVENTION

Prevention entails proper precaution during preoperative, intraoperative, and postoperative period. During preanesthetic checkup, a thorough history should elucidate the presence of any of the risk factors mentioned above. Antiplatelet therapy and heparin have to discontinue prior to surgery. Massive blood loss and dilutional coagulopathy require adequate replacement of plasma and platelets. Intraoperative strict control of blood pressure is mandatory. Smooth emergence and extubation, avoiding coughing and straining are vital for prevention of venous bleeding. Moderate to severe hypothermia causes coagulation disorder and thus patient needs to be rewarmed before surgical hemostasis. Hypertension not only causes failure of autoregulation but may also disrupt hemostatic plug formed. At time of hemostasis, the neurosurgeon usually requests for systolic blood pressure (SBP) 10–20 mmHg above baseline SBP. By achieving hemostasis at a higher BP, one ensures that chance of hemorrhage is low even if BP rises transiently in the immediate postoperative period. Similarly, Valsalva maneuver, often performed at the end of surgery, increases ICP and BP, thus helping in localizing any bleeding points.[4] Epidural tenting sutures prevents development of epidural hematoma. In patients with arterio-venous malformation, the postoperative blood pressure has to be maintained between 90 and 100 mmHg for the prevention of development of bleed or hematoma secondary to phenomenon of normal pressure perfusion breakthrough. Avoidance of upright posture in immediate postoperative period after evacuation of subdural hematoma is also advocated to prevent its reformation.[5]

References

1. Seifman MA, Lewis PM, Rosenfeld JV, Hwang PY. Postoperative intracranial haemorrhage: a review. *Neurosurg Rev.* 2011;34(4):393–407.
2. Koller M, Ortler M, Langmayr J, Twerdy K. Posterior-fossa haemorrhage after supratentorial surgery–report of three cases and review of the literature. *Acta Neurochir Wien.* 1999;141(6):587–592.
3. Fukumachi A, Koizumi H, Nukui H. Postoperative intracerebral haemorrhages: a survey of computed tomographic findings after 1074 intracranial operations. *Surg Neurol.* 1985;23(6):575–580.
4. Taylor WA, Thomas NW, Wellings JA, Bell BA. Timing of postoperative intracranial hematoma development and implications for the best use of neurosurgical intensive care. *J Neurosurg.* January 1995;82(1):48–50.
5. Abouzari M, Rashidi A, Rezaii J, et al. The role of postoperative patient posture in the recurrence of traumatic chronic subdural haematoma after burr-hole surgery. *Neurosurgery.* 2007;61:794–797.

Thromboembolism

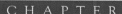

Charu Mahajan[1], Nidhi Gupta[2]

[1]Department of Neuroanaesthesiology and Critical Care, All India Institute
of Medical Sciences, New Delhi, India; [2]Department of Neuroanaesthesia,
Indraprastha Apollo Hospital, New Delhi, India

Deep vein thrombosis (DVT) occurs in deep large veins of lower extremities and rarely in upper limbs. With the enlargement of thrombus, an embolus may get dislodged and be trapped in lungs resulting in pulmonary thromboembolism (PE). This leads to impaired perfusion but normal ventilation resulting in intrapulmonary shunting. The right ventricle, in turn, attempts to maintain the pulmonary perfusion by overcoming the elevated pulmonary vascular resistance. This results in right ventricular strain and in extreme cases right ventricular failure may ensue. The term venous thromboembolism (VTE) incorporates both DVT and PE.

Neurosurgical patients constitute a moderate risk group for development of deep venous thrombosis and pulmonary thromboembolism.[1]

In untreated neurosurgical patients, incidence of DVT is reported to be between 18% and 50%.[2,3] Incidence of PE in neurosurgical patients varies between 8% and 25%.[4] Mechanical prophylaxis reduces the risk of DVT by 10–20%.[2,3] VTE after spine surgery varies between 8.3% and 19% with symptomatic PE in only 0.2% patients.[5,6] The large variation in incidence reported is due to the heterogeneity in the method of diagnosis, inclusion of symptomatic or asymptomatic patients, and whether receiving any prophylaxis or not. While PE is the most commonly recognized in hospital consequence of DVT, venous incompetence and postthrombotic syndrome are a recognized source of morbidity in patients with a history of DVT. Postthrombotic syndrome is estimated to affect 23–60% of patients with DVT.[7]

Risk factors for development of VTE[8] in patients are enumerated in Table 1.

Brain is a rich source of tissue thromboplastin which is an initiator of the coagulation cascade. Patients with brain tumors have been found to have decreased plasmin activity, increased tissue factor, and raised platelet aggregatory action.[9] This all leads to a procoagulant state, more so in malignant tumors. In an observational study by Sawaya et al., incidence of DVT in patients with meningiomas, malignant glioma, and metastatic disease was found to be 72%, 60%, and 20%, respectively.[10] Moreover, restricted mobility or paralysis, osmotic dehydration, long surgical duration, and corticosteroids increase risk of VTE in these patients. In a study done on 4293 neurosurgical patients who were operated for intracranial tumor, 26 (3%) patients developed VTE. The authors found poorer functional status, older age, preoperative motor deficit, high grade glioma, and hypertension each independently increased the risk of perioperative VTE.[11]

Patients with brain tumors, paralytic stroke, subarachnoid hemorrhage, spinal cord injury, or head trauma are thus prone to develop VTE.

TABLE 1   Risk Factors for VTE

Strong risk factors	Moderate risk factors	Weak risk factors
Fracture (hip or leg)	Arthroscopic knee surgery	Bed rest >3 days
Hip or knee replacement	Central venous lines	Immobility due to sitting
Major general surgery	Chemotherapy	Increasing age
Major trauma	Congestive heart or	Laparoscopic surgery
Spinal cord injury	respiratory failure	Obesity
	Hormone replacement therapy	Pregnancy, antepartum
	Malignancy	Varicose veins
	Oral contraceptive therapy	
	Paralytic stroke	
	Pregnancy, postpartum	
	Previous VTE, thrombophilia	

Genetic hypercoagulability syndromes like deficiency of antithrombin C, protein C, protein S, raised antiphospholipid antibodies, and factor V leiden mutation predispose patients to development of thrombosis.

Raslan M et al. suggest that surveillance for DVT should be undertaken in high-risk patients on a biweekly schedule, otherwise individualized surveillance is necessary.[12]

SYMPTOMS/SIGNS

Distal/calf vein DVT is usually clinically asymptomatic. Most of the times, it resolves on its own and rarely extends to proximal veins. Proximal (popliteal and thigh) DVT manifests as pain and tenderness, swelling, redness, warmth, and edema. Positive Homan sign (calf pain on dorsiflexion of foot with leg extended) has poor predictive value for DVT and is not relied upon these days.

PE may manifest as dyspnea, tachypnea, pleuritic chest pain, cough and hemoptysis, fever, and tachycardia. Under anesthesia, hemodynamic instability and sudden decrease in end tidal carbon dioxide should also alert toward PE.

Symptoms of postthrombosis syndrome include pain, venous congestion, edema, skin changes, and ulcers which are difficult to treat and have a significant negative impact on the patient's quality of life.

DIAGNOSIS OF DVT

D-dimer: Cross-linked fibrin on degradation produces D-dimer which can be used for diagnosis of VTE. A negative test excludes DVT and no further testing is required. However, it is nonspecific and is also raised in cases of infection, trauma, recent surgery, malignancy, and pregnancy. Levels more than 0.5 mg/L indicate VTE with a sensitivity of 99.4% and specificity of 38.2%. In postcraniotomy patients, a threshold of 2 mg/L indicates VTE with a high degree of sensitivity and specificity in patients.[13] If D-dimer is raised, next test done is ultrasonography of proximal veins.

Ultrasound: Inability to compress vein lumen, distended vessel lumen, and lack of flow are the features of DVT on ultrasonography. This technique is accurate, noninvasive, and readily available. If proximal ultrasound is positive for DVT, treatment is started and further tests are not required. However, it is difficult to perform in obese patients and cannot always differentiate acute and chronic DVT.

Contrast venograophy: Gold standard test for diagnosing DVT is ascending contrast venography. Presence of intraluminal filling defect, nonfilling of deep venous system, or presence of collateral flow indicate the presence of DVT. The drawbacks of this technique are it is invasive, requires contrast injection, and patient needs to be mobilized.

DIAGNOSIS OF PE

Arterial blood gas will show decrease in PaO_2 and increased arterial–alveolar gradient.

Chest X-ray: Atelectasis and pleural effusion may be seen on chest X-ray, but are nonspecific findings.

Electrocardiogram may show right ventricular strain pattern depicting prominent S wave in lead I, deep Q in lead III, and inverted T wave in lead III (S1Q3T3), right bundle branch block, T inversion, or ST depression in leads V1–4.

D-dimer: Negative test has a high negative predictive value but if test is positive, further diagnostic modalities need to be applied for confirmation.

CT pulmonary angiogram (CTPA) is widely available test which helps in visualization of pulmonary vasculature by noninvasive means and helps in diagnosis of PE. It is now the first line imaging technique for diagnosis of PE. The main disadvantages are radiation exposure and need for contrast.

V/Q scan or scintigram has been widely replaced by CT angiogram. It shows the ventilated and perfused areas of the lung. A normal perfusion scan excludes the diagnosis of PE.

Pulmonary arteriography: When all other tests are inconclusive, gold standard pulmonary arteriography is used to confirm the diagnosis. It is invasive, expensive, requires contrast administration, and is used infrequently these days. An intraluminal filling defect confirms the diagnosis.

Magnetic resonance angiography (MRA): In patients having contraindication for contrast agent or radiation has to be avoided, MRA can be performed. But, it is less sensitive and specific than CTPA for diagnosis of PE.

Other tests such as echocardiography can help in assessing right ventricular dysfunction in hemodynamically unstable patients with PE. Rarely, a thrombus may be directly visualized.

PREVENTION OF DVT

Prevention of DVT is foremost for preventing PE. Early ambulation as soon as possible is ultimate for prevention of venous stasis and DVT formation. DVT prophylaxis can be mechanical, pharmacological, or a combination of both.

Mechanical prophylaxis is especially useful in patients who have high risk of bleeding and pharmacological prophylaxis cannot be given. This can be done by means of intermittent pneumatic compression (IPC) devices, graduated elastic compression stockings (GCS), or venous foot pumps. IPC devices prevent venous stasis by intermittent rhythmic compression of legs in the same way as calf muscles do and by stimulation of intrinsic fibrinolytic system.

GCS apply a circumferential pressure to lower leg, which increases gradually from ankle to thigh, thereby increasing venous outflow and preventing stasis. In the CLOTS 1 trial, GCS failed to show any reduction in risk of DVT in patients after stroke.[14] Later, the CLOTS 3 trial concluded that IPC is an effective method for reducing risk of DVT in these patients.[15]

A Cochrane review on comparison of knee length versus thigh length compression stockings found no difference in the ability of these two modalities in prevention of DVT in postsurgical patients. The quality of evidence was low and requires further multicentric trials.[18] Use of inferior vena cava (IVC) filters as a routine prophylaxis for DVT is not recommended except in select patients who fail anticoagulation or who are not candidates for anticoagulation and/or mechanical devices.[19]

However, in patients with contraindications to or ineffective anticoagulation, IVC filters bear a high risk for complications like thrombus formation, device migration, or penetration of vessels and adjacent organs. A systematic review in trauma patients has described a low rate of filter-associated complications, and a decreased risk of pulmonary embolism and related mortality.[20]

There are few contraindications for the use of sequential pneumatic compression device. These are severe ischemic vascular disease, severe lower-extremity edema, suspected preexisting DVT, postoperative vein ligation, gangrene, dermatitis, recent skin graft, and extreme leg deformity.[16,17]

PHARMACOLOGICAL THROMBOPROPHYLAXIS

A 2013 Cochrane review of thromboprophylaxis in trauma patients found a significant reduction in DVT formation when prophylaxis (mechanical and/or pharmacologic) was implemented and a statistically significant advantage in the reduction of DVT when pharmacological thromboprophylaxis was compared with mechanical prophylaxis.[21]

The initiation of chemoprophylaxis following the demonstration of a stable intracranial hemorrhagic injury has been shown to be safe in numerous studies. Based on an extensive literature review, Foreman et al. provided robust evidence regarding the safety and efficacy of chemoprophylaxis in the setting of traumatic brain injury (TBI) following demonstration of a stable intracranial injury.[22]

Despite being more effective than mechanical devices in preventing DVT, pharmacological thromboprophylaxis is complicated by hemorrhagic manifestations, which may have devastating consequences if situated in intracranial of spinal compartments. This possibility of bleeding has resulted in wide variation in type (mechanical/pharmacological), drug, dose, and even time of commencement of start of prophylaxis for DVT.

Low-dose unfractionated heparin (UFH), 5000 U 8–12 hourly, effectively reduces the risk of DVT. It has a short plasma half-life of 1.5 h and binds extensively to plasma proteins and cells. A regimen of 5000 U subcutaneous twice daily added to mechanical prophylaxis reduced the rate of DVT by 43% when started either 24 or 48 h after surgery. The addition of heparin did not result in any hemorrhagic complications.[3] Another potential benefit of UFH is that its therapeutic effect can be acutely reversed with protamine sulfate in the event of untoward hemorrhage. However, the practical impact of this remains undetermined.

Low molecular weight heparin (LMWH) has a greater ratio of anti-factor Xa/anti-factor IIa activity compared with unfractionated heparin, greater bioavailability, and longer duration of action. The different isoforms like enoxaparin, nadroparin, and dalteparin vary in their potencies. Enoxaparin is commonly used in dose of 40 mg s/c daily or 30 mg s/c twice daily.

Both UFH and LMWH appear to be equally safe for thromboprophylaxis.[23] However, due to the more convenient dosing, LMWH may be chosen as the recommended anticoagulant. Unfractionated heparin should be reserved for patients with renal insufficiency due to its hepatic clearance, compared with the renal clearance of LMWH.

The Brain Trauma Foundation guidelines recommend use of GCS or IPC devices for DVT prophylaxis unless lower-extremity injuries prevent their use. LMWH or low-dose UFH should be used along with mechanical prophylaxis. However, it may increase risk of expansion of intracranial hemorrhage.[24]

In patients with traumatic brain injury (TBI), a parkland algorithm has been proposed on the basis of which VTE prophylaxis can be tailored.[25] According to this algorithm, in patients with low-risk TBI, enoxaparin can be started at 24-h postinjury. In patients with moderate risk TBI, enoxaparin can be started if a repeat CT scan done at 72-h postinjury is stable. In postcraniotomy patients or those having an ICP monitor in situ, prophylactic IVC filter may be considered in this high-risk TBI group. Pastorek et al. proposed a new validated parkland protocol in which TBI patients were categorized into low-risk and high-risk groups.[26] For low-risk groups, the plan remains the same. For high-risk TBI, enoxaparin can be started if a repeat CT scan done at 72-h postinjury is stable. If not, then enoxaparin can be delayed till the hemorrhagic pattern is stable.

The American College of Chest Physicians (ACCP) laid evidence-based clinical practice guidelines for prevention of VTE.[27] These are:

- Recommendations for craniotomy
  - For craniotomy patients, mechanical prophylaxis, preferably with IPC, can be used over no prophylaxis (grade 2C) or pharmacologic prophylaxis (grade 2C).
  - For craniotomy patients at very high risk for VTE (e.g., those undergoing craniotomy for malignant disease), adding pharmacologic prophylaxis to mechanical prophylaxis is suggested, once adequate hemostasis is established and the risk of bleeding decreases (grade 2C).
- Recommendation for spinal surgery
  - For patients undergoing spinal surgery, mechanical prophylaxis, preferably with IPC, over no prophylaxis, unfractionated heparin, or LMWH (grade 2C).
  - For patients undergoing spinal surgery at high risk for VTE (including those with malignant disease or those undergoing surgery with a combined anterior–posterior approach), pharmacologic prophylaxis may be added to mechanical prophylaxis once adequate hemostasis is established and the risk of bleeding decreases (grade 2C).
- Patients with major trauma: traumatic brain injury, acute spinal injury, and traumatic spine injury
  - For major trauma patients, low-dose UFH (grade 2C), LMWH (grade 2C), or mechanical prophylaxis may be started preferably with IPC (grade 2C), over no prophylaxis.
  - For major trauma patients at high risk for VTE (including those with acute spinal cord injury, traumatic brain injury, and spinal surgery for trauma), mechanical prophylaxis may be added to pharmacologic prophylaxis (grade 2C) when not contraindicated by lower extremity injury.

TREATMENT OF VTE

Treatment is started with administration of anticoagulants. Heparin has immediate effect and is the first line of treatment. UFH has a shorter duration of action, requires monitoring, can be rapidly reversed, and carries risk of heparin-induced thrombocytopenia. LMWH is equally effective, has a longer half-life, has more predictable action, and does not require any monitoring.

Fondaparinux is a synthetic pentasaccharide with anti-Xa activity used for initial treatment of VTE. It is administered once daily via subcutaneous route in a dose of 5 mg for body weight <50 kg and 7.5 mg for weight between 50 and 100 kg.

Warfarin is an oral anticoagulant which requires time to take action. It is started simultaneously with heparin, overlapped for 5 days and after achieving international normalized ratio of 2.0–3.0 for 24 h, heparin is stopped and warfarin is continued.

IVC filters are indicated in patients in whom anticoagulation is contraindicated, who have recurrent PE, or are undergoing open embolectomy.

In patients with DVT or PE, systemic thrombolytic therapy and mechanical or surgical embolectomy should be reserved for selected, highly compromised patients on a case-by-case basis and not performed routinely.

Recommendations by APCC regarding antithrombotic therapy for VTE disease[28] include:

- In patients with acute DVT of the leg, LMWH or fondaparinux may be preferred over intravenous UFH (grade 2C) and over subcutaneous UFH (grade 2B for LMWH; grade 2C for fondaparinux).
- In patients with acute proximal DVT of the leg and contraindication to anticoagulation, use of an IVC filter has been suggested (grade 1B).
- In patients with acute PE associated with hypotension (e.g., systolic blood pressure <90 mmHg) who do not have a high risk of bleeding, systemically administered thrombolytic therapy is suggested over no such therapy (grade 2C).
- In most patients with acute PE not associated with hypotension, systemically administered thrombolytic therapy is not recommended (grade 1C).
- In patients with acute PE and contraindication to anticoagulation, use of an IVC filter is recommended (grade 1B).
- For proximal DVT or PE, treatment should be followed for 3 months.

References

1. Geerts WH, Bergqvist D, Pineo GF, et al. Prevention of venous thromboembolism: American College of Chest Physicians evidence-based clinical practice guidelines. *Chest.* 2008;133(suppl 6):381S–453S.
2. Farray D, Carman TL, Fernandez Jr BB. The treatment and prevention of deep vein thrombosis in the preoperative management of patients who have neurologic diseases. *Neurol Clin.* 2004;22:423–439.
3. Khaldi A, Helo N, Schneck MJ, Origitano TC. Venous Thromboembolism: deep venous thrombosis and pulmonary embolism in a neurosurgical population. *J Neurosurg.* 2011;114(1):40–46.
4. Hamilton MG, Hull RD, Pineo GF. Venous thromboembolism in neurosurgery and neurology patients: a review. *Neurosurgery.* 1994;34:280–296.
5. Yoshioka K, Kitajima I, Kabata T, et al. Venous thromboembolism after spine surgery: changes of the fibrin monomer complex and D-dimer level during the perioperative period. *J Neurosurg Spine.* 2010;13(5):594–599.

6. Takahashi H, Yokoyama Y, Lida Y, et al. Incidence of venous thromboembolism after spine surgery. *J Orthop Sci.* 2012;17(2):114–117.
7. Ashrani AA, Heit JA. Incidence and cost burden of post-thrombotic syndrome. *J Thromb Thrombolysis.* 2009;28:465–476.
8. Anderson FA, Spencer FA. Risk factors for venous thromboembolism. *Circulation.* 2003;107:I-9–I-16.
9. Chan AT, Atiemo A, Diran LK, et al. Venous thromboembolism occurs frequently in patients undergoing brain tumor surgery despite prophylaxis. *J Thromb Thrombolysis.* 1999;8:139–142.
10. Sawaya R, Zuccarello M, Elkalliny M, et al. Postoperative venous thromboembolism and brain tumors: part I. Clinical profile. *J Neuro-Oncol.* 1992;14:119–125.
11. Chaichana KL, Pendelton C, Jackson C, et al. Quinones-Hinojosa A. *Neurol Res.* 2013; 35(2):206–211.
12. Raslan AM, Fields JD, Bhardwaj A. Prophylaxis for venous thrombo-embolism in neuro-critical care: a critical appraisal. *Neurocrit Care.* 2010;12:297–309.
13. Prell J, Rachinger J, Smaczny R, et al. D-dimer plasma level: a reliable marker for venous thromboembolism after elective craniotomy. *J Neurosurg.* 2013;119(5):1340–1346.
14. CLOTS Trials Collaboration, Dennis M, Sandercock PA, et al. Effectiveness of thigh length graduated compression stockings to reduce the risk of deep vein thrombosis after stroke (CLOTS trial 1): a multicentre controlled trial. *Lancet.* 2009;373(9679): 1958–1965.
15. CLOTS (Clots in Legs Or sTockings after stroke) Trials Collaboration, Dennis M, sandercock P, et al. Effectiveness of intermittent pneumatic compression in reduction of risk of deep vein thrombosis in patients who have had a stroke (CLOTS 3): a multicentre randomized controlled trial. *Lancet.* 2013;382(9891):516–524.
16. Jeffery PC, Nicolaides AN. Graduated compression stockings in the prevention of post-operative deep vein thrombosis. *Br J Surg.* 1990;77:380–383.
17. Auguste KI, Quinones-Hinojosa A, Berger MS. Efficacy of mechanical prophylaxis for venous thromboembolism in patients with brain tumors. *Neurosurg Focus.* 2004;17(4):E3.
18. Sajid MS, Desai M, Morris RW, Hamilton G. Knee length versus thigh length graduated compression stockings for prevention of deep vein thrombosis in postoperative surgical patients. *Cochrane Database Syst Rev.* May 2012;16:5:CD007162.
19. Dhall SS, Hadley MN, Aarabi B, et al. Deep venous thrombosis and thromboembolism in patients with cervical spinal cord injuries. In: guidelines for the management of acute cervical spine and spinal cord injuries. *Neurosurgery.* 2013;72(suppl 2):244–254.
20. Kidane B, Madani AM, Vogt K, et al. The use of prophylactic inferior vena cava filters in trauma patients: a systematic review. *Injury.* 2012;43:542–547.
21. Barrera LM, Perel P, Ker K, Cirocchi R, Farinella E, Morales Uribe CH. Thromboprophylaxis for trauma patients. *Cochrane Database Syst Rev.* 2013;3:CD008303.
22. Foreman PM, Schmalz PG, Griessenauer CJ. Chemoprophylaxis for venous thromboembolism in traumatic brain injury: a review and evidence-based protocol. *Clin Neurol Neurosurg.* August 2014;123:109–116.
23. Browd SR, Ragel BT, Davis GE, Scott AM, Skalabrin EJ, Couldwell WT. Prophylaxis for deep venous thrombosis in neurosurgery: a review of the literature. *Neurosurg Focus.* 2004;17(4):E1.
24. Brain Trauma Foundation, American Association of Neurological Surgeons, Congress of Neurological Surgeons, et al. Guidelines for the management of severe traumatic brain injury. V. Deep vein thrombosis prophylaxis. *J Neurotrauma.* 2007;24(suppl 1):S-32–S-36.
25. Phelan HA. Pharmacologic venous thromboembolism prophylaxis after traumatic brain injury: a critical literature review. *J Neurotrauma.* 2012;29(10):1821–1828.
26. Pastorek RA, Cripps MW, Bernstein IH, et al. The parkland Protocol's modified Berne-Norwood criteria predict two tiers of risk for traumatic brain injury progression. *J Neurotrauma.* 2014;31(20):1737–1743.

27. Gould MK, Garcia DA, Wren SM, et al. Prevention of VTE in nonorthopedic surgical patients: antithrombotic therapy and prevention of thrombosis, 9th ed.: American College of Chest Physicians evidence-based clinical practice guidelines. *Chest.* 2012;141(suppl 2): e227S–e277S.
28. Kearon C, Akl EA, Comerota AJ, et al. Antithrombotic therapy for VTE disease: antithrombotic therapy and prevention of thrombosis, 9th ed.: American College of chest Physicians evidence-based Clinical Practice guidelines. *Chest.* 2012;141(suppl 2): E419s–E494s.

COMPLICATIONS RELATED TO RESPIRATORY SYSTEM

Hypercapnia

Neus Fabregas[1], Juan Fernández-Candil[2]

[1]Servicio de Anestesiología, Hospital Clínic, Universitat de Barcelona, Barcelona, Spain; [2]Servicio de Anestesiología, Parc de Salut Mar, Barcelona, Spain

O U T L I N E

DEFINITION AND ETIOLOGY

A carbonic dioxide arterial blood level (PCO_2) above 46 mmHg (6.1 kPa) is defined as hypercapnia. The increase in carbon dioxide (CO_2) partial pressure provokes a fall in blood pH, and its clinical features can be arterial hypertension, tachycardia, drowsiness, tachypnea, and skin rush, among other symptoms.

An increase in CO_2 production or a decrease in its excretion can generate hypercapnia; Table 1 details the possible etiologies.[1,2] In the neurosurgical patient, hypoventilation is the main origin of a decrease in CO_2 excretion, leading to different degrees of hypercapnia. During an awake fiber optic intubation, hypercapnia episodes are frequently due to loss of respiratory efforts in a narcotized patient. Bradypnea, secondary to sedation, is a challenge during awake neurosurgery and is the most likely cause of hypercapnia. After posterior cranial fossa procedures, hypoventilation can appear as a consequence of surgical maneuvers besides brain stem

TABLE 1   Causes of Hypercapnia in the Perioperative Management of Neurosurgical Patients

Reduced excretion of CO_2

1. Lungs
    Intraoperative hypoventilation:
        During awake procedures with spontaneous ventilation
        Due to mechanical ventilator settings
        Venous air embolism
        Bronchospasm, asthma, or chronic airway disease
    Postoperative hypoventilation:
        Supraglottic airway obstruction for tissue swelling and edema if in the prone position
        CNS depression (chemical or secondary to brain surgery)
        Involving respiratory muscles (spinal cord injury or residual neuromuscular blockade)
        Bronchospasm, asthma, or chronic airway disease
2. Breathing circuit
    a. Increased dead space (long ventilator tubing)
    b. Inadequate fresh gas flow, incorrect respirator settings, and valve malfunction

Increased production of CO_2

1. Exogenous
    Rebreathing (exhausted soda lime)
    Bicarbonate administration
2. Endogenous
    Increased body temperature (sepsis, malignant hyperthermia, and malignant neuroleptic syndrome)

Adapted from Refs 1 and 2.

structures. Following complex spine surgery in the prone position, edema can produce supraglottic airway obstruction with resulting hypercapnia.

CEREBRAL AND SYSTEMIC EFFECTS

Hypercapnia and Brain Electrical Excitability

Most neurons are highly responsive to changes in pH of the surrounding interstitial fluids. Alkalosis greatly increases neuronal excitability; for instance, a rise in arterial blood pH from 7.4 to 7.8 or 8.0 often causes cerebral epileptic seizures because of increased excitability of some or all of the cerebral neurons. This can be demonstrated especially well by asking a person who is predisposed to epileptic seizures to overbreathe. The overbreathing blows off carbon dioxide and therefore elevates the pH of the blood momentarily, but even in this short time, it can often precipitate an epileptic attack.

Slight elevations of CO_2 cause direct neuronal cortical depression and increase the threshold for seizures. The application of 5% CO_2 has been proven to be effective and safe to suppress febrile seizures in children.[3]

Higher levels of CO_2 (25–30%) stimulate subcortical hypothalamic centers, resulting in increased cortical excitability and seizures. This hyperexcitability is enhanced by adrenal cortical and medullary hormones released secondary to hypercapnia-induced stimulation of the hypothalamus. Further elevation of CO_2 with a fall in pH from 7.4 to below 7.0 usually causes an anesthetic-like state of cortical and subcortical depression. It causes a comatose state, such as in very severe diabetic or uremic acidosis, where coma virtually always develops.[4]

Cerebrovascular Reactivity to Carbon Dioxide

CO_2, not H+, crosses the blood–brain barrier (BBB) and the brain cell membrane affecting the cell metabolism. A sudden change in CO_2 causes a rapid change in cerebrospinal fluid (CSF) pH. Hypercapnia decreases cerebral vascular resistance, causing cerebral blood flow (CBF) to increase. The relationship between CBF and PCO_2 is linear from 20 to 100 mmHg with maximal vasodilatation at approximately 120 mmHg. For each mmHg increase in PCO_2 between 25 and 100 mmHg, CBF increases by 2–4%.[5]

Effect of Hypercapnia on Cerebral Autoregulation

Cerebral autoregulation is a mechanism that maintains a stable CBF for a given cerebral metabolic rate in spite of fluctuation in cerebral perfusion pressure (CPP).[6] It is visualized as a correlation plot of CBF (axis of ordinate) against CPP (axis of abscissas). The three key elements of the autoregulation curve are the lower limit (60mmHg), the upper limit (150mmHg), and the plateau (CBF = 50mL/min/100g). The lower and upper limits are the two sharp inflection points indicating the boundary of pressure-independent flow (the plateau) and the start of pressure–passive flow (see Figure 1 at normocapnia).[7]

Multiple physiological processes are engaged in the regulation of CBF, but its execution relies on the cerebrovascular reactivity that provokes dilation to a decrease in CPP (arterial hypotension) and constriction to an increase in CPP (arterial hypertension).

However, cerebrovascular reactivity (CVR) is not exclusively linked to changes in pressure; changes in other physiological processes, notably CO_2, can also rapidly alter cerebral vasomotor tone and thus regulate CBF.

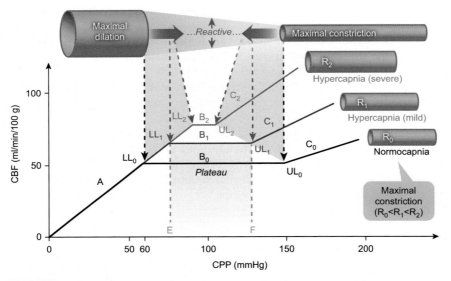

FIGURE 1 **Effect of hypercapnia on cerebral autoregulation.** Autoregulation curves are in black at normocapnia and red at hypercapnia. Cerebral resistance vessels are illustrated in red/pink. The bold solid blue arrows indicate the dynamic shift of the maximally dilated and constricted cerebral resistance vessels at hypercapnia. The dashed black and blue lines/arrows indicate the lower and upper limits at normocapnia and hypercapnia, respectively. A = the curve below the lower limit; B = the plateau at normocapnia (B0), mild hypercapnia (B1), and severe hypercapnia (B2); C = the curve above the upper limit at normocapnia (C0), mild hypercapnia (C1), and severe hypercapnia (C2); CBF = cerebral blood flow; CPP = cerebral perfusion pressure; LL = the lower limit at normocapnia (LL0), mild hypercapnia (LL1), and severe hypercapnia (LL2); R = calibers of cerebral resistance vessels at normocapnia (R0), mild hypercapnia (R1), and severe hypercapnia (R2); UL = the upper limit at normocapnia (UL0), mild hypercapnia (UL1), and severe hypercapnia (UL2). *Figure adapted from Meng et al.[7] with permission.*

Brain vasculature constriction, such as in response to hypocapnia, diminishes CBF and cerebral blood volume (CBV) and can lower intracranial pressure (ICP). The rapid response of hypocapnia in provoking decreases in high ICP values is extensively used during neurosurgical procedures; nevertheless, we need to keep in mind the high risk of brain ischemia that can provoke the lower CBF in response to the vasoconstriction.

Brain vasculature dilation, as in response to hypercapnia, increases CBV and can increase ICP.

If hypercapnia coexists with hypotension, the combined vasodilator effects on brain vasculature could shift the lower limit of autoregulation rightward, then higher arterial pressure values are needed in order to maintain an adequate CBF (Figure 1).

On the opposite end, the dilation induced by hypercapnia could adversely affect the arterial hypertension-induced constriction response on brain vasculature, rendering a leftward shift of the upper limit. In this context, CBF will increase beyond the limits of autoregulation, with elevated arterial pressure levels that would have no effects in a normocapnia setting. In an animal study with dogs, Ekström-Jodal et al.[8] showed that during normocapnia, the upper pressure limit of autoregulation (UPL) was maintained until a mean arterial pressure (MAP) value of 225 mmHg. During mild hypercapnia ($PaCO_2 = 40$–60 mmHg), this UPL had fallen to 150 mmHg and went down to a MAP value less than 125 mmHg, if $PaCO_2 > 60$ mmHg.

We recommend an extensive review on this topic published by Meng et al.[7] showing that during hypercapnia, the plateau of the autoregulation curve is shifted upward and shortened, the lower limit is shifted rightward, and the upper limit is shifted leftward. The extent of these changes depends on the severity of hypercapnia. At severe hypercapnia, when cerebral resistance vessels are maximally dilated, the plateau is lost and the pressure–flow relationship is linear (Figure 1).[7,9]

Cerebrovascular Reactivity to Carbon Dioxide under Anesthesia

Changing the arterial CO_2 levels in order to reduce CBF and ICP is a common practice in neuroanesthesia. Different studies have shown that inhalational and intravenous anesthetic agents have variable effects on CVR to CO_2 variations (CVR–CO_2), and the effects of anesthetic agents on CVR also vary with many physiological and pathological conditions. A qualitative systematic review on this topic has been published by Mariappan et al.[10]; they included 1356 citations and concluded that within the clinical anesthesia concentrations, CVR–CO_2 is maintained under both propofol and inhalational agents. Propofol lowers cerebral metabolic rate of oxygen consumption ($CMRO_2$) and has a net vasoconstriction effect. Relative $CVR–CO_2$ value is higher in the hypercapnia range. Inhalational agents also diminish $CMRO_2$ but have a net vasodilatation effect; relative $CVR–CO_2$ values is lower in the hypercapnia range when anesthetic agents are used. However, most of the available information is on nonneurosurgical patients and is difficult to extrapolate the results to our clinical target.

Hypercapnia and Pulmonary Circulation

Hypercapnia increases pulmonary vascular resistance mainly by the coexisting acidosis. This effect is one of the measurable signs of a venous air embolism and can provoke acute right ventricle dysfunction.

In sleep apnea patients, the chronic hypercapnia develops adaptive mechanisms to diminish the hypoxic negative effects.[11] Plausible explanations to this effect are hyperventilation, increases in the ventilation–perfusion relationship, improvements in tissue oxygen delivery changing the hemoglobin oxygen affinity, increases in CBF due to vasodilation, and so forth. Brain oxygenation can improve when hypercapnia and hypoxemia are combined; nevertheless, this is a controversial topic.[12–15]

Hypercapnia and Oxyhemoglobin Dissociation Curve

Hypercapnia provokes a right shift in the oxyhemoglobin dissociation curve, indicating decreased oxygen affinity and promoting oxygen release at the tissue level. The partial pressure of oxygen, at which the oxygen-carrying protein is 50% saturated (P50), is higher for a right-shifted curve.[16]

Hypercapnia and the Cardiovascular System

An increase in CO_2 concentration causes moderate vasodilation in most tissues but marked vasodilation in the brain. Also, CO_2 in the blood, acting on the brain vasomotor center, has an extremely powerful indirect effect, transmitted through the sympathetic nervous vasoconstrictor system, to cause widespread vasoconstriction throughout the body.[17] Hypercapnia causes profound systemic changes secondary to stimulation of the central nervous and sympathoadrenal systems. The net effect usually includes an increase in cardiac output, heart rate, strength of myocardial contraction, blood pressure, central venous pressure, vasoconstriction in the pulmonary (capacitance) vessels, and a decrease in peripheral resistance. The rise in cardiac output can be up to 50% and exceed the rise in blood pressure. This net stimulatory effect is observed with elevations of PCO_2 up to 90 mmHg. Above this level, further increases in CO_2 cause a marked drop in response.[4]

DIAGNOSIS

Plasma and End-Tidal Values of Carbon Dioxide

Our first step is to identify the status of the patient; for hypercapnia diagnosis, an arterial blood gas analysis (ABG) is usually needed. Given the need to maintain CPP and to avoid increased ICP, an arterial line will allow real-time measurement of blood pressure as well as providing the ability to follow $PaCO_2$ trends during neurosurgical procedures.

The American Society of Anesthesiologists (ASA) included requirements for monitoring exhaled CO_2 in 1986. The use of capnography for increasing patient safety and for applications such as airway management and monitoring has led to its inclusion in practice standards and guidelines of professional societies.[18] The term "capnogram" usually refers to the "time-based" trace of CO_2 in either partial pressure or gas fraction units over time. The slope has three phases associated with the source of the expiratory gases: first, the gas from the dead space; second, the transition between dead space and alveolar gas; and finally, gas from sequential emptying of the alveolar volumes. From this capnogram, estimates of respiratory rate, end-tidal CO_2 ($ETCO_2$), and inspiratory levels of CO_2 are reported.

Capnometers can be side stream (diverted), transporting a portion of the respired gases from the sampling site, through a sampling tube, to the sensor; or mainstream (nondiverted) that does not need to transport gas away from the sampling site.

A number of technologies are known for measuring CO_2 in the breath, including colorimetric, photoacoustic, Raman scattering, mass spectroscopy, and the most frequently used infrared absorption.[19]

The infrared bench comprises an infrared source and filters at two wavelengths, one at which CO_2 is not absorbed and another usually about $4.25\,\mu m$, at which CO_2 is strongly absorbed. Devices also have one or more infrared-sensitive detectors (thermal, microphonic, or photonic). The measured absorption of CO_2 can be altered by cross-interference, the overlapping of absorption bands of other gases[20] due to the presence of nitrogen, nitrous oxide,[21] and oxygen. The use of narrow band filters can eliminate these effects.

$ETCO_2$ globally reflects metabolism, effective circulation, and ventilation. If two of these functions remain still, changes in $ETCO_2$ will warn about variations in the third function.[22]

An initial ABG quantifies $PaCO_2$–$ETCO_2$ difference and can guide the evolution of $PaCO_2$ from $ETCO_2$ noninvasively. $ETCO_2$ to $PaCO_2$ differences can also be followed as a measurement of relative pulmonary dead space.

Oxygen Brain Tissue Saturation

Cerebral oximetry (rSO_2) estimates the oxygenation of regional tissue by transcutaneous measurement of the frontal cerebral cortex. This is accomplished with adhesive pads, applied over the forehead, with two photodetectors with each light source that both emit and capture reflected near-infrared light to different depths, passing through the cranial bone to and from the underlying cerebral tissue. It measures an average of 25% arterial and 75% capillary and venous blood oxygenation. Values of rSO_2 have been reported to be in a range of 60–80%. It is important monitoring trends from baseline values determined on room air when the patient is awake.[23] At the present, there are different devices for rSO_2 measurement, all suggesting that a trend value reductions from baseline greater than 20% is clinically relevant. However, many factors can alter measurements: cardiac output, blood pressure, inspired oxygen concentration, temperature, and hypo- or hypercapnia. A decrease in rSO_2 value may reflect a derangement of systemic perfusion, regional cerebral hypoperfusion, relative hypoxemia, or increased metabolic rate. But a sudden increase in rSO_2 can result in an increase in $PaCO_2$ levels. Hypercapnia immediately provokes an increase in CBF and in venous blood volume; as a consequence, we will observe a simultaneous increase in rSO_2. This response can be detected earlier than the $ETCO_2$ decreases—for example, in venous air embolism.[24]

TREATMENT

Once hypercapnia is diagnosed, it is necessary to check ventilator settings and correct any dysfunction or readapt the minute volume to the CO_2 real production. Treatment will depend on hypercapnia etiology (Table 1), and any hypermetabolic state needs to be detected. If we suspect a venous air embolism, avoiding air entrance will be the main target.

During neurosurgical procedures in an awake patient, hypoventilation is the most frequent cause of hypercapnia. If it is not possible to increase patient spontaneous ventilation, one may plan the need for an assisted ventilation with the aid of a supraglottic device.

PREVENTION

During Induction

If fiber optic intubation in an awake patient is needed, it is preferable to use sedation regimens that can provide sedation and analgesia, such as dexmedetomidine, while maintaining respiratory drive, avoiding hypoventilation, and reducing hypertension.

During Surgery

A continuous control of the $ETCO_2$ is mandatory. In long surgical procedures, it is necessary to repeat ABG in order to be sure that there is no variation in $PaCO_2$–$ETCO_2$ differences and to correct ventilator settings if it is necessary.

If rSO_2 is monitored, any unexpected increase must warn of an increase of CO_2 due to an ongoing venous air embolism.

We want to highlight a specific cause of hyperchloremic metabolic acidosis that can occur in patients on topiramate treatment. It has been reported that it can cause compensated metabolic acidosis by carbonic anhydrase inhibition.[25–27] Patients on topiramate treatment spontaneously hyperventilate to counteract the metabolic acidosis. Acute nonanion gap acidosis is triggered by mechanical ventilation when normocapnia is maintained in these patients. Metabolic acidosis occurred in 60% of patients taking topiramate in a case series.[28]

Acidosis has been related to impaired brain metabolism and CBF. Accordingly, to normalize intraoperative homeostasis, we recommend asking these patients about symptoms on preoperative evaluation and routinely performing ABG before undergoing surgical procedures.

After Surgery

We need to avoid hypoventilation in the immediate postoperative period, as it can increase CO_2, provoke arterial hypertension, and increase CBF and ICP.

There are specific surgeries or intraoperative positions that increase the possibility of postoperative occurrences of hypercapnia. Neuromuscular blockade must be completely reversed (TOF ≥ 90%), with sustained head lift and strong hand grip. Patients with neuromuscular diseases had to be treated according to the evolution of their illness, and a special treatment algorithm must be applied.

Do not extubate patients following complex spine surgery or brain surgery in the prone position if there is an evidence of facial edema and macroglossia, or if pharyngeal and laryngeal edema are detected on flexible fiber optic bronchoscopy. Ensure cranial nerves (IX, X, XII) are intact for airway protection.[29,30] The patient must be able to open eyes and obey commands. Agitation contraindicates extubation. The respiratory efforts must be normal and the O_2 saturation >94% on high-flow O_2. Check adequate spontaneous ventilation with $ETCO_2 < 50\,mmHg$. Normocapnia is defined as $PaCO_2 > 30\,mmHg < 50\,mmHg$.

In some cases, it is recommended to perform a "cuff-leak test"[31] by deflating the tracheal tube balloon, occluding the tracheal tube, and assessing the air movement around the endotracheal tube. Although not specific for predicting stridor, it appears that no- or low-leak volumes of air are reliably associated with an increased risk of upper airway obstruction. In such situations, a decision to delay the extubation is prudent.

CONCLUSION

Hypercapnia needs to be always corrected in neurosurgical or neurocritical patients; a review published by Roberts et al. in patients after brain injury supports this statement.[32]

Moreover, in nonneurocritical patients, hypercapnia can produce neurologic symptoms known as "hypercapnic encephalopathy." It is a heterogeneous and potentially reversible entity with a broad symptom spectrum going from cognitive dysfunction, agitation, and restlessness, and progressing until delirium or coma is reached—all this in the context of a severe hypercapnic respiratory acidosis.[33,34] Its physiopathology is not completely understood, and clinical symptoms are not always related to $PaCO_2$ levels, but acute acidosis of CSF and surrounding tissue may be the explanation.[35–38] Nowadays, pressure support ventilation is the recommended treatment whenever feasible.[39]

In summary, hypercapnia produces changes at the metabolic, cellular, systemic, and brain levels. Increases in CBF, CBV, and ICP can be of special concern in neurosurgical or neurocritical patients as it worsens the expected outcome. It is mandatory to promptly diagnose and treat hypercapnia occurrences, especially in this population.

References

1. Ivashkov Y, Domino K. Airway emergencies after neurosurgery. In: Brambrink AM, Kirsh JR, eds. *Essentials of Neurosurgical Anesthesia & Critical Care*. New York: Springer; 2012:645–655.
2. Staendler S, Fairley-Smith A, Bratteboe G, Whitaker D, Mellin-Olsen J, Borshoff D. Emergency quick reference guide. ESA/EBA. Task force patient safety. "Differ Diagn hypercapnia/high ETCO2": 15. http://html.esahq.org/patientsafetykit/resources/downloads/05_Checklists/Emergency_CL/Emergency_Checklists.pdf.
3. Ohlraun S, Wollersheim T, Weiss C, et al. CARbon DIoxide for the treatment of Febrile seizures: rationale, feasibility, and design of the CARDIF-study. *J Transl Med*. 2013;11:157.
4. Lumb AB. *Nunn's Applied Respiratory Physiology*. 6th ed. Philadelphia: Butterworth-Heinemann; 2005:2328–2330.
5. Fontanella M. LM: intracranial pressure and cerebral blood flow autoregulation. In: Albert RK, Slutsky A, Ranieri M, Takala J, eds. *A Torres Clinical Critical Care Medicine*. Mosby Elsevier; 2006:2383–2393.
6. Koller A, Toth P. Contribution of flow-dependent vasomotor mechanisms to the autoregulation of cerebral blood flow. *J Vasc Res*. 2012;49(5):375–389.
7. Meng L, Gelb AW. Regulation of cerebral autoregulation by carbon dioxide. *Anesthesiology*. 2015;122(1):196–205.

8. Ekstrom-Jodal B, Haggendal E, Linder LE, Nilsson NJ. Cerebral blood flow autoregulation at high arterial pressures and different levels of carbon dioxide tension in dogs. *Eur Neurol*. 1971;6(1):6–10.
9. Harper AM. Autoregulation of cerebral blood flow: influence of the arterial blood pressure on the blood flow through the cerebral cortex. *J Neurol Neurosurg Psychiatry*. 1966;29(5):398–403.
10. Mariappan R, Mehta J, Chui J, Manninen P, Venkatraghavan L. Cerebrovascular reactivity to carbon dioxide under anesthesia: a qualitative systematic review. *J Neurosurg Anesthesiol*. 2015;27(2):123–135.
11. Brzecka A. Role of hypercapnia in brain oxygenation in sleep-disordered breathing. *Acta Neurobiol Exp Wars*. 2007;67(2):197–206.
12. Costello R, Deegan P, Fitzpatrick M, McNicholas WT. Reversible hypercapnia in chronic obstructive pulmonary disease: a distinct pattern of respiratory failure with a favorable prognosis. *Am J Med*. 1997;102(3):239–244.
13. Saryal S, Celik G, Karabiyikoglu G. Distinctive features and long-term survival of reversible and chronic hypercapnic patients with COPD. *Monaldi Arch Chest Dis*. 1999;54(3): 212–216.
14. Nizet TA, van den Elshout FJ, Heijdra YF, van de Ven MJ, Mulder PG, Folgering HT. Survival of chronic hypercapnic COPD patients is predicted by smoking habits, comorbidity, and hypoxemia. *Chest*. 2005;127(6):1904–1910.
15. Oswald-Mammosser M, Weitzenblum E, Quoix E, et al. Prognostic factors in COPD patients receiving long-term oxygen therapy. Importance of pulmonary artery pressure. *Chest*. 1995;107(5):1193–1198.
16. Schumacker P. Cell metabolism and tissue hypoxia. In: Albert RK, Slutsky A, Ranieri M, Takala J, eds. *A Torres Clinical Critical Care Medicine*. Mosby Elsevier; 2006:2041–2050.
17. Hall JE. *Guyton and Hall Textbook of Medical Physiology*. 12th ed. Philadelphia: Saunders Elsevier; 2011:2200.
18. Jaffe M. Time and volumetric capnography. In: Ehrenfeld JM, Cannesson M, eds. *Monitoring Technologies in Acute Care Environment*. New York: Springer Science+Business Media; 2014:2179–2191.
19. Belda J. LJ: Ventilación mecánica en anestesia y cuidados críticos. In: Aran, ed. ; 2009:179–185. [Chapter 6].
20. Carbon dioxide monitors. *Health Devices*. 1986;1915:1255–1985.
21. Kennell EM, Andrews RW, Wollman H. Correction factors for nitrous oxide in the infrared analysis of carbon dioxide. *Anesthesiology*. 1973;39(4):441–443.
22. Trillo G, von Planta M, Kette F. $ETCO_2$ monitoring during low flow states: clinical aims and limits. *Resuscitation*. 1994;27(1):1–8.
23. Ramsingh D. Brain oxygenation. In: Ehrenfeld JM, Cannesson M, eds. *Monitoring Technologies in Acute Care Environment*. New York: Springer Science+Business Media; 2014:2241–2245.
24. Navarro R, Claramunt A, Carrero E, Valero R, Fabregas N. Unexpected bilateral increase of cerebral regional saturation of oxygen as an early warning sign of air embolism. *J Clin Anesth*. 2011;23(5):431–432.
25. Dodgson SJ, Shank RP, Maryanoff BE. Topiramate as an inhibitor of carbonic anhydrase isoenzymes. *Epilepsia*. 2000;41(suppl 1):S35–S39.
26. Groeper K, McCann ME. Topiramate and metabolic acidosis: a case series and review of the literature. *Paediatr Anaesth*. 2005;15(2):167–170.
27. Ozer Y, Altunkaya H. Topiramate induced metabolic acidosis. *Anaesthesia*. 2004;59(8):830.
28. Rodriguez L, Valero R, Fabregas N. Intraoperative metabolic acidosis induced by chronic topiramate intake in neurosurgical patients. *J Neurosurg Anesthesiol*. 2008;20(1):67–68.
29. Tarnal V. KR: extubating the trachea after prolonged prone surgery. In: Mashour GA, Farag E, eds. *Case studies in Neuroanaesthesia and Neurocritical Care*. Cambridge: Cambridge University Press; 2011: 2160–2012.

30. Fabregas N, Bruder N. Recovery and neurological evaluation. *Best Pract Res Clin Anaesthesiol.* 2007;21(4):431–437.

31. Adderley RJ, Mullins GC. When to extubate the croup patient: the "leak" test. *Can J Anaesth.* 1987;34(3(Pt 1)):304–306.

32. Roberts BW, Karagiannis P, Coletta M, Kilgannon JH, Chansky ME, Trzeciak S. Effects of $PaCO_2$ derangements on clinical outcomes after cerebral injury: a systematic review. *Resuscitation.* 2015;91:32–41.

33. Young GB. DD: metabolic encephalopathies. In: Young GB, Ropper AH, Bolton CF, eds. *Coma and Impaired Consciousness: A Clinical Perspective.* New York, USA: McGraw-Hill Companies; 1998:1307e1992.

34. Scala R. NM: Expanding indications of non-invasive mechanical ventilation: hypercapnic encephalopathy. In: Esquinas AME, Scala R, eds. *Year Book of Noninvasive Mechanical Ventilation.* Almeria (Spain): Fotomecanica Indalo c/Santa Ana; 2008. p. 2244e2052.

35. Meissner HH, Franklin C. Extreme hypercapnia in a fully alert patient. *Chest.* 1992;102(4):1298–1299.

36. Scala R, Turkington PM, Wanklyn P, Bamford J, Elliott MW. Effects of incremental levels of continuous positive airway pressure on cerebral blood flow velocity in healthy adult humans. *Clin Sci Lond.* 2003;104(6):633–639.

37. Kilburn KH. Neurologic manifestations of respiratory failure. *Arch Intern Med.* 1965;116:409–415.

38. Posner JB, Swanson AG, Plum F. Acid-base balance in cerebrospinal fluid. *Arch Neurol.* 1965;12:479–496.

39. Scala R. Hypercapnic encephalopathy syndrome: a new frontier for non-invasive ventilation? *Respir Med.* 2011;105(8):1109–1117.

21

Hypoxia

Pirjo H. Manninen, Zoe M. Unger

Department of Anesthesia, Toronto Western Hospital, University Health
Network, University of Toronto, Toronto, ON, Canada

OUTLINE

Hypoxia is a serious complication that continues to be a leading cause of morbidity and mortality, especially in anesthesia-related events.[1–3] There are many potential causes of perioperative hypoxia, and airway management is one of the most common. To diagnose, treat, and prevent these events, it is necessary to understand the various causes and effects of hypoxia, especially on the neurological system. Monitoring for diagnosis and prevention of hypoxia is routinely done, and there are also specialized monitors for the assessment of oxygenation of the brain.[4] This chapter will review the causes, treatment, monitoring, and prevention of hypoxia in the perioperative period.

DEFINITION

Hypoxia is a condition in which tissues of the body do not receive sufficient oxygen (O_2) supply.[1,2] The imbalance between tissue O_2 supply and consumption results in an insufficient O_2 supply to maintain cellular function. Hypoxia is defined as an O_2 saturation (SpO_2) < 90%. Hypoxemia is a decrease in oxygen tension in the arterial blood (PaO_2) and is defined as a PaO_2 < 60 mmHg. A SpO_2 < 90% or a PaO_2 < 60 mmHg places a patient on the "steep" area of the oxygen–hemoglobin dissociation curve, where small changes in PaO_2 cause large changes in SpO_2 and rapid clinical deterioration (Figure 1).

CAUSES

There are various causes of hypoxia, including hypoxic hypoxia, pulmonary hypoxia, anemic hypoxia, stagnant hypoxia, cellular hypoxia, or increased oxygen consumption due to a hypermetabolic state, or any combination of these (Table 1).[2]

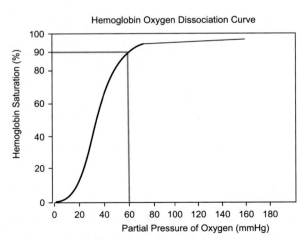

FIGURE 1   This graph illustrates the oxygen–hemoglobin dissociation curve, where a small change in the partial pressure of oxygen will result in large changes in the oxygen saturation.

Hypoxic hypoxia can result from a low fraction of inspired oxygen (FiO_2) or hypoventilation. A low FiO_2 can be due to high altitude or, during anesthesia, the failure of delivery systems such as incorrect flowmeter settings, faulty tank or hose connections, a central gas distribution failure, or an excessive inspired concentration of nitrous oxide. Hypoventilation may occur due to a low respiratory rate and/or decreased tidal volume with reduced minute ventilation. Reduced minute ventilation also results in reduced carbon dioxide (CO_2) elimination from the alveoli. As CO_2

TABLE 1   Causes of Hypoxia and Treatment

Hypoxic hypoxia	
Hypoventilation	Decrease/reverse sedation or analgesia
	Encourage patient to breathe
	Secure airway
	Increase ventilation
Low-inspired oxygen	Increase inspired oxygen
Airway obstruction/loss	Immediate maneuvers to identify, correct problem, or secure airway
Pulmonary hypoxia	
Ventilation/perfusion mismatch	Increase inspired oxygen
	Correct etiology of mismatch
Shunt	Correct shunt
	Cardiovascular support (vasopressors and/or inotropes)
Stagnant hypoxia	Augment cardiac output with volume resuscitation
	Add vasopressors ± inotropes
Cellular hypoxia	
Cyanide	Hydroxycobalamin, sodium thiosulfate, sodium nitrite
Methanol	Nasogastric evacuation
	Hemodialysis
Anemic hypoxia	
Carbon monoxide	100% Oxygen
	Hyperbaric oxygen therapy
Methemoglobinemia	100% Oxygen
	Methylene blue

V. COMPLICATIONS RELATED TO RESPIRATORY SYSTEM

accumulates, there is increasingly less physical space for O_2 molecules in the alveoli; therefore, alveolar partial pressure of oxygen (P_AO_2) decreases, while O_2 consumption by the body continues, and hypoxia ensues. The P_AO_2 can be calculated using the alveolar gas equation [$P_AO_2 = F_IO_2$ ($P_{ATM} - P_{H20}$) − $PaCO_2$], where P_{ATM} is the atmospheric pressure, which at sea level is 760 mmHg, P_{H20} is the saturated vapor pressure of water at body temperature, $PaCO_2$ the arterial partial pressure of CO_2, and 0.8 is the respiratory exchange ratio under resting conditions. Alveolar hypoventilation may be caused by underlying lung and airway pathology, chronic obstructive pulmonary disease (COPD), obesity hypoventilation syndrome, neuromuscular diseases (such as myasthenia gravis, Guillain–Barré syndrome, muscular dystrophy, amyotrophic lateral sclerosis), acute neurological processes, or deformities of the chest or spine.[5]

Pulmonary hypoxia may result from shunting, ventilation/perfusion (V/Q) mismatch, or impaired diffusion. A shunt refers to blood reaching the left side of the heart without participating in ventilation and by extension in oxygenation or CO_2 removal. There are two types of shunts: anatomic or physiologic. The anatomic shunt, present in healthy subjects, is formed by thebesian veins from the myocardium that empty directly into the left atrium and bronchial veins that empty directly into the pulmonary veins, both of which bypass gas exchange in the pulmonary bed. Approximately 2–3% of cardiac output is part of this anatomic shunt. A physiologic shunt occurs when there is a pathological condition in the lung parenchyma that leads to complete collapse or dense consolidation, resulting in zero ventilation across that region of lung. These pathological conditions include events that can easily occur during the perioperative period such as atelectasis, pulmonary edema, venous air embolism, pneumonia, aspiration, and pneumothorax.

The V/Q ratio provides information about the relationship between ventilation (the amount of air that reaches the alveoli) and perfusion (the amount of blood that passes by the alveoli). The ideal V/Q ratio is 1. In the supine position, V/Q equals 1 only in the middle lung zones. At the apex of the lung, ventilation exceeds perfusion (V/Q > 1); at the base, perfusion exceeds ventilation (V/Q < 1). In a healthy supine individual, the V/Q equals 0.8. A low V/Q ratio is found in the setting of a number of pathological conditions, including COPD, asthma, and bronchitis. The decreased V/Q in these conditions is due to bronchospasm and/or the destruction of alveoli, both of which reduce the surface area across which ventilation can take place.[6] By contrast, an embolism (venous air, pulmonary, fat, or amniotic fluid) results in occlusion of the vascular bed. These occlusions are of various sizes and result in increased perfusion to another region of the lung while ventilation to that region remains the same, thus resulting in a decreased V/Q.

During general anesthesia, the functional residual capacity decreases due to a change in the balance between outward forces, respiratory muscle tone, and inward forces such as lung elastic recoil. Overall, the loss of respiratory muscle tone leads to a decreased compliance of the lung and atelectasis, both of which contribute to a shunt effect. Furthermore, a redistribution of inspiratory gas from dependent to nondependent regions of the lungs, some of which are not perfused, leads either to a V/Q mismatch or dead space ventilation.

Diffusion impairment occurs when the alveolar–capillary membranes thicken. This thickening occurs in interstitial lung diseases such as pulmonary fibrosis, sarcoidosis, hypersensitivity pneumonitis, and connective tissue disorders.[6] Early in the disease process, the impaired diffusion is offset by the transit time of the pulmonary capillary system; later in the disease, the severity of the diffusion abnormality outstrips the transit time, and hypoxemia ensues.

Stagnant hypoxia occurs when blood flow to the lung is abnormally low, such as during shock states, cardiac arrest, severe congestive heart failure, or abdominal compartment syndrome. The primary disturbance lies within the cardiovascular system. Despite a severe reduction in perfusion, the PaO_2 often does not fall because the peripheral tissue increases the amount of O_2 it extracts from the blood; however, the mixed venous O_2 (PvO_2) falls.

Cellular hypoxia occurs when there is a normal delivery of O_2 but cells are unable to extract the O_2 from the hemoglobin. Cyanide poisoning causes hypoxia by inhibiting cytochrome c oxidase, an enzyme required for the utilization of O_2 in mitochondria cellular respiration. Cyanide poisoning can be due to prolonged exposure to high doses of sodium nitroprusside or to the inhalation of burning polyurethane or vinyl. Methanol poisoning results in the metabolism of methanol to numerous by-products, including formic acid, which inhibits mitochondrial cytochrome oxidase and, similar to cyanide, inhibits cellular utilization of O_2. Cellular hypoxia can be overlooked because it does not affect the SpO_2 or the PaO_2 since there is neither an impairment of the lungs' ability to delivery O_2 nor of hemoglobin's ability to bind and carry O_2. Clinical symptoms of cellular hypoxia, however, are present and include physiological changes and metabolic perturbations.

Anemic hypoxia is a "relative" anemia caused by the decreased O_2-carrying capacity of compromised hemoglobin. While anemic hypoxia can be due to massive blood loss, the two most common causes of anemic hypoxia are carbon monoxide (CO) poisoning and methemoglobinemia. With CO poisoning, the CO binds to the same receptor site on hemoglobin as O_2 does but with 200 times the affinity. This prevents O_2 from binding to the receptors, thus impairing O_2 delivery to the body. This impairment results in a shift of the O_2–Hb curve to the left and impedes the unloading of O_2 at the tissue. Methemoglobinemia is a change in the hemoglobin molecule from a ferrous ion (Fe^{2+}) to a ferric ion (Fe^{3+}). The Fe^{3+} has a decreased ability to bind free O_2 and an increased affinity for bound O_2 which, like CO, causes a left shift in the O_2–Hb curve. Methemoglobinemia can be either congenital or acquired. The acquired form is caused by medications (chloroquine, benzene, nitrites) and by local anesthetics (benzocaine).

PERIOPERATIVE HYPOXIC EVENTS

The critical times for perioperative acute hypoxic events are during induction and emergence from anesthesia, but hypoxic events may also occur during the maintenance phase as well as during the postoperative recovery phase. During induction of anesthesia, the major concerns leading to hypoxia are the inability to ventilate the patient adequately after they become unconscious and/or the ability to secure an airway. After securing of the airway (with endotracheal tube or laryngeal mask), the correct positioning and maintaining of the airway device is critical. During the maintenance phase of anesthesia, potential causes of hypoxia include endobronchial intubation, atelectasis, or obstruction of the airway due to malpositioning, kinking, or secretions. The position of the patient, such as in the prone position, or when there is limited access to the airway as during a posterior fossa craniotomy, further increases the risk of airway-related episodes of hypoxia. Emergence from anesthesia is often overlooked, but there are many situations that may result in hypoxia, including premature extubation, decreased respiratory effort from residual effects of anesthetic agents (especially opioids and muscle relaxants), obstructed airway, laryngospasm, and excessive secretions. Hypoxia may be the cause of a restless, agitated, or combative patient during the emergence phase from anesthesia. In the postanesthetic care unit (PACU), other common causes of hypoxia relate to prolonged effects of anesthetic agents and over sedation from treatment of any pain. These are all made worse in patients with comorbidities (obesity, COPD).

SIGNS AND SYMPTOMS

At the onset of acute hypoxia, the body makes physiological attempts to maintain adequate oxygenation as body stores of O_2 are limited. If O_2 delivery to cells is insufficient, anaerobic metabolism initially occurs, and then lactic acid will accumulate in tissues and blood due to inadequate mitochondrial oxygenation. When prolonged or severe, this leads to cell death. Hypoxia is detected by chemoreceptors in the carotid body, which results in increased ventilation in an awake patient. However, it is important to remember that the body's defense mechanisms are impaired by general anesthetic agents, muscle relaxants, and opioids.

Acute hypoxia results in increased sympathetic nervous system discharge. Common symptoms include shortness of breath, tachypnea, tachycardia, cyanosis, sweating, and neurological symptoms such as speech difficulty and confusion. During general anesthesia, the occurrence of hypoxia is most frequently noted by a change in SpO_2. Other signs include a change in the patient's color, the color of the blood in the surgical field, or blood gas results.

DIAGNOSIS

The initial management of hypoxia requires a rapid diagnosis and, simultaneously, treatment. The situation in which the hypoxia occurs determines the exact process of diagnosis. The history of the events leading to the onset of hypoxia, the patient's medical comorbidities, and the surgical events are helpful to determine the cause of perioperative hypoxia. Two common scenarios are (1) the onset of acute hypoxia with decreasing SpO_2, and/or airway pressure changes in the operating room during general anesthesia, and (2) the gradual decline in SpO_2 in a patient in the PACU following surgery.

In the operating room during general anesthesia, possible airway/respiratory causes of hypoxia include inadequate oxygen flow, unintentional esophageal or endobronchial intubation, unintentional extubation, airway obstruction, bronchospasm, pneumothorax, pulmonary edema, or laryngospasm (when using a supraglottic airway). The diagnosis is determined by a thorough and systematic examination of the O_2 and gas flows, anesthesia circuit, patency of the airway, and auscultation of the chest. Further assessment may require bronchoscopy, chest X-ray, and blood gases. Cardiovascular parameters (blood pressure, heart rate and rhythm, and electrocardiogram) may also help in finding the cause of hypoxia.

In the postoperative awake patient, examination should begin with vital signs and level of consciousness including neurological assessment. To rule out an airway obstruction, assessment of the patient's airway is needed, including an examination of the neck for swelling and tracheal deviation. The respiratory system examination may identify residual anesthesia drug effects such a paradoxical breathing pattern or signs of restrictive lung disease with use of accessory muscles of breathing. Auscultation of the lungs provides information about the quality and symmetry of breath sounds, such as wheezes, rhonchi, rales, or dullness. Decreased breath sounds may be an indication of an airway obstruction, pneumothorax, or consolidation, while wheezes or rales may indicate congestive heart failure, COPD, or asthma exacerbation. Examination of the cardiovascular system may also be helpful in assessing signs of the patient's volume status (vital signs, jugular venous pressure), or signs of congestive heart failure. Auscultation of the heart sounds can indicate aortic stenosis or valvular insufficiencies due to stenotic or regurgitant lesions. The focus of the neurological examination is to assess the patient's level of consciousness to ensure that the patient is alert enough to protect their airway.

Depending on the circumstances, other different diagnostic modalities may be needed to evaluate the hypoxia. A complete blood count can rule out acute blood loss, and arterial blood gases will indicate the acid-base status and quantify the hypoxia. Blood work for cyanide and methanol levels should be requested if cellular hypoxia is suspected based on patient history. Likewise, if CO poisoning is suspected, a CO-oximeter can be used to accurately measure SpO_2 in the setting of CO poisoning (standard pulse oximeters cannot distinguish between O_2 and CO bound to hemoglobin); alternatively, blood work can be sent to measure blood CO concentration by infrared spectroscopy.

PREDISPOSING FACTORS

During anesthesia, factors that may predispose to the onset of hypoxia include the patient's comorbidities of respiratory disease (asthma, restrictive or obstructive lung disease, and smoking), cardiovascular disease (heart failure, congenital heart), and acute illness (sepsis). The patient's weight (obesity), potentially difficult mask ventilation and/or airway, and positioning for surgery (prone) will increase the risk of hypoxia. In situations where there is a "shared airway" with surgery (head and neck, transphenoidal, oral surgery), there is an increased chance of obstruction or dislodgement of the airway. Emergency situations are well-recognized sources of hypoxic events as there is often lack of time or ability to do a thorough preoperative assessment or examination, especially of the patient's airway, or preparation of the operating room. But overall, induction and emergence from anesthesia during airway manipulation remain the most critical periods for hypoxia in the operating room.

TREATMENT

The goals of treating hypoxia are to rapidly identify the underlying cause(s) and to treat the cause(s). The successful management of a patient with hypoxia requires a systematic approach. There are basic maneuvers that must be performed immediately to treat hypoxia and to stabilize the patient, even as the medical history and intraoperative events are reviewed and the patient examined. In the operating room during anesthesia, the first step is to place the patient on 100% high-flow O_2, scan the patient's monitors, and assess the patient's airway, breathing circuit, airway pressure, presence of end-tidal CO_2 ($ETCO_2$), and ventilator settings. Auscultation of the lung fields is performed to confirm equal and bilateral breath sounds and to rule out crackles or wheezes. A suction catheter should be passed into the endotracheal tube to confirm its patency and to remove any mucus plugs. If bronchospasm is present, treatment with bronchodilators (salbutamol) may be helpful. Finally, if none of these evaluations establish the cause of hypoxia, bronchoscopy should be performed to evaluate location of the endotracheal tube and perform segmental suctioning of the lung fields and/or a chest X-ray obtained to help clarify the situation. Blood gas analysis may also be useful. For the postoperative patient in the PACU, the systematic approach to treat hypoxia is similar to that above, though the patient will generally be awake and have no airway device in place. If hypoxia continues and worsens, securing of the airway may be required. Physiotherapy may be helpful for some patients.

PREVENTION

The prevention of perioperative hypoxia begins with a thorough preoperative assessment and preparation of the patient for surgery. All comorbidities should be noted and optimized. Patients are encouraged to quit smoking and to continue on any respiratory medications such as those for asthma or COPD. Being well prepared for and aware of the critical periods of anesthesia (intubation, extubation, positioning) will help to decrease the incidences of hypoxia. The patient with a known difficult airway may need extra attention and adjunct devices, including an extra pair of hands, for safe intubation. The continuous perioperative monitoring of SpO_2 can detect hypoxia and reduce the incidence of hypoxemia and its possible consequences. During general anesthesia, this monitoring is mandatory, but all patients who are sedated for surgery or for a procedure in or outside of the operating room, and patients in the PACU, should also be continuously monitored with SpO_2.[4] The monitoring of $ETCO_2$ and respiratory rate is also valuable in sedated patients to detect early any changes in respiratory function. During anesthesia, there are a number of maneuvers that may be of benefit in preventing hypoxia such as preoxygenation, recruitment maneuvers, and the use of positive end-expired pressure. During transfer to the PACU and initially in the PACU, all patients should receive submental O_2 by mask or nasal prongs. Postoperatively, patients with a history of sleep apnea should be treated with their continuous positive pressure devices, if indicated. Chest physiotherapy along with a good analgesia may be useful in patients with excessive secretions or difficulty in maintaining optimal breathing.

A common event when signs of hypoxia (decreasing SpO_2) occur is to question the validity of the monitor. There can be many reasons for the misreading of monitors, such as artifacts from movement, cold extremities, or poor positioning of the SpO_2 probe. However, while the situation is being evaluated, treatment should immediately be undertaken in order to prevent injury to the patient.

CEREBRAL PHYSIOLOGY

Hypoxia has devastating consequences for the brain.[7] Although the brain represents a small fraction of total body weight (2%), it consumes a disproportionate percentage of total body O_2 consumption (20%) because of the high cellular metabolic demands that are fueled with ATP from the Krebs cycle. The production of ATP through mitochondrial respiration requires O_2 as the electron acceptor. In a conscious person, the cerebral metabolic rate for oxygen is 3.5 mL/100 g tissue/min to maintain an average brain tissue partial pressure of oxygen ($PbtO_2$) of 20–40 mmHg. According to the Brain Trauma Foundation, a $PbtO_2$ less than 15–20 mmHg is considered the critical threshold in which to initiate treatment to raise $PbtO_2$. Cerebral autoregulation maintains cerebral blood flow (CBF) across a wide range of PaO_2 and cerebral perfusion pressures (CPP) via myogenic, neurogenic, and metabolic mechanisms. During physiological conditions, increased O_2 demand or decreased supply is quickly matched by increased CBF. Acute hypoxia ($PaO_2 < 50$ mmHg) is a potent cerebral vasodilator and leads to a rapid increase in CBF as well as increases in the cellular production of nitric oxide and adenosine, both of which cause vasodilation.

MONITORS OF CEREBRAL OXYGENATION

Standard monitors will aid in the diagnosis and treatment of hypoxia (SpO_2, gas vapor analyzer, capnography, measurement of arterial blood gases, blood pressure, and heart rate). In situations where ongoing concerns are present for the possible occurrence of inadequate cerebral oxygenation, more specific brain monitors are used. These include jugular venous oximetry, brain tissue oxygen tension, near infrared spectroscopy, and cerebral microdialysis.

Jugular venous oxygen saturation ($SjvO_2$) measures the balance between cerebral oxygen supply and demand.[8] The $SjvO_2$ can be monitored either intermittently with blood samples taken from the internal jugular vein, or continuous by insertion of an oximetric catheter into the jugular bulb (located in the jugular vein immediately below the skull base). Because venous drainage of the brain tends to be asymmetric and to favor drainage into the right jugular vein, the access to $SjvO_2$ via the right jugular vein is most frequently used. However, in the setting of a focal injury, ipsilateral placement of the catheter increases the sensitivity to regional ischemia of the pathological side. Normal $SjvO_2$ is 55–75%. A drop in this value suggests an increase in O_2 extraction and necessitates a search for decreased O_2 supply or increased cerebral metabolic rate. While data to support routine monitoring of $SjvO_2$ is lacking, it may be useful to help direct management of hyperventilation and CPP in patients following traumatic brain injury, postsubarachnoid vasospasm monitoring, and intraoperatively during cardiopulmonary bypass, intracranial neurosurgical (aneurysm clipping), and pediatric procedures.

Brain tissue oxygen tension ($PbtO_2$) directly measures the partial pressure of O_2 in the extracellular fluid of the brain.[9,10] Sensors can be inserted at the bedside via a burr hole or intraoperatively during a craniotomy. A number of variables influence the $PbtO_2$, including FiO_2, hemoglobin, mean arterial pressure, and CPP. The $PbtO_2$ measurements are taken directly from brain tissue, thus providing information about local diffusion of O_2. Normal $PbtO_2$ values range from 37 to 48 mmHg. A value less than 20 mmHg is consistent with moderate brain hypoxia and less than 15 mmHg signals a critical threshold. This monitoring modality is used in the management of posttraumatic brain injury and subarachnoid hemorrhage (SAH) secondary to cerebral aneurysms, but may have the greatest value in comatose patients who cannot be followed using serial neurological examinations.

Near-infrared spectroscopy (NIRS) is a noninvasive measurement of regional oxygen saturation (rSO_2) at the capillary–venous level of brain tissue.[11] This measurement is based on the relative absorption of near infrared light by oxygenated and deoxygenated hemoglobin. For NIRS, transcutaneous probes are placed bilaterally on the patient's forehead. In the clinical setting, a reading of rSO_2 less than 50–55% or a decline more than 20% of baseline is usually accepted as a threshold alerting for cerebral ischemia. Clinically, NIRS is best used to monitor trends rather than isolated readings. Clinical uses of the NIRS include neurovascular procedures such as carotid endarterectomy and for estimation of CBF and cerebral oxygenation in patients with traumatic head injury.

Cerebral microdialysis is a minimally invasive technique used for continuous sampling and monitoring of brain tissue biochemistry.[12] It measures the concentrations of free unbound analytes in the extracellular fluid such as neurotransmitters, glucose, glycogen, glutamate, and exogenous molecules such as medications. A microdialysis catheter is inserted into the extracellular fluid of cerebral tissue at risk for secondary brain injury. This technology has been primarily used in patients with acute brain injury or SAH.

References

1. Ward DS, Karan SB, Pandit JJ. Hypoxia: developments in basic science, physiology and clinical studies. *Anaesthesia*. 2011;66(suppl 2):19–26.
2. Wilson WC, Shapiro B. Perioperative hypoxia: perioperative hypoxia the clinical spectrum and current oxygen monitoring methodology. *Anesthesiol Clin NA*. 2001;19(4): 769–812.
3. Cook TM, MacDougall-Davis SR. Complications and failure of airway management. *BJA*. 2012;109(suppl 1):i68–i85.
4. Pedersen T, Nicholson A, Hovhannisyan K, Møller AM, Smith AF, Lewis SR. Pulse oximetry for perioperative monitoring. *Cochrane Database Syst Rev*. 2014;17(3):CD002013.
5. Sivak ED, Shefner J, Sexton J. Neuromusclar disease and hypoventilation. *Cur Opin Pul Med*. 1999;5(6):355–362.
6. Wallis A, Spinks K. The diagnosis and management of interstitial lung disease. *BMJ*. May 2015;350:2072.
7. Masamoto K, Tanishita K. Oxygen transport in brain tissue. *J Biomech Eng*. 2009;131(7):74–82.
8. Schell RM, Cole DJ. Cerebral monitoring: jugular venous oximetry. *Anesth Analg*. 2000;90(3):559–566.
9. Scheufler KM, Röhrborn HJ, Zentner J. Does tissue oxygen-tension reliably reflect cerebral oxygen delivery and consumption? *Anesth Analg*. 2002;95(4):1042–1048.
10. Maloney-Wilensky E, Le Roux P. The physiology behind direct brain oxygen monitors and practical aspects of their use. *Childs Nerv Syst*. 2010;26(4):419–430.
11. Ghosh A, Elwell C, Smith M. Review article: cerebral near-infrared spectroscopy in adults: a work in progress. *Anesth Analg*. 2012;115(6):1373–1383.
12. Tisdall MM, Smith M. Cerebral microdialysis: research technique or clinical tool. *BJA*. 2006;97(1):18–25.

Neurogenic Pulmonary Edema

Prasanna Udupi Bidkar[1], Hemanshu Prabhakar[2]

[1]Department of Anaesthesiology and Critical Care, JIPMER, Puducherry, India; [2]Department of Neuroanaesthesiology and Critical Care, All India Institute of Medical Sciences, New Delhi, India

O U T L I N E

Complications in Neuroanesthesia
http://dx.doi.org/10.1016/B978-0-12-804075-1.00022-5

INTRODUCTION

Pulmonary edema is characterized by an accumulation of fluid in the air spaces and interstitium of the lung. It may be due to intrinsic pathology of the lung or due to systemic factors. Hence, pulmonary edema has been traditionally classified into cardiogenic and noncardiogenic causes. Cardiogenic pulmonary edema ensues due to acute left ventricular failure, following a variety of insults like myocardial infarction. Noncardiogenic pulmonary edema may be caused by acute lung injury or adult respiratory distress syndrome (ARDS). Cardiogenic pulmonary edema is caused by increased pulmonary hydrostatic pressure, secondary to elevated pulmonary venous pressure.

NEUROGENIC PULMONARY EDEMA (NPE)

Neurogenic pulmonary edema (NPE), a relatively rare form of pulmonary edema, follows central nervous system (CNS) insult. It is caused by an increase in pulmonary interstitial and alveolar fluid. It has the potential to increase the secondary injury to the brain and can often be fatal. A number of CNS insults like subarachnoid hemorrhage (SAH), traumatic brain injury (TBI), cervical spinal cord injury (SCI), and intracerebral hemorrhage are associated with NPE.[1-5]

EPIDEMIOLOGY

The exact number of NPE incidences is not clear, as most of the data are derived from case reports or studied with a few patients or with different diagnostic criteria. The reported incidences of NPE range from 2% to 42% in patients with SAH.[1,6,7] The SAH patients with NPE have higher mortality approaching 10%.[1] Increasing age, delay in surgery, and clinical and radiological presentations (poor-grade SAH) were associated with higher incidences of NPE.[7,8] In TBI patients, reports of development of NPE is as high as 20%.[9] In a large autopsy series by Rogers et al., the incidence of NPE was 32% in TBI patients who died at the scene, and it increased to 96% within 96 h following TBI.[2] The incidence of NPE following status epilepticus is not clear. However, it is estimated that nearly one-third of patients with status epilepticus develop NPE.[10]

PATHOPHYSIOLOGY OF NPE

The pathophysiology of NPE following CNS insult is poorly understood. The common finding in these cases is the severity of the CNS insult and sudden increases in intracranial pressure (ICP).[11,12] The raised ICP

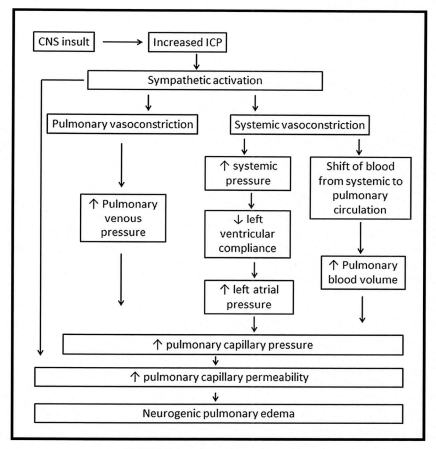

FIGURE 1   Pathophysiology of NPE.

level in these patients correlates with extravascular lung water (EVLW) and occurrence of NPE[13] (Figure 1). There are two probable mechanisms by which NPE develops following CNS injury:

1. Damages to the neurons directly or indirectly affects the pulmonary vascular bed, leading to increased permeability and hence pulmonary edema.[1,14]
2. Overstimulation of the vasomotor center inflicts changes in autonomic function. [15,16]

The sudden increase in ICP leads to neuronal compression or damage, which follows an intense activation of the CNS. The increased secretion of catecholamines lead to systemic vasoconstriction and shift of blood from systemic to pulmonary circulation. This, in association with increased pulmonary vascular permeability, increases EVLW and NPE.

TABLE 1   NPE Trigger Zones

1. Hypothalamus
2. Area 1
3. Area 5
4. Nuclei of solitary tract
5. Area postrema
6. Medial reticulated nucleus
7. Dorsal motor vagal nucleus

NPE TRIGGER ZONES

The precise source in the brain that triggers sympathetic outflow has not been identified. Certain areas of the brain have been identified and are called "NPE trigger zones" (Table 1). These trigger zones include the hypothalamus, brain stem, and upper cervical spinal cord.[4] The important centers for triggering NPE are A1, A5 nuclei, nuclei of solitary tract, and area postrema. The A1 nuclei are present in ventrolateral aspect of the medulla and project into the hypothalamus. The neurons of A5 are located in the upper brain stem and project into centers for sympathetic flow in the spinal cord. Any injury to the area A1 or disruption of the pathway from A5 to sympathetic outflow is associated with the development of pulmonary edema.[17] In the experimental animal models, destruction of the hypothalamus led to the evolution of NPE.[18–20] in animal experiments, stimulation of the solitary tract and unilateral area postrema also lead to hypertension and NPE.[17]

PATHOGENESIS

The sudden increase in ICP, in association with sympathetic discharge, has been associated with the development of NPE, but it is not clear by which mechanism pulmonary edema develops. Four mechanisms have been proposed.

1. Traditionally, NPE is classified under noncardiogenic pulmonary edema. But the available evidence suggests that in some subset of patients with neurological insult, NPE directly inflicts myocardial injury, which in turn leads to pulmonary edema. It is characterized by a cardiomyopathy with diastolic dysfunction, decreased contractility, and global hypokinesia. In the histopathology,

myocytolysis and contraction-band necrosis are observed.[21,22] In the echocardiography regional wall, motion abnormality can be seen.[23] The sudden surge of catecholamines is the causative factor in this form of NPE. Hence, this form of NPE is also known as neurocardiac NPE.

2. In the neurohemodynamic theory of NPE, alteration in the ventricular compliance is believed to cause abrupt increases in pulmonary and systemic pressures after a CNS injury. The sudden increase in afterload causes altered left ventricular function, thus shifting blood from a systemic to a low-resistance pulmonary vascular system. The increased pressure in the pulmonary circulation forms hydrostatic pulmonary edema.[24]

3. The proposed above mechanisms relate to the formation of hydrostatic edema, but they fail to explain the presence of red blood cells (RBCs) and exudative fluid in alveolar space.[25] "Blast theory" proposes that the shift in the blood from systemic circulation to pulmonary circulation causes altered permeability and forms the exudative pulmonary edema.[26] The sudden increase in pulmonary circulation also leads to damage of alveolar–capillary membrane, which explains the presence of RBCs and protein-rich pulmonary edema.

4. There can be adrenergic hypersensitivity of pulmonary venules to catecholamines. This catecholamine surge leads to endothelial injury irrespective of systemic changes.[27]

CLINICAL FEATURES

Following a neurologic injury, NPE can develop within minutes to hours. Depending on the onset of symptoms and signs, two forms of NPE have been identified.[4]

1. Early onset: onset of symptoms within minutes to hours.
2. Delayed onset: delayed onset NPE is seen following 12–24 h of CNS insult.

Generally, the severity of the neurologic insult determines the severity of NPE. Typically, the patient may complain of difficulty in breathing. Acute onset dyspnea, tachypnea, and hypoxia characterize the onset of NPE. On auscultation, bilateral crackles will be present. Pink, frothy sputum can be observed through the endotracheal tube. In addition, sympathetic hyperactivity is seen, characterized by tachycardia, hypertension, and fever spikes. The CNS catastrophes that lead to NPE are described in Table 2.

TABLE 2   Causes of NPE

Common causes

1. SAH[29,30]

2. Cerebral hemorrhage[31]

3. Head injury[32]

4. Seizures

Other less common causes

1. Brain tumors

2. Cervical SCI

3. Endovascular embolization

4. Air embolism

5. Nonhemorrhagic strokes[33]

6. Following electroconvulsive therapy

TABLE 3   Tests to Look for Other Pathologic Causes

Diagnostic test	Findings
Chest X-ray	• Typically shows bilateral infiltrates • May show presence of pneumonia (aspiration pneumonitis) • Other traumatic lung pathologies like pneumothorax/hemothorax
Electrocardiography	• Changes associated with SAH • Associated myocardial ischemia/infarction • Presence of tachy/bradyarrhythmias
Transthoracic echocardiography	• May show myocardial stunning • Regional wall motion abnormalities • Reduced ejection fraction and impaired contraction
Cardiac output monitoring	• Reduced cardiac index with increased SVR • Increased pulmonary capillary wedge pressure

DIAGNOSIS

There is no specific diagnostic test that confirms the diagnosis of NPE. The pulmonary edema due to neurologic origin is a diagnosis of exclusion. The electrocardiographic changes and increased cardiac enzymes may be associated with SAH. A high degree of suspicion should be exercised to rule out cardiogenic pulmonary edema. The diagnostic tests that can be helpful in the diagnosis of NPE are enumerated in Table 3.

DIFFERENTIAL DIAGNOSIS

The diagnosis of NPE is difficult and relies largely on the history of neurological insult. The left ventricular failure, community-acquired pneumonia, aspiration pneumonia, and pulmonary contusion will have clinical features similar to NPE. Sometimes it is possible that more than one condition may coexist. These conditions should be ruled out before confirming the diagnosis of NPE.

MANAGEMENT

The treatment of NPE is mainly supportive care. The focus should be on the management of the CNS disorder and its associated complications. Generally, neurologic pulmonary edema resolves in 48–72 h.

General Supportive Care

1. Airway and breathing: The management of the airway using endotracheal intubation is most often decided by the patient's neurologic condition. Supplemental oxygen by mask is often necessary. If the patient is in severe respiratory distress, endotracheal intubation and mechanical ventilation may be required. In conscious patients who are not at risk of aspiration, noninvasive positive pressure ventilation may be tried. The patients with desaturation and hypoxia may require higher levels of positive end-expiratory pressure (PEEP). Lung protective ventilation is essential in patients with ARDS. Higher levels (>10 cmH$_2$O) should be avoided in patients with signs of raised ICP. In cases where higher PEEP is essential, ICP should be monitored using intraventricular catheters. Permissive hypercapnia should be avoided in patients with raised ICP. In patients with refractory hypoxemia high frequency oscillatory ventilation may be used.
2. Circulation: The hemodynamic management of NPE patients is a challenging one. The choice of drug depends on the associated injuries and preexisting pathology. The cardiac index should be maintained >2.5 L/min/M^2 and systemic vascular resistance (SVR) <1000 dyn. s/cm^5. Dobutamine is the first line of drug for maintenance of cardiac index and SVR. Additionally, β1 agonists and alpha-adrenergic blocking drugs have been tried.

Specific Therapy

1. Pharmacological agents are not routinely used in the management of NPE. Beta blockers and alpha-adrenergic blockers have been tried

with variable results. Generally, NPE is self-limiting and resolves spontaneously. Care must be taken to ensure adequate cerebral perfusion pressure.

2. Efforts to reduce ICP, like decompression, hematoma evacuation, antiepileptics, tumor resection, and steroids, have all been associated with improvement in patient oxygenation.[1,18,28]

CONCLUSIONS

Despite the developments in modern medicine, the diagnosis and management of NPE remains controversial and challenging. Though several mechanisms have been proposed, the exact pathology and pathophysiology are still not very clear. The sudden onset of hypoxemic respiratory failure in association with a CNS catastrophe, which cannot be attributed to any other known cause, generally points toward the diagnosis of NPE. While there are no specific therapies available, supportive care of the patient to prevent the hypoxia is the mainstay of the treatment in this group of patients.

References

1. Fontes RB, Aguiar PH, Zanetti MV, Andrade F, Mandel M, Teixeira MJ. Acute neurogenic pulmonary edema: case reports and literature review. *J Neurosurg Anesthesiol.* 2003;15:144–150.
2. Rogers FB, Shackford SR, Trevisani GT, Davis JW, Mackersie RC, Hoyt DB. Neurogenic pulmonary edema in fatal and nonfatal head injuries. *J Trauma.* 1995;39:860–866.
3. Kaufman HH, Timberlake G, Voelker J, Pait TG. Medical complications of head injury. *Med Clin North Am.* 1993;77:43–60.
4. Colice GL. Neurogenic pulmonary edema. *Clin Chest Med.* 1985;6:473–489.
5. Davison DL, Terek M, Chawla LS. Neurogenic pulmonary edema. *Crit Care.* 2012;16:212.
6. Friedman JA, Pichelmann MA, Piepgras DG, et al. Pulmonary complications of aneurysmal subarachnoid hemorrhage. *Neurosurgery.* 2003;52:1025–1031.
7. Solenski NJ, Haley Jr EC, Kassell NF, et al. Medical complications of aneurysmal subarachnoid hemorrhage: a report of the multicenter, cooperative aneurysm study. Participants of the Multicenter Cooperative Aneurysm Study. *Crit Care Med.* 1995;23:1007–1017.
8. Ochiai H, Yamakawa Y, Kubota E. Deformation of the ventrolateral medulla oblongata by subarachnoid hemorrhage from ruptured vertebral artery aneurysms causes neurogenic pulmonary edema. *Neurol Med Chir (Tokyo).* 2001;41:529–534.
9. Bratton SL, Davis RL. Acute lung injury in isolated traumatic brain injury. *Neurosurgery.* 1997;40:707–712.
10. Simon RP. Neurogenic pulmonary edema. *Neurol Clin.* 1993;11:309–323.
11. Ducker TB, Simmons RL. Increased intracranial pressure and pulmonary edema. 2. The hemodynamic response of dogs and monkeys to increased intracranial pressure. *J Neurosurg.* 1968;28:118–123.
12. Kosnik EJ, Paul SE, Rossel CW, Sayers MP. Central neurogenic pulmonary edema: with a review of its pathogenesis and treatment. *Childs Brain.* 1977;3:37–47.

13. Gupta YK, Chugh A, Kacker V, Mehta VS, Tandon PN. Development of neurogenic pulmonary edema at different grades of intracranial pressure in cats. *Indian J Physiol Pharmacol*. 1998;42:71–80.
14. Baumann A, audibert G, mcdonnel J, mertes PM. Neurogenic pulmonary edema. *Acta Anaesthesiol Scand*. 2007;51:447–455.
15. Leal filho MB, Morandin RC, De Almeida AR, Cambiucci EC, Metze K, Borges G, et al. Hemodynamic parameters and neurogenic pulmonary edema following spinal cord injury: an experimental model. *Arq Neuropsiquiatr*. 2005;63:990–996.
16. Demling R, Riessen R. Pulmonary dysfunction after cerebral injury. *Crit Care Med*. 1990;18:768–774.
17. Blessing WW, West MJ, Chalmers J. Hypertension, bradycardia, and pulmonary edema in the conscious rabbit after brainstem lesions coinciding with the A1 group of catecholamine neurons. *Circ Res*. 1981;49:949–958.
18. Brown Jr RH, Beyerl BD, Iseke R, Lavyne MH. Medulla oblongata edema associated with neurogenic pulmonary edema. Case report. *J Neurosurg*. 1986;64:494–500.
19. Imai K. Radiographical investigations of organic lesions of the hypothalamus in patients suffering from neurogenic pulmonary edema due to serious intracranial diseases: relationship between radiographical findings and outcome of patients suffering from neurogenic pulmonary edema. *No Shinkei Geka*. 2003;31:757–765.
20. Nathan MA, Reis DJ. Fulminating arterial hypertension with pulmonary edema from release of adrenomedullary catecholamines after lesions of the anterior hypothalamus in the rat. *Circ Res*. 1975;37:226–235.
21. Bahloul M, Chaari AN, Kallel H, et al. Neurogenic pulmonary edema due to traumatic brain injury: evidence of cardiac dysfunction. *Am J Crit Care*. 2006;15:462–470.
22. Connor RC. Myocardial damage secondary to brain lesions. *Am Heart J*. 1969;78:145–148.
23. Mayer SA, Lin J, Homma S, et al. Myocardial injury and left ventricular performance after subarachnoid hemorrhage. *Stroke*. 1999;30:780–786.
24. Sarnoff SJ, Sarnoff LC. Neurohemodynamics of pulmonary edema. II. The role of sympathetic pathways in the elevation of pulmonary and systemic vascular pressures following the intracisternal injection of fibrin. *Circulation*. 1952;6:51–62.
25. van der Zee H, Malik AB, Lee BC, Hakim TS. Lung fluid and protein exchange during intracranial hypertension and role of sympathetic mechanisms. *J Appl Physiol*. 1980;48:273–280.
26. Theodore J, Robin ED. Speculations on neurogenic pulmonary edema (NPE). *Am Rev Respir Dis*. 1976;113:405–411.
27. McClellan MD, Dauber IM, Weil JV. Elevated intracranial pressure increases pulmonary vascular permeability to protein. *J Appl Physiol*. 1989;67:1185–1191.
28. Phanthumchinda K, Khaoroptham S, Kongratananan N, Rasmeechan S. Neurogenic pulmonary edema associated with spinal cord infarction from arteriovenous malformation. *J Med Assoc Thai*. 1988;71:150–153.
29. Lee VH, Oh JK, Mulvagh SL, Wijdicks EF. Mechanisms in neurogenic stress cardiomyopathy after aneurysmal subarachnoid hemorrhage. *Neurocrit Care*. 2006;5:243–249.
30. Wartenberg KE, Mayer SA. Medical complications after subarachnoid hemorrhage: new strategies for prevention and management. *Curr Opin Crit Care*. 2006;12:78–84.
31. Goncalves V, Silva-Carvalho L, Rocha I. Cerebellar haemorrhage as a cause of neurogenic pulmonary edema – case report. *Cerebellum*. 2005;4:246–249.
32. Qin SQ, Sun W, Wang HB, Zhang QL. Neurogenic pulmonary edema in head injuries: analysis of 5 cases. *Chin J Traumatol*. 2005;8:172–174. 178.
33. Rochester CL, Mohsenin V. Respiratory complications of stroke. *Semin Respir Crit Care Med*. 2002;23:248–260.

SECTION VI

COMPLICATIONS RELATED TO AIRWAY

Intraoperative Increased Airway Pressure

Prasanna Udupi Bidkar[1], Hemanshu Prabhakar[2]

[1]Department of Anaesthesiology and Critical Care, JIPMER, Puducherry, India; [2]Department of Neuroanaesthesiology and Critical Care, All India Institute of Medical Sciences, New Delhi, India

INTRODUCTION

Monitoring of the airway pressure is important during neurosurgical operations. Due to a variety of positions used during neurosurgery, there is a high risk of kinking endotracheal tubes (ETTs). Often, a slight increase in the airway pressure is the only sign that denotes recovery from neuromuscular blocking agents, necessitating the additional dose of these agents. Clinically, it presents as a tight bag, where it is difficult to maintain ventilation.[1]

NORMAL VENTILATION IN NEUROSURGICAL OPERATIONS

Controlled ventilation with profound neuromuscular blockade is commonly used in neurosurgical patients. Tidal volume and respiratory rate is adjusted to have mild to moderate hyperventilation ($PaCO_2$ 30–34 cm H_2O). With a tidal volume of 8–10 mL/kg, the airway pressures will be around 15–20 cm H_2O. Any airway pressures >25 cm H_2O will be clinically significant. In neurosurgical patients, higher airway pressures can have deleterious effects on intracranial pressure due to impaired venous return. Also, the associated increases in carbon dioxide levels can increase the cerebral blood flow, leading to cerebral edema.

ETIOLOGY

The causes of increased airway pressure can be anticipated or unanticipated. For example, in morbidly obese patients, there can be increased airway pressures. It is stressful and challenging for the anesthesiologist when the increases in airway pressures are unanticipated. The increased airway pressures can be observed in the following ways:

1. Immediately after endotracheal intubation (Table 1)
2. During maintenance of anesthesia (Table 2)
3. During recovery from anesthesia (Table 3)

For the purpose of understanding, all the causes can be divided into mechanical and pathological causes. Some of the causes of increased airway pressure, unique to the neuroanesthesia, are discussed in this chapter.

TABLE 1   Increased Airway Pressures Following Endotracheal Intubation

Mechanical causes	Pathologic causes
1. Obstruction in tube	1. Bronchospasm
2. Kinking of tube	2. Bronchial asthma
3. High flows due to active oxygen flush	3. Anaphylaxis
4. Smaller tube	4. Aspiration pneumonia
5. Malfunctioning inspiratory/expiratory valves	5. Endobronchial intubation
	6. Light anesthesia
6. Foreign bodies, e.g., mucous plug	7. Obesity, smoking
	8. NPE

TABLE 2   Causes During Maintenance of Anesthesia

Anticipated causes	Unanticipated causes
1. Recovery from muscle relaxants	1. Venous air embolism
2. Light anesthesia	2. NPE
3. Tube abutting the carina	3. Aspiration pneumonia
4. NPE	4. Pneumothorax
5. Cardiogenic pulmonary edema	5. Anaphylaxis
6. Precipitation of bronchial asthma	6. Mechanical causes
7. Drug injection, e.g., nonsteroidal antiinflammatory drugs	a. Kinking of tube
	b. Obstruction by mucous plug
8. Venous air embolism during sitting position craniotomy	c. Malfunctioning valves
	d. Kinking/obstruction of breathing circuit

TABLE 3   During Recovery from Anesthesia

1. Bucking patient

2. Biting of ETT

3. Breath holding

4. Bronchospasm

5. Aspiration

MECHANICAL CAUSES

Mechanical causes of an increase in airway pressure are not uncommon in neurosurgical anesthesia, owing to the unique positions in neurosurgical operations. Immediately following intubation, either higher flows or accidentally active oxygen flush may be the common cause of abnormal airway pressure.[2] Partial or complete obstruction of the ETT may occur due to mucous plug or blood clot. The ETT should be carefully positioned in the middle trachea to prevent endobronchial migration of ETT following extreme flexion used in neurosurgical operations. Most of the mechanical causes are unanticipated, and obstruction of the ETT by kinking is one of the common causes of increased airway pressures,[3] this is more common in prone,[4,5] lateral, and park bench positions. Some of the unique positions, such as the Concorde position, increase the risk of airway obstruction.

The kinking of the ETT can be intraoral or outside the oral cavity.[6] There is still debate regarding the ideal type of ETT for neurosurgical anesthesia. Both polyvinyl chloride (PVC) and flexometallic (reinforced or spirally

TABLE 4   Merits and Demerits of ETTs

	PVC tubes	Flexometallic tubes
Advantages	• Cheap and commonly used • Easy to insert • Takes the shape of the airway • Obstruction is relieved, after additional dose of neuromuscular blockers • Do not require change of ETT in postoperative period, if patient requires mechanical ventilation	• Spirally reinforced using metal • Resistant to kinking by extreme flexion of the neck
Disadvantages	• Can easily kink with extreme flexion and rotation of the neck	• Costly and difficult to insert • If the patient bites the tube intraoperatively, it will lead to permanent obstruction • Need to change ETT to PVC tubes if patient requires postoperative ventilation

embedded) tubes are commonly used. Plenty of literature is available on the merits and demerits of each of these ETTs (Table 4). It appears a matter of subjective comfort of the individual anesthesiologist in selecting ETTs. We routinely use PVC tubes in clinical practice for all neurosurgical operations.

Several case reports of permanent obstruction of the lumen of flexometallic tubes intraoperatively have been reported due to the patient biting the tube.[7–10] This can lead to autostrangulation of the patient and hypoxia intraoperatively.[9] In patients with prolonged neurosurgical procedures in prone position, significant vocal cord and soft tissue edema will occur. Postoperatively changing of these tubes to PVC tubes is challenging when the patient requires mechanical ventilation.

Kinking of the PVC-made ETTs has also been reported in the literature.[12] Because of the ease of insertion and stability, PVC-made ETTs are more popular than reinforced tubes. The kinking of PVC tubes is reversible when it happens due to the patient biting the ETT while recovering from neuromuscular blockade.

Prevention of Tube Kink

The baseline airway pressures should be noted in all neurosurgical patients. In patients requiring extreme flexion and rotation, a simulatory position can be adapted in supine position itself, and auscultation for bilateral equal air entry and changes in the airway pressures should be noted. The final airway pressures should be recorded after final positioning. Generally, if the suction catheter can be easily passed through the ETTs, kinking is absent or not significant. Several other methods, like tube-over-tube techniques or use of an oral airway,[11] have been described to prevent intraoral kinking of ETTs. A neuromuscular monitor should be used to guide the use of muscle relaxants to avoid the patient biting the ETT.

Malfunctioning of the Valves

Due to prolonged nature of the neurosurgical operations, condensation of the water vapors in the circle absorber system can make the valve stuck into the inspiratory system, allowing total rebreathing and increased airway pressures. In intraoral surgeries on odontoid process, introduction of a mouth gag may compress the ETT, leading to a narrowing of the airway.

Pathologic Causes

1. **Aspiration**: Patients with severe traumatic brain injury lose the ability to maintain and protect the airway.[13] These patients are at a high risk of aspiration of gastric contents. The initial event following aspiration is chemical reaction of the trachea and bronchi leading to mucosal edema and bronchospasm. Gastric fluid pH of <2.5 or volume >25 mL lead to severe injury of the mucosa. The injury to alveolar–capillary membrane results in leakage of fluids, proteins, and cellular components. All patients with a Glasgow coma scale score <8 require immediate endotracheal intubation. Neurological patients with bulbar palsy are also at high risk of aspiration due to impaired coughing ability. The aspiration can happen before or after induction of anesthesia. Hence, aspiration prophylaxis and rapid sequence intubation are advocated in these patients.

2. **Neurogenic pulmonary edema (NPE)**: NPE is a relatively rare form of pulmonary edema that follows central nervous system insult. It is due to a sudden adrenergic response following acute increases in intracranial pressure.[14] The details of NPE, diagnosis, and management are described elsewhere in this book (Chapter 22).

3. **Venous air embolism**: The use of sitting position is drastically reduced in modern-day neurosurgery. But in some institutions it is still being used for posterior cranial fossa surgeries. The incidence of venous air embolism varies from 40% to 76% in various studies. Small amounts of air entrained may not have pulmonary manifestations. Moderate amounts of air entrained (0.5–2 mL/kg) will lead to reflex vasoconstriction and release of immune mediators, leading to bronchospasm and higher airway pressures (Figure 1).

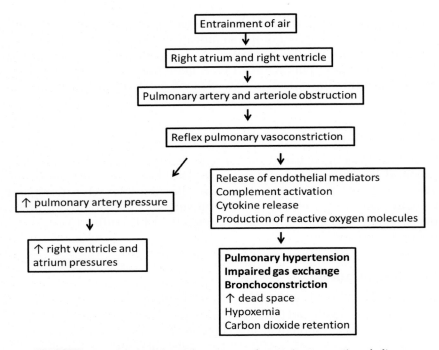

FIGURE 1   Pathophysiology of respiratory changes in venous air embolism.

4. **Anaphylaxis**: Anaphylaxis can happen during anesthesia.[15] Allergic reactions can come in two types: (1) minor anaphylactoid type of reaction with edema of airways or (2) major reactions such as hypotension and bronchospasm. Intraoperatively, anaphylaxis can be seen following administration of drugs like neuromuscular blocking drugs,[16–18] morphine, and other histamine-releasing drugs. Anaphylaxis can also occur following colloid infusion.[19] The drug adenosine, used for transient cardiac arrest in complex neurovascular procedures, has the potential to induce bronchospasm.[20] The effect is more pronounced in asthmatic patients. The topical papaverine, used for relieving vasospasm, can cause anaphylaxis with hypotension and bronchospasm.

5. **Bronchospasm, bronchial asthma, and chronic pulmonary obstructive diseases**: These conditions cause obstructive airway disease. The diagnosis of these conditions may be missed in the preoperative evaluation. Exposure to allergens like dust and smoke cause a release of inflammatory mediators, which lead to bronchoconstriction. Patients get sensitized over a period of time. Even a trivial stimulus later in the process intraoperatively can cause an episode of severe increases in airway resistance.

Thirty percent of relatives of patients with bronchial asthma will have hyperreactive airway disease. Neostigmine administration may lead to bronchospasm.[21]

6. **Other extrinsic factors**: Intubation in the light plane of anesthesia, bucking of the patient, or recovery from neuromuscular relaxants intra- or postoperatively can lead to reflex narrowing of the airway due to increases in pleural pressure. The sustained expiratory muscle contractions and reduced compliance leads to increases in intrapleural pressures and reduced chest wall compliance.

Another condition that produces extrinsic compression is pneumothorax.[22] Subclavian central vein catheterization is commonly performed during neurosurgical operations. It is associated with a 5% risk of pneumothorax. Massive pleural effusions also reduce the compliance.[23] A bedside ultrasound can aid in the diagnosis and management of both of these conditions.

CONCLUSIONS

The unanticipated abnormal airway pressures can lead to unsatisfactory ventilation, adding considerable stress for the anesthesiologist. Mechanical causes should be kept in mind before considering the pathologic causes of increased airway pressures. Tube kinking is a matter of concern in the intraoperative period and should be avoided with careful positioning and monitoring of the airway pressures. Drug-induced bronchospasm or anaphylaxis should be suspected when increased pressures are seen following drug administration. Finally, extrinsic factors like pneumothorax should be suspected, particularly when a subclavian central venous line is placed.

References

1. Parthasarathy S, Ravishankar M. Tight bag. *Indian J Anaesth*. 2010;54:193–198.
2. Brockwell RC, Andrews JJ. Understanding your anesthesia machine. *ASA Refresh Courses Anesthesiol*. 2002;30:41–59.
3. Sprung J, Bourke DL, Harrison C, Barnas GM. Endotracheal tube and tracheobronchial obstruction as causes of hypoventilation with high inspiratory pressures. *Chest*. 1994;105:550–552.
4. Inada T, Shingu K, Yamanouchi Y, Katoh A. Delayed kinking of the tracheal tube during neck flexion in a paediatric neurosurgical patient. *Paediatr Anaesth*. 1998;8:364.
5. Korn S, Schubert A, Barnett G. Endotracheal tube obstruction during stereotactic craniotomy. *J Neurosurg Anesthesiol*. 1993;5:272–275.
6. Leissner KB, Ortega R, Bodzin AS, Sekhar P, Stanley GD. Kinking of an endotracheal tube within the trachea: a rare cause of endotracheal tube obstruction. *J Clin Anesth*. 2007;19(1):75–76.
7. Kumar A, Dash HH. Dynamic intraoperative kinking of flexometallic tube. *J Neurosurg Anesthesiol*. 2001;13:243–245.

8. Tose R, Kubota T, Hirota K, Sakai T, Ishihara H, Matsuki A. Obstruction of an reinforced endotracheal tube due to dissection of internal tube wall during total intravenous anesthesia. *Masui*. 2003;52:1218–1220.
9. Azim A, Matreja P, Pandey C. Desaturation with flexometallic endotracheal tube during lumbar spine surgery—a case report. *Indian J Anaesth*. 2003;47:48–49.
10. Bruce D. Spices: complete airway obstruction of armoured endotracheal tubes. *Anesth Analg*. 1991;73:95–96.
11. Ogden LL, Bradway JA. Maneuver to relieve kinking of the endotracheal tube in a prone patient. *Anesthesiology*. 2008;109:159.
12. Hübler M, Petrasch F. Intraoperative kinking of polyvinyl endotracheal tubes. *Anesth Analg*. 2006;103:1601–1602.
13. Chowdhury T, Kowalski S, Arabi Y, Dash HH. Pre-hospital and initial management of head injury patients: an update. *Saudi J Anaesth*. 2014;8:114–120.
14. Davison DL, Terek M, Chawla LS. Neurogenic pulmonary edema. *Crit Care*. 2012;16:212.
15. Fisher M, Baldo BA. Anaphylaxis during anaesthesia: current aspects of diagnosis and prevention. *Eur J Anaesthesiol*. 1994;11:263–284.
16. Yoon Y, Lee B, Seo HS, Bang J, Ha SI, Song JG. Anaphylactic reactions after cisatracurium administration in two patients – a report of two cases. *Korean J Anesthesiol*. 2013;65(2): 147–150.
17. Brusch AM, Clarke RC, Platt PR, Phillips EJ. Exploring the link between pholcodine exposure and neuromuscular blocking agent anaphylaxis. *Br J Clin Pharmacol*. November 20, 2013. http://dx.doi.org/10.1111/bcp.12290.
18. Sadleir PH, Clarke RC, Bunning DL, Platt PR. Anaphylaxis to neuromuscular blocking drugs: incidence and cross-reactivity in Western Australia from 2002 to 2011. *Br J Anaesth*. June 2013;110(6):981–987.
19. Polyzois I, Lampard A, Mohanlal P, Tsiridis E, Manidakis N, Tsiridis E. Intraoperative anaphylaxis due to gelofusine in a patient undergoing intramedullary nailing of the femur: a case report. *Cases J*. 2009;2:12.
20. Coli S, Mantovani F, Ferro J, Gonzi G, Zardini M, Ardissino D. Adenosine-induced severe bronchospasm in a patient without pulmonary disease. *Am J Emerg Med*. 2012;30:2082. e3–2082.e5.
21. Hazizaj A, Hatija A. Bronchospasm caused by neostigmine. *Eur J Anaesthesiol*. 2006;23:85–86.
22. Lee JY, Kim JU, An EH, Song E, Lee YM. Bilateral tension pneumothorax caused by an abrupt increase in airway pressure during cervical spine surgery in the prone position – a case report. *Korean J Anesthesiol*. 2011;60:373–376.
23. Hori G, Akatsu M, Nemoto C, Iida H, Isosu T, Murakawa M. A case of respiratory distress due to massive pleural effusion after surgery for ovarian tumor. *Masui*. March 2013;62(3):362–364. [Article in Japanese].

Difficult Airway in the Neurosurgery Patient

Eckhard Mauermann, Luzius A. Steiner

Anesthesiology, University Hospital Basel, Basel, Switzerland

DEFINITION

Airway management is a core competency in anesthesiology, and a number of philosophies, algorithms, and tools have been established. Furthermore, airway management is influenced by the interaction between the clinical setting, patient factors, and practitioners' skills.[1]

A common definition is that a *difficult airway* is one in which a conventionally trained anesthesiologist experiences difficulty with mask ventilation, tracheal intubation, or both. Although we are aware that an increasing number of surgeries can be performed with supraglottic airways, we will focus on endotracheal tubes (ETTs) to ensure controlled ventilation of the neurosurgery patient. *Difficulty in mask ventilation* has been defined as an inability to maintain oxygen saturation above 90%. Some estimates state that such "cannot ventilate situations" occur approximately one in 700 times.[2] Although no universal definition exists for *difficult tracheal intubation*, it has been defined as one requiring multiple attempts or requiring a change in plan. The incidence of a *difficult airway* in the general surgical population has been estimated to be between 5% and 15% based on the classical laryngoscopy,[a] with a higher incidence occurring outside of the operating room.[3,4] The "failed airway"—one requiring an alternative instrument or operator—has been estimated to be 3–5%.[5,6]

In addition, we must also consider the largely neglected topic of extubating a difficult airway. After all, it is fair to say that in the majority of cases, a difficult airway has not become any easier through intubation. Furthermore, and often forgotten, is that nondifficult airways may, in fact, have become difficult intraoperatively as illustrated by the fact that some 80% of laryngeal injuries occur in nondifficult intubations.[7] The Difficult Airway Society (DAS) has labeled extubation a "high-risk phase of anesthesia"[8] as also evident in large national surveys[9] and closed claims.[10] While the definition of a *difficult extubation* refers to difficulty in removing the tube (e.g., due to a surgical stitch), *at-risk of extubation failure*, or simply *at-risk extubation*, refers to the risk of losing airway patency and/or ventilation.[11] As a transition from a proactive and controlled situation to a somewhat uncontrolled and somewhat reactive situation, tracheal extubation is especially challenging in neurosurgery patients who often are a vulnerable and unpredictable population.

---

[a] Given the increase in number and availability in video assisted tools and fiber optics, implementation of the Cormack and LeHane criteria based on classical laryngoscopy may be becoming increasingly antiquated.

CAUSES OF DIFFICULT AIRWAY

The American Society of Anesthesiologists (ASA) describes a number of difficult issues in airway management: patient cooperation and consent, difficult mask ventilation, difficult laryngoscopy, difficult intubation, difficult supraglottic airway placement, and difficult surgical airway access. We will ignore the last two points for neurosurgery but add difficult airway maintenance and causes of the at-risk extubation.

Difficulty in patient cooperation and consent may be a major factor in neurosurgery patients, who may range from cooperative elective patients to aggressive emergency patients. This may be challenging not just from a legal perspective, but also from the standpoint of adequate preoxygenation or feasibility of induction techniques (e.g., awake fiber optic intubation). Difficult mask ventilation may occur in any patient but is particularly detrimental in neurosurgery patients. Not only may this cause suboptimal induction conditions in terms of oxygenation, but also in terms of inducing hypercarbia. Causes include poor mask seal, loss of airway tonus, and increased airway reactivity (e.g., laryngospasm, bronchospasm, obstruction through aspiration, etc.). Difficult laryngoscopy is generally caused by factors impeding access to the airway or proper placement of the laryngoscope. For this reason, a fiber optic or video laryngoscopy may be a prudent first choice. Difficult intubation is largely dependent upon laryngoscopy, although problems may occur with tube placement (use a stylet!), tube size, or airway obstruction. Difficult airway maintenance can be caused by a number of factors in neurosurgery patients, including altered and changing consciousness affecting both the neurological aspect of respiration as well as airway tonus. This is particularly challenging in neurosurgery due to the unpredictability of drug effects in more sensitive patients as well as limited access to the patient's head (see the excursion topic awake craniotomy and the stereotactic frame). Finally, the causes of at-risk extubation must be considered. Basically, all of the above mentioned causes during induction and during the operation also apply to extubation. Additional causes for the at-risk extubation include further changes in vigilance, residual drug concentrations affecting airway patency and respiratory reflexes as well as any intraoperative factors inhibiting airway function such as edema of the base of the tongue, pharynx, and/or larynx after prolonged surgery in the prone position.

DIAGNOSIS

The diagnosis of a difficult airway is by definition one requiring actual difficulty in one of the relevant aspects, e.g., bag-mask ventilation or intubation/extubation. Because we would rather be safe than correct, we suggest diagnosing the *suspected* difficult airway. Unfortunately, there are no firm diagnostic criteria for the suspected difficult airway. We advise using individual judgment—preferably conducted by the anesthesiologist/intensivist directly involved in airway management—on the basis of the predisposing factors.

PREDISPOSING FACTORS AND SIGNS

One way of structuring predisposing factors is to review general preoperative and intra/postoperative factors. Although current guidelines clearly state that an anesthesiologist should perform an intubation history in addition to a general history and also perform a physical examination of the airway, they remain vague about specific examples, and evidence is limited to observational studies and case reports. Even more neglected is the topic of extubating the difficult airway. For neurosurgery patients, a number of additional patient and procedural factors can complicate the management of securing the airway. Additionally, the potential consequences of even relatively commonplace fluctuations in physiology during induction or extubation (e.g., in blood pressure, in ventilation, increases in intracranial pressure (ICP) due to coughing, stress, etc.) may be tolerated poorly in neurosurgical patients on account of their underlying pathologies.

General Factors

A great deal of attention has been placed on a patient's history and on identifying anatomical factors associated with a difficult airway (see Table 1). Particular focus has been on difficult mask ventilation and intubation. However, prediction remains poor at best with a cohort analysis of over 188,000 patients showing that 94% of difficult mask ventilations and 93% of difficult intubation were unanticipated, and when anticipated, only 22% and 25% actually had difficult mask ventilation and difficult intubation, respectively.[12] Even when patients had had a difficult or failed intubation using direct laryngoscopy in the past, an analysis of 15,000 patients showed this to be a predictor of a subsequent difficult or failed intubation in only 30% of patients.[13]

The identification of factors associated with difficult mask ventilation has led to the mnemonic MOANS®, which refers to mask seal, obstruction/obesity, age, no teeth, and stiffness of lungs.[14]

Predictors of a difficult intubation have been summarized by the mnemonic LEMON®, which refers to look externally, evaluate (3-3-2 rule), Mallampati, obstruction/obesity, and neck mobility.[15] "Look externally" includes abnormal anatomy of the patient, trauma, and evidence of surgical scars. "Evaluate (3-3-2)" refers to three patient

TABLE 1 Factors Associated with a Difficult Airway in Neurosurgical Patients

General preoperative factors and signs	General intra/postoperative factors
History of • Obstructive sleep apnea and snoring • Previous difficult laryngoscopy and/or intubation • Potential mediastinal mass (e.g., lymphoma, goiter) • Acquired conditions (e.g., degenerative osteoarthritis, rheumatoid arthritis, ankylosing spondylitis, acromegaly) • Congenital conditions (e.g., Down-, Marfan-, or Pierre-Robin syndromes, achondroplasia) **Physical Characteristics** • Long incisors ("buckteeth") and reduced interincisor distance • Micro- or retrognathia ("overbite")/poor voluntary protrusion of mandible • Poor visibility of uvula (Mallampati grade) • Gothic palate • Short thyromental distance (<6 cm) • Short, thick neck ("no neck") • Limited range of motion of head and neck • Small mouth and decreased jaw mobility • Previous neck surgery or irradiation • Space-occupying lesions in oropharynx/larynx • Poor mask seal/facial hair • Age • Obesity/obstruction • Male sex	**Most preoperative factors unchanged postoperatively!** **Additionally** • Exaggerated laryngeal reflexes (e.g., breath holding, coughing, bucking, laryngospasm, biting) • Reduced laryngeal reflexes (residual anesthetics, opioids, or muscle relaxants) • Airway occlusion (internal clots, accumulation of respiratory secretion) • Airway injury or edema due to anesthesia (laryngoscopy, placement of tube or adjuncts, transesophageal echocardiography, nasogastric tubes, larger tubes, excessive cuff pressure, incorrect tube placement) • Airway injury or edema due to surgery (nerve damage or hematomas from carotid of head/neck procedures, prone or prolonged Trendelenburg position, long surgical duration, fluid overload)

Factors specifically related to neurosurgery

Patient factors
- Potentially lacking or difficult preoperative assessment
- Emergency situations
- Uncooperative or even combative behavior, reduced communicability
- Problems in head and neck mobility or facial trauma
- Less predictable response to drugs (e.g., anesthetics, opioids, local anesthetics)
- Difficulty in attaining optimal preoxygenation
- Problems in swallowing, decreased laryngeal reflexes (risk of aspiration and potentially a full stomach)
- Clinical signs of increased cranial pressure or traumatic brain injury
- Patients often either older, polymorbid, and taking antithrombotic/antiplatelet drugs or younger polytrauma patients
- Tendency to tolerate changes in physiology much more poorly and with graver consequences
- Spinal injury with rising lesion

Procedural Factors
- Challenges of awake craniotomy, asleep-awake-asleep craniotomy, and variations thereof (see excursion 1)
- Restricted access to the head and airway (transsphenoidal surgery, stereotactic halo; see excursion 2)
- In the event of difficulties, additional help and equipment may be far away (e.g., if in the angiography suite, CT/MRI)

finger widths between maxillary and mandibular incisors when maximally opening the mouth, three finger widths from the chin to the hyoid bone, and two finger widths from the larynx to the base of the tongue. The Mallampati grade refers to observable structures in the pharynx without phonation. Obstruction/obesity and neck mobility are self-explanatory.

The Cormack and Lehane score, another classical score for a difficult intubation, is based on visibility under standard laryngoscopy. This score no doubt rather late.

Factors During Neurosurgery

A number of factors during neurosurgery can change airway-relevant factors even to the point of inhibiting extubation. Patients may also be required to remain intubated for neuroprotective reasons.

Similarly, there may be concerns regarding vital neural structures and their influence on functional gas exchange. Specifically, preoperative lower cranial nerve dysfunction, hydrocephalus, tumor location, duration of surgery >6 h, blood loss >1000 ml were all found to be independent factors of delayed intubation in a trial of 800 patients undergoing infratentorial craniotomy.[16] In this study, 49.8% underwent delayed extubation and those patients remaining intubated exhibited significantly higher rates of pneumonia, longer intensive care unit (ICU) and hospital stays, and higher costs.

Furthermore, a secured airway, whether difficult or not, may have to remain in place to prevent secondary brain damage. Classical examples of this are patients with traumatic brain injury (TBI) or intracranial hemorrhage. While they may have to remain intubated due to decreased vigilance or to optimize ventilation, sedation, or even muscle relaxants may have to be administered to lower ICP. Even once extubated, some 10% of TBI patients may require reintubation.[17]

In trials examining multilevel spine surgery in the prone position, nearly half of all patients were not extubated at the end of the procedure due to factors such as total crystalloid, colloid, and blood volume administered, procedure duration, extent of surgery, age, ASA class, and case end time.[18,19] Although most patients were extubated within 24 h, the risk of postoperative pneumonia was three times higher in this group (10.3% vs 3.1%; $p = 0.0146$).

Excursion 1: Awake Craniotomy as an Extreme Example of a Procedural Factor

A number of interventions in neurosurgery require a vigilant anesthesiologist continually assessing the airway and its patency, even in the absence of airway instrumentation. The most striking example of this is the awake craniotomy, asleep-awake-asleep craniotomy, or variations thereof. The main benefit of these techniques is maximizing tumor resection in eloquent brain regions while minimizing functional sequelae. The main challenges for an anesthesiologist in this setting, which may occur under local anesthesia, conscious sedation, or general anesthesia, are titrating medication to reduce patient discomfort and stress while ensuring airway patency or managing its loss.[20] Additionally, seizures represent a potentially serious complication and may also require securing the airway. Depending on the variation of awake craniotomy employed, the anesthesiologist may or may not have to instrument the airway in an appropriate way. For example, if a seizure is not abruptly terminated by cold water irrigation, a flexible laryngeal mask should quickly be placed (recall that these patients are starved and hypercarbia/ICP are not major issues). However, regardless of the planned procedure, the anesthesiologist will constantly have to assess airway patency and have a plan of how to cope with a loss of the airway.

Excursion 2: Reduced Neck Mobility and the Stereotactic Frame In Situ

Reduced neck mobility due to a cervical pathology or protective collar may severely impede classical intubation. Furthermore, excessive force may result in lasting spinal damage. However, generally speaking, reduced neck mobility per se is not a major problem if a protective collar is in place, as fiber optic or video-assisted intubation can be easily performed.[21,22]

The stereotactic frame may be another matter. While local anesthetic may suffice for some patients, a great deal may also require small intraoperative dosages of a hypnotic or analgesic drug. Complications occurring may include seizures, loss of airway patency, and changes in the neurological state. The need to emergently intubate with a stereotactic frame in situ poses greater challenges. In addition to full immobilization, the frame is bulky and cannot generally be opened without a key. Furthermore, immediate access to the head of the patient will be limited intraoperatively, limiting the use of video-assisted laryngoscopy. We recommend keeping a fiber optic bronchoscope nearby and ready, having a supraglottic airway device with intubation option (e.g., intubating laryngeal mask airway) available, and a key to open the stereotactic frame if need be. Additionally, more predictable drug delivery by target-controlled infusion may avoid excess sedation or at least avoid longer periods of excess sedation than bolus administration.

TREATMENT

As with many important processes and situations in medicine, a checklist or algorithm provides a sensible basis to appropriately treat most patients. A number of factors influence management including urgency, patient-related factors, the clinical situation, the experience and preferences of the treating physicians, as well as local conditions. Consequently, any difficult airway algorithms may have to be adapted locally in addition to being modified for neurosurgical patients. For example, a preclinical, crash airway of a patient in respiratory arrest lying on the floor with a suspected intracranial hemorrhage is very different from a planned, daytime induction in theater, with all tools, personnel, and preoperative assessments available. Similarly, immediate postoperative extubation in theater of patient undergoing uncomplicated lower segment laminectomy is very different from nighttime extubation in the ICU of an obtunded patient just having undergone prolonged and complicated surgery in the posterior fossa. In other words, management must be dependent not only upon evidence and guidelines, but also on experience, local algorithms, and situations.

We first present special considerations for the neurosurgical patient and then apply this knowledge to two algorithms: the ASA Difficult Airway Algorithm® and the DAS Extubation Guidelines: "at-risk" algorithm®.

Special Consideration for the Neurosurgical Patient

Obviously, the adage that what kills the patient is hypoxia and not a missing ETT is true in neurosurgery patients as well. However, while a "cannot intubate, cannot ventilate" situation certainly trumps all other problems, the goals of airway management must also consider the underlying pathologies involved in the neurosurgical patient and merit special mention as they influence patient outcome and our management.

Our general aim in many neurosurgical settings is to limit secondary brain damage. In TBI, intracerebral hemorrhage, subarachnoid hemorrhage, and stroke, the penumbra is much more susceptible to damage than an elective neurosurgery patient's brain. Consequently, in terms of management goals, we must rigorously avoid hypoxia and maintain cerebral perfusion pressure (CPP) by ensuring hemodynamic stability and reducing ICP. In other words, not only hypoxia and hypotension, but also hypercarbia, coughing, bucking, and so forth may harm viable brain tissue. Furthermore, excessive hypertension may increase bleeding in patients with an already increased propensity to bleed, be it due to medication or due to vascular frailty.

Combining general factors of a difficult airway with both specific neurosurgical factors increasing the difficulty of the airway, as well as the potentially detrimental effects of not maintaining ventilation and CPP, makes successful management even more challenging.

Intubation of the Difficult Airway: the ASA Difficult Airway Algorithm®

Originally created in 1993, the ASA Difficult Airway Algorithm® (Figure 1) has become a standard in difficult airway management. Especially appealing is its early consideration of potential problems (Point 1), consideration of management choices (Point 3), and developing and communicating first-, second-, and third-line mangement plans (Point 4). For example, while awake fiber optic intubation is generally the gold standard, it will not always be possible. For a patient with a TBI and neck injuries without excessive bleeding, an alternative may be a fiber optic intubation with a jaw thrust after the loss of consciousness.[23] Especially in case of excessive bleeding, another option would be to use any of a number of video laryngoscopes,[24] many of which have been shown to improve Cormack and Lehane grading and provide excellent intubation rates even in patients with cervical spine immobilized by a semirigid collar.[21]

Addressing the initial points of the algorithm may require even more thought, planning, and communication in neurosurgery patients, as also illustrated in Figure 1. Many of the generally available options in either avoiding or reversing "point of no return" situations in the general population may not be applicable (e.g., spontaneous breathing, predictable minimal drug doses, reversing agents, awakening the patient, etc.). Furthermore, even if these should be feasible they may return the patient to a deranged and worsening physiological state requiring intubation in addition to all other problems posed by inducing neurosurgery patients. As always, general preparation, such as having sufficient help and all required materials, as well as optimizing intubation conditions, are essential, especially in a remote in-hospital locations.

Extubation of the Difficult Airway: The DAS Extubation Guidelines: "At-Risk" Algorithm®

Nearly 20 years after the publication of the difficult airway intubation guideline, the DAS difficult airway extubation guidelines were published.[8] As in the intubation guidelines, the extubation algorithm (Figure 2) begins with a stepwise approach: (1) planning extubation, (2) preparing for extubation, (3) performing extubation, and (4) postextubation care.

In step one, an extubation plan should be in place prior to induction and reviewed throughout and immediately before performing extubation. Determining whether or not the patient may have an at-risk intubation is

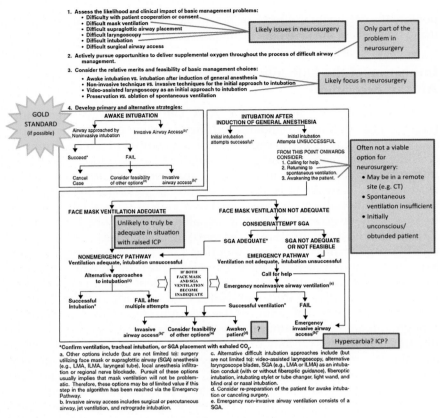

FIGURE 1   ASA Difficult Airway Algorithm® adapted for Neurosurgery.

made on the basis of preexisting airway difficulties, perioperative airway deterioration, and restricted airway access.

In step two, the airway itself must be reassessed on the basis of the expected feasibility of spontaneous breathing, bag-mask ventilation, and reintubation. This may include assessing potential problems of the lower airway (e.g., excess secretions, poor gas exchange, splinting of diaphragm by gastric distention, etc.), of the larynx (consider a cuff leak test or inspection), and of the neurological state of the patient (e.g., compression of brain and spinal cord regions responsible for respiration by edema, hematoma, ascending paraplegia, etc.). Neurological drive may be assessed by intraoperative tidal volumina and negative pressure in spontaneous respiration. Following a final evaluation and optimization of general factors (e.g., reversal of neuromuscular blockade, cardiovascular stability, temperature, acid-base status, adequate analgesia, etc.) and logistic factors (e.g., full monitoring, sufficient time,

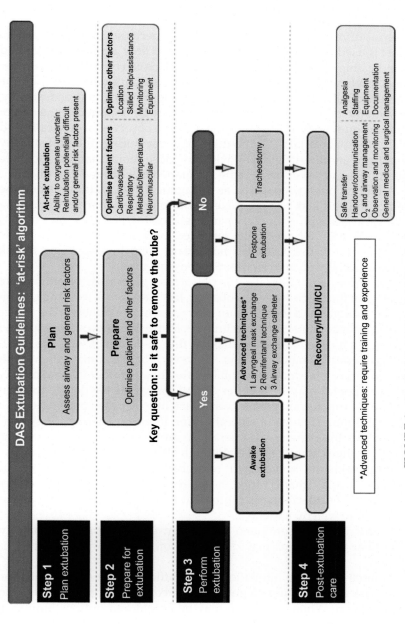

FIGURE 2 The DAS Extubation Guidelines for the at-risk airway.

communication with ICU for postoperative care, etc.), the fundamental questions, "Is it safe to remove the tube?" and "Should we attempt to remove the tube?" must be answered. In the ICU setting, a tracheostomy may be an alternative.

In terms of management, the cuff leak test merits some extra attention. This test is used to assess whether or not air can flow around the uncuffed tube, indicating open space around the ETT. This can be done in a number of ways, preferably one after another. While still anesthetized, the tube can be uncuffed and a leak observed on the monitor and acoustically. Next, with the tube still uncuffed, the tube may be occluded at the end of inspiration, and the flow of air around the tube observed acoustically and clinically (e.g., chest falls). If these are both reassuring, the patient may emerge from anesthesia—ideally with low-dose remifentanil to facilitate cooperation—and asked to breathe spontaneously around the uncuffed tube. Although often propagated as a diagnostic tool, data regarding the benefit of the cuff leak test are mixed, with one metaanalysis examining six clinical trials with over 3000 patients showing an odds ratio of 2.09 (95% CI 1.28–2.89) for predicting laryngeal edema.[25] In summary, while potentially useful, this test does not greatly help in identifying at-risk patients, especially given the potential consequences.

In step three, extubation itself is performed. A number of options are advocated by the DAS: awake extubation, laryngeal mask exchange, remifentanil technique, and the use of an airway exchange catheter. The choice of technique or combination of techniques to use depends on the expected difficulty. An awake extubation may be fine in a patient who has a difficult preoperative anatomy alone. However, for the same patient with suspected laryngeal edema, the combination of a remifentanil and airway exchange catheter may be a better option, provided we decide to extubate at all. In this second scenario, a sufficient effect site concentration of remifentanil may facilitate a smooth, calm, low oxygen–requiring emersion in which the patient will tolerate an airway exchange catheter. The airway exchange catheter itself—although also not without risks and also not guaranteeing 100% successful reintubation[26,27]—generally allows us to quickly place a (smaller) tube in the event that reintubation becomes necessary.[28–30] Furthermore, it can be left in place for some time and is tolerated quite well by patients.

Step four involves continued assessment of the patient and airway, as a number of problems may occur later on, and reintubation may be necessary.

In summary, both the intubation of the difficult airway and extubation of the at-risk airway require a good deal of consideration, planning, and communication. While intubation may be urgent and options limited in neurosurgery, extubation is elective but must additionally consider that the airway and neurological status may have changed.

PREVENTION

Difficult airways may largely be unpreventable as many causes and predisposing factors cannot be changed. Equally frustrating is the poor prognostic values of patients' history and certain anatomical features that may predict difficulties. Consequently, we suggest adopting the term suspected difficult airway, according to the philosophy that we would rather be safe than right. This has several benefits:

1. A real difficult airway is less likely to be unexpected, meaning that appropriate equipment and personnel will already be at hand and ready.
2. Sufficient practice in the tools and algorithms will take place to allow for calm management during a real emergency.
3. Additional information may be gained regarding the airway (e.g., via a fiber optic or video-assisted intubation).
4. Damage to the airway may be reduced if we do not try to initially intubate everyone conventionally.

Additionally, suspected laryngeal edema due to trauma may be treated with steroids. Although somewhat controversial, early treatment with corticosteroids several hours prior to extubation has been successful in reducing laryngeal edema and reintubation,[31] especially in ICU patients with long-term intubation.[32,33]

In terms of the difficult airway at extubation, it helps to remember that this is not an emergency and that we can invest time into optimizing conditions. This may include calling for more experienced personnel and additional equipment or assessing the airway fiber-optically, by video-assisted laryngoscopy, and/or by cuff leak test. If the decision is made to extubate, an intubating bougie or airway exchange catheter may be used to facilitate reintubation.

References

1. Apfelbaum JL, et al. Practice guidelines for management of the difficult airway: an updated report by the American Society of Anesthesiologists Task Force on Management of the Difficult Airway. *Anesthesiology*. 2013;118(2):251–270.
2. Kheterpal S, et al. Prediction and outcomes of impossible mask ventilation: a review of 50,000 anesthetics. *Anesthesiology*. 2009;110(4):891–897.
3. Martin LD, et al. 3,423 emergency tracheal intubations at a university hospital: airway outcomes and complications. *Anesthesiology*. 2011;114(1):42–48.
4. Burkle CM, et al. Airway management after failure to intubate by direct laryngoscopy: outcomes in a large teaching hospital. *Can J Anaesth*. 2005;52(6):634–640.
5. UptoDate. Available from: www.uptodate.com Accessed on 07.07.15.
6. Practice guidelines for management of the difficult airway. A report by the American Society of Anesthesiologists Task Force on Management of the Difficult Airway. *Anesthesiology*. 1993;78(3):597–602.

7. Domino KB, et al. Airway injury during anesthesia: a closed claims analysis. *Anesthesiology*. 1999;91(6):1703–1711.
8. Popat M, et al. Difficult Airway Society Guidelines for the management of tracheal extubation. *Anaesthesia*. 2012;67(3):318–340.
9. Cook TM, Woodall N, Frerk C. Major complications of airway management in the UK: results of the Fourth National Audit Project of the Royal College of Anaesthetists and the Difficult Airway Society. Part 1: anaesthesia. *Br J Anaesth*. 2011;106(5):617–631.
10. Peterson GN, et al. Management of the difficult airway: a closed claims analysis. *Anesthesiology*. 2005;103(1):33–39.
11. Cavallone LF, Vannucci A. Review article: extubation of the difficult airway and extubation failure. *Anesth Analg*. 2013;116(2):368–383.
12. Norskov AK, et al. Diagnostic accuracy of anaesthesiologists' prediction of difficult airway management in daily clinical practice: a cohort study of 188 064 patients registered in the Danish Anaesthesia Database. *Anaesthesia*. 2015;70(3):272–281.
13. Lundstrom LH, et al. A documented previous difficult tracheal intubation as a prognostic test for a subsequent difficult tracheal intubation in adults. *Anaesthesia*. 2009;64(10):1081–1088.
14. Murphy M, Walls RM. Identification of the difficult and failed airway. In: Murphy M, Walls RM, Luten RC, eds. *Manual of emergency airway management*. Philadelphia: Lippincott Williams & Wilkins; 2004:70.
15. Reed MJ, Dunn MJ, McKeown DW. Can an airway assessment score predict difficulty at intubation in the emergency department? *Emerg Med J*. 2005;22(2):99–102.
16. Cai YH, et al. Factors influencing delayed extubation after infratentorial craniotomy for tumour resection: a prospective cohort study of 800 patients in a Chinese neurosurgical centre. *J Int Med Res*. 2013;41(1):208–217.
17. Karanjia N, et al. A clinical description of extubation failure in patients with primary brain injury. *Neurocrit Care*. 2011;15(1):4–12.
18. Anastasian ZH, et al. Factors that correlate with the decision to delay extubation after multilevel prone spine surgery. *J Neurosurg Anesthesiol*. 2014;26(2):167–171.
19. Li F, et al. Risk factors for delayed extubation in thoracic and lumbar spine surgery: a retrospective analysis of 135 patients. *J Anesth*. 2014;28(2):161–166.
20. Conte V, et al. Awake neurosurgery: an update. *Minerva Anestesiol*. 2008;74(6):289–292.
21. Bathory I, et al. Evaluation of the GlideScope for tracheal intubation in patients with cervical spine immobilisation by a semi-rigid collar. *Anaesthesia*. 2009;64(12):1337–1341.
22. Krugel V, et al. Comparison of the single-use Ambu((R)) aScope 2 vs the conventional fibrescope for tracheal intubation in patients with cervical spine immobilisation by a semirigid collar. *Anaesthesia*. 2013;68(1):21–26.
23. Albrecht E, Schoettker P. Images in clinical medicine. The jaw-thrust maneuver. *N Engl J Med*. 2010;363(21):e32.
24. Theiler L, et al. SWIVIT–Swiss video-intubation trial evaluating video-laryngoscopes in a simulated difficult airway scenario: study protocol for a multicenter prospective randomized controlled trial in Switzerland. *Trials*. 2013;14:94.
25. Zhou T, et al. Cuff-leak test for predicting postextubation airway complications: a systematic review. *J Evid Based Med*. 2011;4(4):242–254.
26. Heininger A, et al. Complications using a hollow fiber airway exchange catheter for tracheal tube exchange in critically ill patients. *Acta Anaesthesiol Scand*. 2008;52(7):1031.
27. McLean S, et al. Airway exchange failure and complications with the use of the Cook Airway Exchange Catheter(R): a single center cohort study of 1177 patients. *Anesth Analg*. 2013;117(6):1325–1327.
28. Karthik S, Subramaniam B. A method of avoiding loss of airway control during tracheal tube change using an airway exchange catheter. *Anesth Analg*. 2007;105(4):1173–1174.

29. Mort TC. Continuous airway access for the difficult extubation: the efficacy of the airway exchange catheter. *Anesth Analg*. 2007;105(5):1357–1362. Table of contents.
30. Neustein SM. The safe use of an airway exchange catheter. *Anesth Analg*. 2014;119(1):216.
31. Fan T, et al. Prophylactic administration of parenteral steroids for preventing airway complications after extubation in adults: meta-analysis of randomised placebo controlled trials. *BMJ*. 2008;337:a1841.
32. Francois B, et al. 12-h pretreatment with methylprednisolone versus placebo for prevention of postextubation laryngeal oedema: a randomised double-blind trial. *Lancet*. 2007;369(9567):1083–1089.
33. Lee CH, Peng MJ, Wu CL. Dexamethasone to prevent postextubation airway obstruction in adults: a prospective, randomized, double-blind, placebo-controlled study. *Crit Care*. 2007;11(4):R72.

The Difficult Pediatric Airway

Shobana Rajan[1], Melissa Ehlers[2], Laura Leduc[3]

[1]Department of Anesthesiology, Cleveland Clinic, Cleveland, OH, USA;
[2]Associate Professor of Anesthesiology, Albany Medical Center,
Albany, NY, USA; [3]Department of Anesthesiology, Albany Medical Center,
Albany, NY, USA

OUTLINE

PEDIATRIC AIRWAY ANATOMY AND IMPLICATIONS

The pediatric airway is both anatomically and physiologically different from the adult airway in many ways. These differences are most important in children under two years of age[1] and decrease as the child matures. Understanding of pediatric airway anatomy is crucial to the safe care of children under anesthesia.

Anatomic differences in the pediatric airway include the fact that children have a larger head relative to their body size and a prominent occiput, which can impact visualization of the airway if proper positioning is not obtained. This may be further complicated by the shorter neck and less-developed mandible. As a result, positioning may be more difficult. Many practitioners will place a shoulder roll to assist with neck flexion. Alternatively, other practitioners prefer a flat surface with an extended neck. Occasionally, the airway may be best visualized with some flexion, which is obtained by gently lifting and supporting the head. In general, it is prudent to try a different position if one encounters unusual difficulty.

The larynx is relatively higher in the neck in children as opposed to adults. Whereas the adult larynx is located at the junction of the fourth and fifth cervical vertebrae (C4-5), the neonate/infant larynx is at least one level higher, typically located at C3-4,[2] and may even be as high as C2-3.[3] This superior position creates a more acutely angled view of the vocal cords during direct laryngoscopy.

Additionally, the epiglottis in children is longer, floppier, and omega shaped as compared with adults. The epiglottis also sits at a greater angle to the anterior pharyngeal wall. Both issues make visualization of the vocal cords difficult. Traditionally, miller blades have been used for intubation in infants and small children with placement of the blade either in the vallecula or more commonly using the tip to lift the epiglottis to obtain an adequate view. School-aged children may be more easily intubated with an appropriately sized Macintosh blade, placed in the vallecula and used to lift the epiglottis out of view.

Until recently the pediatric airway was considered to be funnel shaped with the narrowest portion of the airway located at the level of the cricoid. Adult airways were considered to be more cylindrical with the narrowest portion of the airway at the glottis. However, evidence seems to support that the narrowest part of the pediatric airway may actually be at the level of the vocal cords; the nondistensibility of the complete cricoid ring can predispose the infant to more potential edema at this level of the airway,[4] and functionally, it is reasonable to consider the airway in a more traditional fashion.

For this reason, uncuffed endotracheal tubes were traditionally used in children in order to minimize the risk of tracheal ischemia and subglottic stenosis from a tightly fitting endotracheal tube. However, increasing literature supports the safe and effective use of cuffed endotracheal tubes in children and neonates because contemporary endotracheal tubes have a low-pressure, high-volume cuff. It is still prudent to confirm and document the presence of a leak around the endotracheal tube at less than $20\,cm\,H_2O$ and to recheck the pressure of the cuff frequently, especially in circumstances where nitrous oxide is used.

The lymphoid tissue in the airway reaches the greatest size in school-aged children, and during this time many patients present for pediatric ENT procedures. Adenotonsillar hypertrophy can significantly impact the airway obstruction to which children are prone under anesthesia, and early placement of oral airways may be helpful during inhalation induction. Alternatively, many prefer to use a jaw-thrust technique to relieve airway obstruction during induction until the patient is sufficiently deep to tolerate placement of an oral airway.

The major physiologic difference noted in children undergoing anesthesia is that they are more susceptible to hypoxemia than adults. There are a few contributing factors to this phenomenon. Pediatric patients have an elevated metabolic rate, leading to a rate of oxygen consumption double that of the adults ($6\,mL/kg/min$ compared with $3\,mL/kg/min$ in adults).

The infants' respiratory muscles are primarily composed of type II fibers, which have lower stores of glycogen and fat, allowing them to become easily fatigued after short periods of exertion or labored breathing. Additionally, children have a lower functional residual capacity in the supine position and elevated closing volumes.[5] Therefore, thorough preoxygenation prior to intubation is critical, especially if nitrous oxide has been used for induction with the resultant decrease in inspired oxygen concentration.

In managing the pediatric airway, it is prudent to remember that any swelling can have catastrophic effects. This is explained by Poiseulle's law, $R = 8\eta L/\pi r^4$, which states that resistance to flow is inversely related to the radius of the airway raised to the fourth power. As the radius of the airway decreases due to edema from manipulation, the resistance to airflow is increased by a power of four.

CLINICAL SCENARIOS ASSOCIATED WITH DIFFICULT AIRWAYS

A difficult airway for children and adults is defined as the clinical situation in which a conventionally trained anesthesiologist experiences difficulty with mask ventilation of the upper airway, tracheal intubation, or both.[6] As in adults, difficult airways in children may be anticipated or unanticipated. The following clinical scenarios are most pertinent to the pediatric neurosurgical population.

Hydrocephalus

Hydrocephalus is commonly found in premature infants who have sustained an intraventricular hemorrhage. Additionally, patients with meningomyelocele, Arnold–Chiari malformation, aqueductal stenosis, and Dandy–Walker malformation are at an increased likelihood of developing hydrocephalus. Hydrocephalus generally leads to macrocephaly, which is where the airway difficulty is most likely to be encountered. Proper positioning may be challenging but is important to facilitate intubation (see Figure 1). Patients with hydrocephalus often present for anesthesia for imaging and ventriculoperitoneal shunts.

Craniosynostosis

Craniosynostosis is a condition in which the sutures of a child's skull fuse prematurely. This can result in asymmetry as well as an abnormally enlarged head. As with hydrocephalus patients, positioning for intubation is crucial for success. Additionally for craniosynostosis children, the head may require support on either side to prevent movement during intubation.

Encephalocele

Encephalocele is a neural tube defect in which there is a sac-like protrusion of the brain and membranes through openings in the skull. There may be associated craniofacial abnormalities, and patients may present with hydrocephalus, spastic quadriplegia, microcephaly, ataxia, and developmental delay, in addition to other conditions. Mask ventilation and intubation of patients with encephalocele may be particularly challenging due to positioning and access. If the encephalocele is anterior, obtaining an adequate mask seal may be impossible. Patients may have to be induced and intubated in the lateral position with the encephalocele supported by a gel doughnut or by placing the child's head beyond the edge of the table with support of an assistant. Additionally, needle decompression of the encephalocele sac may need to be performed, under sterile conditions, to facilitate tracheal intubation.[2,7]

Macroglossia

Macroglossia, defined as a disproportionately large tongue, has the potential to create a difficult airway through posterior migration of the tongue after induction. This can cause obstruction to the airway, causing difficulty with mask ventilation and obtaining an adequate view of the vocal cords during laryngoscopy. Congenital disorders such as mucopolysaccharidosis (MPS; namely Hurler's and Hunter's syndromes), Beckwith–Wiedemann syndrome and Down syndrome can be associated with macroglossia. Airway obstruction from a large tongue can be managed by placement of an oral airway. Pulling the tongue forward with padded forceps or using a suction to pull the tongue forward can aid in visualization of the vocal cords. Macroglossia can also be acquired due to an allergic reaction to drugs or due to placement of an oral airway during surgery that obstructs the venous drainage of the tongue.

Mandibular Hypoplasia and Micrognathia

Mandibular hypoplasia and micrognathia lead to a difficult intubation due to poor visualization of the laryngeal inlet. This situation is commonly associated with the Pierre Robin sequence (PRS). The clinical triad of this syndrome consists of micrognathia, cleft palate, and glossoptosis. Mandibular hypoplasia and micrognathia are also seen in the Treacher–Collins and Goldenhar syndromes. Difficult airway tools should be available whenever intubating patients with mandibular hypoplasia or micrognathia.

Maxillary/Midfacial Hypoplasia

Maxillary hypoplasia is seen with several congenital malformations like Apert syndrome, Crouzon syndrome, Pfeiffer syndrome, and Saethre–Chotzen syndrome. These patients may pose difficult bag mask ventilation as well as difficult intubating conditions similar to micrognathia.

Midfacial hypoplasia typically consists of a hypoplastic nasal bone, maxilla, and zygomas. Due to underdeveloped facial bones forcing the tongue to a more posterior position, airway obstruction is a common problem resulting in obstructive sleep apnea, which may complicate extubation and should be anticipated.[8]

Cleft Palate

Cleft palate can be isolated or associated with a number of different syndromes. For patients with bilateral cleft palates, the premaxilla is angled forward, causing the upper incisors to obstruct the line of sight during direct laryngoscopy. During direct laryngoscopy in a patient with a unilateral left or bilateral cleft palate, the laryngoscope blade tends to drop into the left cleft palate, further obstructing the view.[9] This can be remedied by gently packing the cleft palate with gauze before intubation or by using a plastic tooth guard to span the cleft, which also helps to protect these mucous membranes from trauma during intubation.

Cervical Spine Instability

Cervical spine instability may be acute or chronic. Children with Down syndrome have an increased risk of chronic cervical spine instability. Atlantooccipital or atlantoaxial instability may be a consequence of a generalized ligamentous laxity. It is hypothesized that laxity of the cervical ligaments can be acquired or worsened by inflammation that is precipitated by upper respiratory infections, whereby inflammatory mediators travel retrograde via the common lymphatics.[10]

Bony anomalies can also contribute to instability at the atlantooccipital or atlantoaxial joints. Flattening or hypoplasia of the occipital condyles, anomalies of the atlas, and anomalies of C2 (which include an odontoid process that is absent, hypoplastic, or incompletely fused to the body of C2) result in instability. The most common screening test for AAI involves lateral flexion, extension films, and odontoid views, and should be requested for any patient who exhibits classic symptoms such as neck pain and gait disturbance.[11] Regardless of symptomatology, most practitioners attempt to use airway management in these patients that requires minimal neck extension.

Acute presentations of cervical spine instability may be due to trauma. Pediatric patients have a higher incidence of spinal cord injury without radiographic abnormality (SCIWORA).[12] Patients with cervical instability are at risk of compression of the cervical spinal cord during laryngoscopy due to movement of the cervical vertebrae during laryngoscope manipulation. Immobilization of a patient with suspected cervical injury is crucial so that further damage to the cord is prevented. In-line stabilization is of utmost importance, and the neck and head should remain in as neutral a position as possible throughout the entire procedure with a specific person assigned to perform the manual in-line stabilization. A hard collar, spine board, and soft-spacing devices between the head and securing straps may be helpful.

Another potential acute presentation of cervical instability is in the case of infection or neoplasm. Because neurologic impairment is usually present at the time of diagnosis, these children are particularly vulnerable to spinal cord injury during intubation. Therefore, every effort should be made to maintain a neutral position.

Cervical Spine Immobility

In general, cervical spine immobility is either congenital or chronic and progressive. Congenital fusion (or surgical fusion) of the cervical spine may be seen in patients with Arnold–Chiari malformation, where there is herniation of part of the brain through the foramen magnum. Of note, there is a high incidence of sleep apnea in patients with Arnold–Chiari malformation.

Patients with symptomatic basilar impression may need odontoid decompression and cervicooccipital fusion to maintain the stability of the cervical spine. Due to limited mobility, these patients may be extremely difficult to intubate.

Klippel–Feil syndrome is characterized by fusion of two or more cervical vertebrae. Other features include short neck, a low posterior hairline, scoliosis, and congenital heart disease. Difficulty with airway management usually arises in the latter half of the first decade of life. The degree of difficulty with airway management depends on the severity of neck fixation.

Goldenhar syndrome, also known as oculo-auriculo-vertebral (OAV) syndrome, is a congenital defect in the development of the first and second branchial arches resulting in incomplete development of the ear, nose, soft palate, lip, and mandible on one side of the face. Difficulties in airway management result from mandibular hypoplasia, cleft or high-arched palate, cervical vertebral anomalies, and scoliosis.[13]

Patients with juvenile rheumatoid arthritis may have temporomandibular ankylosis, mandibular hypoplasia, and cricoarytenoid arthritis leading to a difficult airway. Mouth opening may be severely limited due to chronic inflammation of the temporomandibular joint and is a major factor in forming the anesthetic plan.

Neck tumors such as cystic hygroma or teratoma may limit mobility of the neck and cause significant airway obstruction which can make induction of anesthesia extremely difficult. If any difficulty with mask ventilation is anticipated, awake fiber optic intubation may be the only option.[14] If mask ventilation is possible, alternative methods can be cautiously employed, recognizing that a rescue tracheostomy is frequently not an option since the mass typically sits directly in front of the trachea. Ideally, these patients will be intubated with pediatric ENT specialists available as a rigid bronchoscope may be required to facilitate intubation past the mass.

There are numerous conditions that may cause the pediatric airway to become acutely difficult to secure, such as inflammatory and infectious conditions like acute epiglottitis, laryngotracheobronchitis, peritonsillar abscess, and retropharyngeal abscess. Airway hemangiomas, papillomatosis, lingual tonsillar hypertrophy or neurofibromatosis of the airway are other conditions that can lead to difficult intubation and ventilation. A thorough airway plan with multiple back-up maneuvers is essential in these patients; transtracheal jet ventilation, emergency cricothyroidotomy, or tracheostomy may be life-saving rescue maneuvers to consider if the patient's condition suddenly deteriorates while attempting airway manipulation.

PREOPERATIVE EVALUATION OF THE DIFFICULT AIRWAY

There are few studies for predictors of difficult intubation in children. Physical examination to predict the potentially difficult airway should be guided from the knowledge of normal anatomy and the associated syndromes. The evaluation of the pediatric airway should begin with a history and physical examination of the head and neck followed by imaging when indicated. An important question to consider is whether ventilation by face mask is likely to be difficult as this will significantly impact the number of options available for successful intubation, and may also impact the plan for postoperative extubation.

A clear history should be obtained to look for respiratory problems such as snoring, noisy breathing, change of voice, recurrent croup or sleep apnea, a history of feeding problems, and prior surgery to the face and neck. If available, prior anesthetic records can provide invaluable information regarding mask ventilation and intubation difficulties.

Physical examination should be performed and should include assessment of the presence or severity of respiratory distress as well inspiratory or expiratory stridor.

The airway examination should assess:

- Adequacy of mouth opening
- Presence of loose or protruding teeth
- Size of the tongue
- Presence of soft tissue masses such as cystic hygroma in the neck or cysts in the mouth
- Mandibular size
- Neck mobility
- Temporomandibular joint movement

Many evaluations used to predict the difficult airway in adults have not been validated in the pediatric population. Cooperation of the patient is necessary for precise evaluation. In the young or uncooperative child, appropriate evaluation is limited. Preliminary data indicate that the Mallampati classification may be an insensitive predictor of difficult intubation in the pediatric population,[15] although certainly a Mallampati score of 1 is reassuring. Although mandibular space assessment is most useful in older children to predict difficult airways, it still should be examined in all patients. Careful clinical evaluation of the patient is essential, particularly examination of the child from the side to assess for micrognathia.[16]

Vigilant preoperative evaluation of patients with limited cervical mobility must be done before anesthetic induction. Previous anesthetic records, if available, should be reviewed for any relevant information. Once a difficult airway is suspected, preparation for management must be made, which typically would involve an airway cart with multiple modalities to choose from as the case warrants.

THE ANESTHETIC PLAN

Management of difficult airways in general will vary depending upon the resources available and an individual practitioner's skill set. Ideally, a difficult airway cart should be available anywhere anesthesia is provided, and that cart should have multiple tools for use.

The gold standard of awake fiber optic intubation for a difficult airway has limited use in the pediatric population where cooperation cannot reasonably be expected.

Preinduction intravenous access should be considered in cases where a difficult airway is anticipated.

Premedication with oral or intravenous atropine (0.01–0.02 mg/kg) may be useful due to its antimuscarinic effects.

Induction can be done via inhalation with sevoflurane and oxygen; maintenance of spontaneous ventilation during induction of the difficult pediatric airway is key.

Sevoflurane has been used in the management of the difficult airway with great success.[17,18] The low blood–gas solubility of sevoflurane and consequent rapid smooth induction and emergence as well as the absence of airway irritation are advantageous when managing the difficult airway.

For pediatric patients who can tolerate an awake intubation technique, judicious sedation with adequate topicalization is reasonable. One could use midazolam, fentanyl, ketamine, remifentanil infusion or dexmedetomidine for sedation, depending on the experience and personal preference of the anesthesiologist. The key is to make sure the patient is sedated but breathing spontaneously. Sedatives should not be given to any patient in acute respiratory distress or with the potential for acute airway obstruction, and should be used cautiously in any patients with a potential increase in intracranial pressure. In pediatric patients, topicalization may be obtained by nebulizing, spraying, or swabbing local anesthetic solution or by applying viscous gel to a gloved finger. The suction port of all but the smallest fiber optic bronchoscopes can be used to spray local anesthesia on the vocal cords under direct vision. The maximum dose of local anesthetic allowed should be calculated before topicalization. The drug of choice is lidocaine because it has the best safety profile. Maximum doses of lidocaine are 5 mg/kg. Agents containing benzocaine should be avoided in infants and young children because of the risk of methemoglobinemia.

DIFFICULT AIRWAY TOOLS

Direct laryngoscopy: Laryngoscope blades in different sizes and shapes (i.e., straight and curved) should be available before induction of anesthesia. *Straight* laryngoscope blades are often recommended for use in neonates and infants to lift the epiglottis. The most common straight blades include the Miller, Wisconsin, Wis–Hipple, and Wis–Foregger blades. *Curved blades* may be more suitable for older children as they are potentially less likely to dislodge deciduous teeth. The total number of intubation attempts with **direct laryngoscopy** should be limited because the "cannot intubate cannot ventilate" situation may develop quickly as the airway becomes edematous and bloody (Figure 1).

The flexible fiber optic bronchoscope is the gold standard for difficult airway management in the pediatric population. This can be done either awake (rare in pediatric practice) or after inhalation induction. Ultra-thin fiber optic bronchoscopes (2.7 mm) with a flexible tip are available (Figure 2) which can accommodate a 3.0 mm endotracheal tube.[7,19] For older children, a pediatric fiber optic bronchoscope is utilized that can accommodate a size 4.5 endotracheal tube or higher. If only an adult scope is available, then a flexible wire may be passed through the suction port to be used as a guide to pass the endotracheal tube.

Fiber optic intubation is a technique that requires a great deal of skill. It is less useful when there is blood or secretions obscuring the airway. The ultrathin fiber optic scope has been found to be useful in situations like cystic hygroma,[14] PRS, and Klippel–Feil syndrome. In a retrospective analysis of 33 PRS newborns, 63% had failed intubation with direct

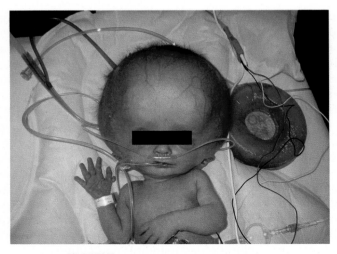

FIGURE 1   Neonate with hydrocephalus

laryngoscopy but were successfully intubated with a flexible fiber optic bronchoscope. This series demonstrated that flexible fiber optic bronchoscopy was a reliable alternative method when direct laryngoscopy was not possible.[20]

The laryngeal mask airway (LMA) is a critical component of difficult airway management in children and is part of the pediatric difficult airway algorithm (Figures 3–5). It is a potential rescue device in emergent situations, although it clearly doesn't protect against laryngospasm or

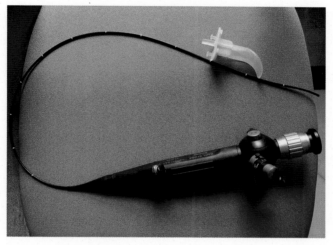

FIGURE 2   Pediatric fiberoptic scope

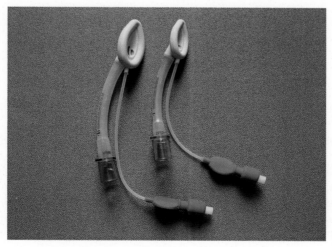

FIGURE 3   Laryngeal mask airway-pediatric sizes

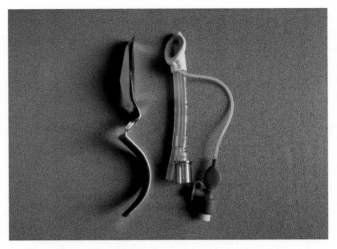

FIGURE 4   LMA-pediatric and introducer for proseal LMA

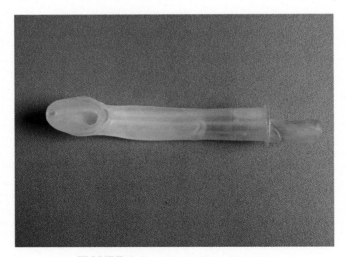

FIGURE 5   Igel laryngeal mask airway

aspiration. It can be used to maintain the airway during inhalation anesthesia or as a conduit for intubation along with the fiber optic bronchoscope. It is also extremely useful in the "cannot ventilate cannot intubate" situation. LMAs are available down to a size 1 and have been used in infants as small as 2kg (authors' personal experience). Determination of LMA size is typically by weight, although other factors such as mandibular size may be a factor as well. The LMA may be used as a conduit for blind intubation or for fiber optic intubation.[21–25] Awake placement of the

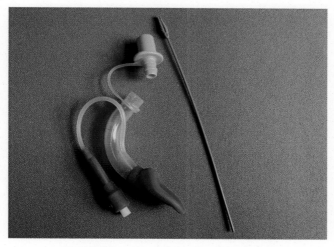

FIGURE 6   The Air-Q intubating LMA-SP

LMA has been described in infants with PRS and then FOB intubation can occur through the LMA.

The self-pressurized Air-Q ILA (ILA-SP) is a first-generation supraglottic airway for children with a self-adjusting cuff and lack of a pilot balloon (Figure 6). It is used both for airway maintenance during routine anesthesia and as a conduit for tracheal intubation for patients with a difficult airway. The Air-Q ILA is available in six sizes (1, 1.5, 2, 2.5, 3.5, and 4.5) for single use and in four sizes (2.0, 2.5, 3.5, and 4.5) for reuse. Sizing of the pediatric Air-Q ILA is similar to the LMA, in that it is weight-based (size 1 for patients <5 kg; size 1.5 for 5–10 kg; size 2 for 10–20 kg).

Video Laryngoscopes

1. The GlideScope (Cobalt/Verathon)
2. The Truview
3. The Storz DCI
4. The Airtraq optical laryngoscope
5. The Bullard

1. **The GlideScope** video laryngoscope (GVL) is a device for intubation that has a digital camera located at the distal end of the blade (Figure 7). Improvement in the glottis view of GVL compared with direct laryngoscopy is considered to be due to its 60° blade angulation. The camera on the blade provides a more anterior laryngeal view that may be invisible using a direct laryngoscope (DL). Although the GVL rarely worsens an easy laryngeal view in children, it makes tracheal intubation more awkward and slower with an increased first attempt

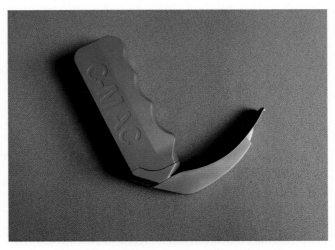

FIGURE 7   The blade of the C-MAC laryngoscope

failure rate and longer time to intubation especially in patients with an easy laryngoscopic view. According to the study, lack of familiarity with the GVL and not angulating the stylet properly was the potential explanation for the longer intubation time.[26] A meta-analysis demonstrates that compared to DLs, pediatric video laryngoscopes were associated with improved glottis visualization in children either with normal airways or with potentially difficult intubations.[27] A study by Lee et al. reported that in pediatric patients with Cormack and Lehane grade ≥3 under direct laryngoscopy, using a GVL with a smaller blade significantly improved the laryngoscopic view when compared with direct laryngoscopy or GVL using the blade size based on weight.[27] According to the authors, a smaller blade can be introduced into the mouth deeper. By sliding above the tongue, the blade tip can be rotated more anteriorly and cephalad in the vallecular, improving the ability to view the glottis. The GVL (weight-based blade selection) is not easy to insert deeper, resulting in possible inability to visualize the glottis structures.

2. **The Truview (Truphatek International, Netanya, Israel)** is a rigid laryngoscope that has an angulated tip and an optical assembly that provides an illuminated and magnified view of the larynx. The tip of the device is narrow to accommodate small mouth openings and angulated 46° anteriorly. This laryngoscope also has a side port that allows for oxygen insufflation. A study compared the Truview laryngoscope with a C-MAC video laryngoscope and DL and showed that all devices allowed excellent visualization of the vocal cords, but the time to intubation was prolonged when the Truview

EVO2 was used. The absence of a decline in oxygen saturation may be due to apneic oxygenation via the Truview scope and may provide a margin of safety. The use of the Truview by a well-trained anesthetist may be an alternative for difficult airway management in pediatric patients.[28]

3. **The Storz DCI video laryngoscope system** is one of the several airway devices on the market that incorporate video capability into the standard Macintosh laryngoscope blades by integration of a fiber optic bundle. A charge-coupled device camera housed in the laryngoscope handle produces the images. The Storz DCI video laryngoscope has been used successfully in difficult airways in pediatric surgeries.[29]

4. **The Airtraq optical laryngoscope (AOL; Prodol, Vizcaya, Spain)** is a single-use indirect laryngoscope for tracheal intubation (Figure 5). The AOL comes in two pediatric sizes: infant (size 0) for ETT 2.5–3.5 and pediatric (size 1) for ETT sizes 3.5–5.5. Both sizes require a mouth opening of 12–13 mm. The rubber eyepiece may be used or a camera may be attached. Images from the distal tip of the blade are projected to the proximal eyepiece. The AOL is inserted midline, and the tip may be placed in the vallecula or used to lift the epiglottis. Once the glottis is visualized, the ETT is slowly advanced. For intubation, it is important to lubricate the ETT so that the tube advances easily. There is a built-in antifoaming system which prevents fogging of the image. Two case reports documented the use of the AOL in pediatric patients with difficult airways: a 9-year-old child with Treacher Collins syndrome who weighed 23 kg,[30] and a 4.8-kg infant with PRS.[31]

5. **The Bullard laryngoscope** is a rigid fiber optic laryngoscope that aids with visualization of the glottic opening even when there is an inability to align the oral, pharyngeal, and laryngeal axes. Compared to conventional direct laryngoscopy, the rigid fiber optic laryngoscopes only require minimal head manipulation and positioning.[32,33] In addition, the Bullard laryngoscope can be used in patients with a mouth opening of as little as 6 mm and a patient size as small as 1.2 kg has been described.[34] The Bullard laryngoscope is a good option for certain scenarios where conventional direct laryngoscopy might prove to be very difficult such as patients with an anterior larynx, unstable cervical spine fracture, upper-body burns, trauma, TMJ immobility, and micrognathia.

Lighted Stylets and Video Stylets

There are various types of stylets available as adjuncts to endotracheal intubation, including the traditional malleable stylet, lighted stylets, and optical stylets.

Light wands: Pediatric versions are available for use with ETTs as small as 2.5. The use of the lighted stylet to guide blind endotracheal intubation relies on the principle of transillumination. The presence of a well-defined glow in the neck indicates tracheal placement. Esophageal placement is indicated by the absence of a glow in the neck. Several different reports describe successful intubation of pediatric patients with the light wand in routine pediatric patients[35] and in situations of cervical spine immobility[36] although it seems unlikely that this would be a viable option in any emergency airway situation. Factors contributing to successful intubation included: (1) use of a shoulder roll and *slight* head extension; (2) conscientious alignment of airway axes; (3) anterior jaw lift to elevate the epiglottis; and (4) gentle handling of the light wand to avoid displacing soft tissue. Inability to advance the light wand despite correct glow is caused by entrapment in the vallecula, hang up of the light wand on the aryepiglottic folds, subglottic narrowing, or vocal cord closure.

Video stylets: The Shikani optical stylet (Clarus Medical) is a portable video stylet. It is inserted into the endotracheal tube after lubrication with silicon spray. The fiber optic cable can be connected to a video monitor. The mandible is lifted with the left hand and displaced anteriorly, and the stylet with the loaded endotracheal tube is advanced into the trachea under direct vision. The Bonfils fiberscope (also a video stylet) seems to be a reliable option to use in the pediatric difficult airway. A study conducted by Kaufman et al.[37] tested the hypothesis that children with difficult airways can be intubated faster with the Bonfils than with the fiber optic bronchoscope. The ease of intubation was rated excellent with good image quality with the Bonfils. The time required to view the glottis was comparable with the fiber optic bronchoscope and the time to intubation was shorter with the Bonfils. The Bonfils has the advantage of allowing visualization as the tube passes through the larynx.

EXTUBATION OF THE DIFFICULT PEDIATRIC AIRWAY

Planning for extubation of a difficult airway is as important as the plan for intubation. Careful consideration should be given to delayed extubation especially in circumstances of a traumatic intubation. It may be prudent to place a guidewire through an ETT prior to removal to facilitate reintubation if necessary. In the smallest patients, a guidewire may be the only adjunct that can be used without significant obstruction of the airway; however, in patients as small as full term neonates, a small ureteral stent may be used as a stylet with the added advantage that oxygen can be passively infused if there are difficulties with reintubation after a failed extubation. Older children may have a large enough airway to accommodate a cook exchange catheter or a small pediatric bougie (Figure 8). An awake extubation is generally indicated for any patient with a difficult airway. Administration of dexamethasone 0.25–0.5 mg/kg IV (maximum 8 mg)

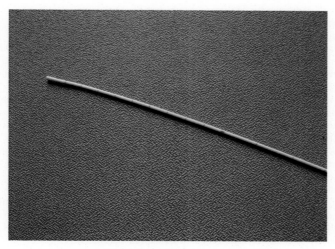

FIGURE 8   Pediatric bougie

after the airway is secured should be considered if there are any worries about airway edema, and may even need to be continued every 8 h until the patient is extubated. One might even consider a period of postoperative ventilation in prolonged surgeries to get the patient fully awake and allow airway edema to subside.

CONCLUSION

Management of the difficult pediatric airway should be performed by a highly skilled pediatric anesthesiologist. The most critical patients may require interdisciplinary management between anesthesiologists, intensivists, pediatric otorhinolaryngologists, and surgeons. Careful planning can help to avoid dire situations, but clinical scenarios can evolve quickly, and anticipation and vigilance are key to maintaining airway safety. The best technique in any given situation may vary depending on provider preference and individual skill. The difficult airway algorithm is as relevant in children as it is in adults, and it is essential to move through the algorithm and not fixate on any one method if it is not working.

References

1. Morray JP, Geiduschek JM, Caplan RA, Posner KL, Gild WM, Cheney FW. A comparison of pediatric and adult anesthesia closed malpractice claims. *Anesthesiology*. 1993;78(3):461–467.
2. Mahajan C, Rath GP, Dash HH, Bithal PK. Perioperative management of children with encephalocele: an Institutional experience. *J Neurosurg Anesthesiol*. October 2011;23(4): 352–356.
3. Walker R. Management of the difficult airway in children. *J Roy Soc Med*. 2001;94 (suppl 7):341–344.

4. Litman RS, Weissend EE, Shibata D, Westesson PL. Developmental changes of laryngeal dimensions in unparalyzed, sedated children. *Anesthesiology*. 2003;98:41–45.
5. Lerman J, Steward D, Cote CJ. *Manual of Pediatric Anesthesia*. 6th ed. ; 2009:22.
6. American Society of Anesthesiologists Task Force on Management of the Difficult Airway. Practice guidelines for management of the difficult airway: an updated report by the American Society of Anesthesiologists Task Force on Management of the Difficult Airway. *Anesthesiology*. 2003;98:1269.
7. Kleeman PP, Jantzen J-PAH, Bonfils P. The ultra-thin bronchoscope in management of the difficult paediatric airway. *Can J Anaesth*. 1987;34:606–608.
8. Infosino A. Pediatric upper airway and congenital anomalies. *Anesthesiol Clin North Am*. 2002;20(4):747–766.
9. Xue FS, Zhang GH, Li P, et al. The clinical observation of difficult laryngoscopy and difficult intubation in infants with cleft lip and palate. *Paediatr Anaesth*. 2006;16(3):283–289.
10. Menezes AH, Ryken TC. Craniovertebral abnormalities in Down's syndrome. *Pediatr Neurosurg*. 1992;18:24–33.
11. Hata T, Todd MM. Cervical spine considerations when anesthetizing patients with Down syndrome. *Anesthesiology*. March 2005;102(3):680–685.
12. Martz DG, Schreibman DL, Matjasko MJ. Neurologic diseases. In: Benumof JL, ed. *Anesthesia and Uncommon Diseases*. 4th ed. Philadelphia: Saunders; 1998.
13. Frei FJ, Ummenhofer W. A special mask for teaching fiber-optic intubation in pediatric patients. *Anesth Analg*. 1993;76:458–459.
14. Bryan Y, Chwals W, Ovassapian A. Sedation and fiberoptic intubation of a neonate with a cystic hygroma. *Acta Anaesthesiol Scand*. January 2005;49(1):122–123.
15. Kopp VJ, Bailey A, Valley RD, et al. Utility of the Mallampati classification for predicting difficult intubation in pediatric patients. *Anesthesiology*. 1995;83:A1147.
16. Gupta S, Sharma R, Jain D. Airway assessment: predictors of difficult airways. *Indian J Anaesth*. 2005;49(4):257–262.
17. Kandasamy R, Sivalingam P. Use of sevoflurane in difficult airways. *Acta Anaesthesiol Scand*. 2000;44:627–629.
18. Wang CY, Chiu CL, Dellkan AE. Sevoflurane for difficult intubation in children. *Br J Anaesth*. 1998;80:408.
19. Biban P, Rugolotto S, Zoppi G. Fiber optic endotracheal intubation through an ultra-thin bronchoscope with suction channel in a newborn with difficult airway. *Anesth Analg*. 2000;90:1007.
20. Marston AP, Lander TA, Tibesar RJ, Sidman JD. Airway management for intubation in newborns with Pierre Robin sequence. *Laryngoscope*. June 2012;122(6):1401–1404. Epub 2012 Mar 27.
21. Steward DJ, Lerman J. Techniques and procedures of pediatric anesthesia. In: Steward DJ, Lerman J, eds. *Manual of Pediatric Anesthesia*. 5th ed. New York: Churchill Livingstone; 2001.
22. Ellis DS, Potluri PK, O'Flaherty JE, et al. Difficult airway management in the neonate: a simple method of intubating through a laryngeal mask airway. *Paediatr Anaesth*. 1999;9:460–462.
23. Patel A, Venn PJH, Barham J. Fiber optic intubation through a laryngeal mask airway in an infant with Robin sequence. *Eur J Anaesthesiol*. 1998;15:237–239.
24. Rabb MF, Minkowitz HS, Hagberg CA. Blind intubation through the laryngeal mask airway for management of the difficult airway in infants. *Anesthesiology*. 1996;84:1510–1511.
25. Selim M, Mowafi H, Al-Ghamdi A, et al. Intubation via LMA in pediatric patients with difficult airways. *Can J Anaesth*. 1999;46:891–893.
26. Sun Y, Lu Y, Huang Y, Jiang H. Pediatric video laryngoscope versus direct laryngoscope: a meta-analysis of randomized controlled trials. *Pediatr Anesth*. 2014;24:1056–1065.
27. Lee JH, Park YH, Byon HJ, et al. A comparative trial of the GlideScope(R) video laryngoscope to direct laryngoscope in children with difficult direct laryngoscopy and an evaluation of the effect of blade size. *Anesth Analg*. July 2013;117(1):176–181.

28. Mutlak H, Rolle U, Rosskopf W, et al. Comparison of the TruView infant EVO2 PCD™ and C-MAC video laryngoscopes with direct Macintosh laryngoscopy for routine tracheal intubation in infants with normal airways. *Clinics (Sao Paulo)*. January 2014;69(1):23–27.
29. Weiss M, Hartmann K, Fischer J, Gerber AC. Video-intuboscopic assistance is a useful aid to tracheal intubation in pediatric patients. *Can J Anaesth*. 2001;48:691–696.
30. Agro F, Hung OR, Catalda R, et al. Lightwand intubation using the Trachlight: a brief review of current knowledge. *Can J Anaesth*. 2001;48:592–599.
31. Alfrey DD, Ward CF, Harwood IR, et al. Airway management for a neonate with congenital fusion of the jaws. *Anesthesiology*. 1979;51:340–342.
32. Hastings RH, Vigil AC, Hanna R, Yang BY, Sartoris DJ. Cervical spine movement during laryngoscopy with the Bullard, Macintosh, and Miller laryngoscopes. *Anesthesiology*. 1995;82:859–869.
33. Watts ADJ, Gelb AW, Bach DB, Pelz DM. Comparison of the Bullard and Macintosh laryngoscopes for endotracheal intubation of patients with a potential cervical spine injury. *Anesthesiology*. 1997;87:1335–1342.
34. Borland LM, Casselbrant M. The Bullard laryngoscope: a new indirect oral laryngoscope (pediatric version). *Anesth Analg*. 1990;70:105–108.
35. Fisher QA, Tunkel DE. Lightwand intubation of infants and children. *J Clin Anesth*. June 1997;9(4):275–279.
36. Berns SD, Patel RI, Chamberlain JM. Oral intubation using a lighted stylet vs direct laryngoscopy in older children with cervical immobilization. *Acad Emerg Med*. January 1996;3(1):34–40.
37. Kaufmann J, Laschat M, Engelhardt T, Hellmich M, Wappler F. Tracheal intubation with the Bonfils fiberscope in the difficult pediatric airway: a comparison with fiber optic intubation. *Pediatr Anesth*. 2015;25:372–378.

Further Reading

1. Vialet R, Nau A, Chaumoître K, Martin C. Effects of head posture on the oral, pharyngeal and laryngeal axis alignment in infants and young children by magnetic resonance imaging. *Pediatr Anaesth*. 2008;18(6):525–531.
2. Westhorpe RN. The position of the larynx in children and its relationship to the ease of intubation. *Anaesth Intensive Care*. 1987;15(4):384–388.
3. Dickison AE. The normal and abnormal pediatric upper airway: recognition and management of obstruction. *Clin Chest Med*. 1987;8(4):583–596.
4. Hudgins PA, Siegel J, Jacobs I, Abramowsky CR. The normal pediatric larynx on CT and MR. *Am J Neuroradiol*. 1997;18(2):239–245.
5. Holm-Knudsen R. The difficult pediatric airway—a review of new devices for indirect laryngoscopy in children younger than two years of age. *Paediatr Anaesth*. 2011;21(2):98–103.
6. Semine AA, Ertel AN, Goldberg MJ, Bull MJ. Cervical-spine instability in children with Down syndrome (trisomy 21). *J Bone Joint Surg Am*. 1978;60(5):649–652.
7. Zamora JE, Nolan RL, Sharan S, Day AG. Evaluation of the Bullard, GlideScope, Viewmax, and Macintosh laryngoscopes using a cadaver model to simulate the difficult airway. *J Clin Anesth*. 2011;23(1):27–34.
8. Ono S, Takeda K, Nishiyama T, Hanaoka K. Endotracheal intubation with a lighted stylet in a patient with difficult airway from the first and second branchial arch syndrome. *Masui*. 2001;50:1239–1241.
9. Chen PP, Cheng CK, Abdullah V, Chu CP. Tracheal intubation using suspension laryngoscopy in an infant with Goldenhar's syndrome. *Anaesth Intensive Care*. 2001;29:548–551.
10. Kim J-T, Na H-S, Bae J-Y, et al. *Br J Anaesth*. 2008;101(4):531–534.

1

Stridor

Prasanna Udupi Bidkar[1], Hemanshu Prabhakar[2]
[1]Department of Anaesthesiology and Critical Care, JIPMER, Puducherry, India; [2]Department of Neuroanaesthesiology and Critical Care, All India Institute of Medical Sciences, New Delhi, India

OUTLINE

INTRODUCTION

The term stridor is derived from the Latin word *stridere*, meaning a harsh creaking or grating sound. It is a manifestation of a disordered airway due to air flow changes within the larynx, trachea, and bronchus.[1] The frequency and quality of sound may vary from case to case. However, it should be differentiated from other voluntary or involuntary vocalizations such as bubbling of the secretions in the pharynx and larynx.

DEFINITION

Stridor is a manifestation of a partially obstructed airway. The resulting turbulent flow produces harsh, vibratory sounds. Hence, stridor can be defined as "a high-pitched sound produced by turbulent flow of air through a narrowed segment of the respiratory tract." It denotes the underlying airway obstruction with potential/imminent life-threatening obstruction of the airway.[2–4] Due to a narrower diameter of the airway, children are more susceptible to partial airway obstruction, thus producing stridor.[5]

GRADING OF STRIDOR

Stridor has been classified into varying grades. Depending on the onset of symptoms, it is classified into acute stridor due to an abrupt onset of symptoms, and chronic, prolonged stridor due to a permanent narrowing of the air flow tract. Stridor is always a symptom of an underlying disease (Table 1).

TABLE 1   Types of Stridor

Type	Lesion location	Conditions
Inspiratory stridor	Extrathoracic	• Laryngomalacia • Supraglottic mass • Glottic lesions • Vocal cord paralysis
Expiratory stridor	Intrathoracic	• Tracheomalacia • Bronchomalacia • Extrinsic compression of the airway
Biphasic stridor	Fixed lesions	• Bilateral vocal cord paralysis • Laryngeal web • Vocal cord papillomas • Subglottic stenosis • Epiglottitis • Croup

Acute onset stridor in children is generally due to causes such as viral and bacterial infections of the larynx and/or trachea, and it is the most life-threatening type of stridor.

Based on the appearance of the stridor in the respiratory cycle it is divided into the following grades:

Grade 1: Inspiratory stridor
Grade 2: Expiratory stridor
Grade 3: Inspiratory and Expiratory (Biphasic) stridor, plus pulsus paradoxus
Grade 4: Respiratory arrest

ETIOLOGY

Depending on the onset of symptoms, the stridor is divided into acute and chronic stridor.

Acute Stridor

1. Infectious causes
   a. Acute viral laryngitis
   b. Laryngotracheobronchitis
   c. Acute bacterial tracheitis
   d. Acute bacterial epiglottitis
2. Other causes
   a. Laryngeal diphtheria
   b. Laryngeal foreign body
   c. Laryngospasm
   d. Laryngeal edema

Chronic Stridor

1. Congenital chronic stridor
   a. Laryngomalacia
   b. Tracheomalacia
   c. Laryngeal web
   d. Laryngeal cyst
2. Acquired chronic stridor
   a. Laryngeal stenosis
   b. Tracheal stenosis
   c. Laryngeal tumors
   d. Laryngeal paralysis

TABLE 2   Neurological Conditions Associated
with Stridor

---

1. Arnold–Chiari malformation[6–10]

2. Cerebral palsy[11,12]

3. Hydrocephalus[13,14]

4. Myelomeningocele[7,9,14,15]

5. Spina bifida

6. Hypoxia[16]

7. Intracranial hemorrhage[17–19]

STRIDOR IN NEUROSURGICAL PATIENTS

Though rare, various neurological and neurosurgical conditions are associated with stridor (Table 2). Stridor is frequently seen in patients with Arnold–Chiari malformation, cerebral palsy, hydrocephalus, myelomeningocele, and spina bifida. It is also seen in patients with hypoxic ischemic encephalopathy and intracranial hemorrhage. In these groups of patients, bilateral vocal cord palsy is tipped to be the common mechanism. The development of vocal cord palsy is due to downward displacement of the brain stem secondary to raised intracranial pressure. This leads to compression of the fourth ventricle and stretching of vagus nerve, leading to recurrent laryngeal nerve palsy. The treatment of the primary condition often leads to a resolution of stridor symptoms. Tracheal stenosis following prolonged tracheostomy can also lead to stridor in patients with traumatic brain injury. Tracheomalacia and laryngomalacia can also be present in patients with prolonged ventilation.

POSTEXTUBATION STRIDOR

Endotracheal intubation and positive pressure ventilation is frequently used in intensive care units (ICU). The intubation/extubation may cause vocal cord and tracheal mucosal injury leading to laryngeal edema and stridor following extubation of patients.[20,21] The level of laryngeal edema may vary, but >50% of the luminal narrowing is needed before respiratory symptoms develop.[21,22] In adults, the most common location of edema-causing stridor is at the level of vocal cords. Neurosurgical patients with poor neurological condition (e.g., severe traumatic brain injury, stroke) are at a high risk of prolonged ventilation, thus increasing the risk of laryngeal and tracheal mucosal edema. The severity of edema increases with the duration of mechanical ventilation.[23] The incidence of postextubation stridor (PES) varies from 15% to 40% of mechanically ventilated in ICUs.[20,24] The PES is one of the important causes of reintubation in mechanically ventilated ICU patients. Reintubation increases the risk of morbidity and mortality. The associated morbidity includes increased duration of mechanical ventilation, increased length of stay, and increased risk of acquired infections.[25,26] Reintubation-associated mortality can be as high as 30–40%.[25,27]

CLINICAL FEATURES

Stridor is always a symptom or sign of underlying disease. An acute onset of stridor always indicates partial obstruction of the airway and a chance of a life-threatening emergency situation.[21,22] Careful history and examination of the respiratory system gives an idea of the degree of obstruction. Signs of increased airway resistance such as flaring of the nares, suprasternal, subcostal, and intercostal retractions should be looked for, as they indicate significant airway obstruction. Irritability, altered level of consciousness, and in children not accepting feeds are good indicators of severe stridor. Rising pulse rate is the consistent sign of increasing distress. Depending on the presenting symptom, stridor is divided into four grades (Table 3). Patients with severe stridor (grade 3 and 4) require immediate hospitalization and emergency management of the airway.

TABLE 3   Clinical Grades of Stridor

Grade	Classification	Symptoms
Grade 1	Exertional stridor	• At rest—no symptoms • Stridor appears during exercise or crying
Grade 2	Stridor at rest	• Stridor is present at rest • Symptoms worsen with physical activity or crying
Grade 3	Stridor with signs	• Stridor is present at rest • Decreased air entry • Continuous stridor with suprasternal and supraclavicular retractions • Irritable patient with dyspnea (air hunger) • Arterial saturation may be normal or decreased
Grade 4	Stridor with hypoxia	• Minimal air exchange • In addition to grade 3, patient is cyanotic, and altered level of consciousness

DIAGNOSIS

In children, acute onset of stridor along with additional signs like fever and runny nose points to the diagnosis of infectious etiology of bacterial or viral causes. But onset of stridor in the absence of antecedent signs should warrant a search for other causes of central nervous system pathology. Rarely persistent hiccup or stridor can be the presenting symptoms in patients with Arnold–Chiari malformation and hydrocephalus. Flexible fiber-optic bronchoscopy (FFB) is helpful in the diagnosis of vocal cords movements, tracheal mucosal edema, and tracheal stenosis. The FFB can also be easily performed in children. A 30° nasendoscope is a good instrument for the visualization of false and true vocal cords. Using FFB, tracheomalacia and laryngomalacia can be easily diagnosed.

CUFF LEAK TEST

The visualization of complete vocal cords and the underlying subglottic area is not always possible due to the presence of endotracheal tube. Cuff leak tests aim to find the magnitude of the leak around the endotracheal tube, when the cuff is deflated (Table 4). The amount of expired tidal volume is noted on the mechanical ventilator. The difference between the inspiratory and expiratory volumes gives "the cuff leak volume." In one study, none of the patients developed PES with the cuff leak volume >110 mL with specificity of 99%, and the negative predictive value for absence of stridor was 98%.[28] The cuff leak volume, which predicts the presence or absence of PES, varies in the available literature. However, it is a simple and useful bedside test to predict PES and is commonly practiced in ICUs.

TABLE 4   Steps to Measure the Cuff Leak Volume[28]

Step 1	For thorough oral and endotracheal suction, set the ventilator in assist control mode.
Step 2	Monitor and record the inspiratory and expiratory volumes (with inflated cough) to ensure both the volumes are similar.
Step 3	Deflate the cough.
Step 4	Record the expiratory volumes for the next 6–8 cycles.
Step 5	Average of the least three volumes.
Step 6	Cuff leak volume is the difference between the inspired and the average of the least three expired tidal volumes.

LARYNGEAL ULTRASONOGRAPHY

Laryngeal ultrasound has been used as an alternative to cuff leak test for the prediction of PES. It is useful in assessing vocal cord morphology, movement, and the air column width surrounding the endotracheal tube with or without deflated cuff.[29,30] The images obtained by laryngeal ultrasound have a good correlation with the images obtained from flexible fiber-optic bronchoscopy. The difference in air column width with cuff-inflated and deflated determines the occurrence of stridor.

TREATMENT

Treatment of stridor includes humidified respiratory gases, oxygen, corticosteroids, and epinephrine nebulization (Figure 1).

1. Humidification of the airway: Inhalation of humidified respiratory gases and oxygen can loosen the dry, clogged-up secretions and helpful in airway suctioning, thus clearing the airway obstruction. Humidification soothes the inflamed mucosa and provides comfort to the patient. In patients with higher amounts of secretions, N-acetyl cysteine nebulization can be used to loosen the secretions.
2. Nebulized epinephrine: Nebulized racemic epinephrine is by far the most commonly used and most effective treatments to reduce mucosal edema. The racemic mixture of epinephrine contains equal volumes of L- and D-isomers. The L-isomer is supposed to be 30 times more active than its D-isomer. The usual dose used is 0.5 mL of 2.25% of racemic epinephrine in a 4 mL normal saline.[31] This nebulization can be repeated hourly. The proposed mechanism of action of epinephrine is the reduction of mucosal edema by alpha adrenergic vasoconstriction of the inflamed mucosa. It is indicated in patients with stridor at rest and a need for intubation (Grades 2, 3, and 4 stridor). In places where the racemic epinephrine is not available, regular epinephrine (1:1000) 0.5 mL/kg up to a maximum of 5 mL can be used, and can be repeated hourly if required.
3. Corticosteroids: Corticosteroids are the mainstay therapy for the prevention of PES. Steroids reduce the mucosal edema by anti-inflammatory action. In a meta-analysis comprising of six randomized trials of 1923 patients, it was shown that steroids are effective in reducing PES in high-risk patients when given before extubation.[32] They significantly reduced the risk of reintubation and stridor in high-risk patients, as determined by the cuff leak test.[33] A multidose regimen is superior to a single-dose regimen for the prevention of PES.[32] Aerosolized budesonide has been used in the management of stridor. In one study, it was as equally effective as an aerosolized L-epinephrine.[34]

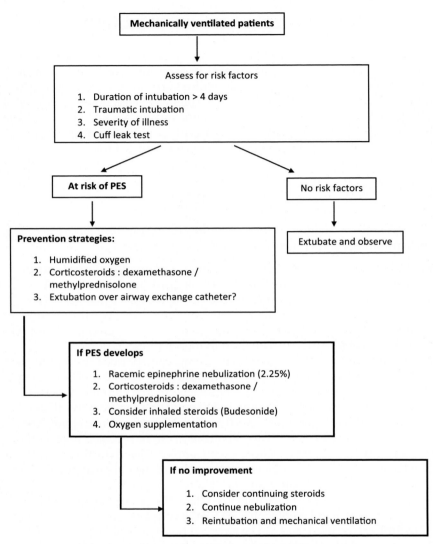

FIGURE 1 Management of postextubation laryngeal edema.

4. Oxygen: Oxygen is important to relieve hypoxia. It can be easily administered using a face mask. However, a struggling child may not accept a face mask, and it delays the appearance of cyanosis.
5. Sedatives: Though sedatives can calm the anxious patient, the use of these is contraindicated in patients with stridor due to the high risk of impaired consciousness and respiratory failure.

6. Endotracheal intubation: Endotracheal intubation is indicated in patients with moderate to severe respiratory distress. Endotracheal intubation using an FFB appears to be the method of choice. The size of the endotracheal tube should be carefully planned so it can pass through the narrowing of the airway. In patients with failed intubation, an emergency tracheostomy may be indicated. Emergency tracheostomy can be lifesaving for patients with severe stridor, and it also provides additional advantages such as reduction dead space, better airway suctioning, and faster weaning from mechanical ventilation.

7. Heliox and oxygen mixture: A mixture of heliox and oxygen (70:30) is less dense than air and oxygen. This reduced density facilitates the laminar flow in narrowed segments of the airway. In a randomized controlled trial, use of a heliox and oxygen mixture was as effective as racemic epinephrine nebulization.

8. Treatment of the cause of raised intracranial pressure leads to improvement in the symptoms within 24–48 h. In patients with Arnold–Chiari malformation, posterior decompression of foramen magnum improves the symptoms.[6,7] A ventriculo-peritoneal shunt also reduces stridor by relieving hydrocephalus.

References

1. Cotton RT, Reilly JS. Stridor and airway obstruction. In: Bluestone C, Stool S, Kenna M, eds. *Pediatric Otolaryngology*. 3rd ed. Philadelphia, PA: WB Saunders Co.; 1995:1275–1286.
2. Rashkin MC, Davis T. Acute complication of endotracheal intubation. *Chest*. 1986;89: 165–167.
3. Colice GL, Stukel TA, Dain B. Laryngeal complication of prolonged intubation. *Chest*. 1989;96:877–884.
4. Torres A, Gatell JM, Aznar E, et al. Re-intubation increases the risk of nosocomial pneumonia in patients needing mechanical ventilation. *Am J Respir Crit Care Med*. 1995;152:137–141.
5. Mandal A, Kabra SK, Lodha R. Upper airway obstruction in children. *Indian J Pediatr*. June 25, 2015. [Epub ahead of print].
6. Yamada H, Tanaka Y, Nakamura S. Laryngeal stridor associated with the Chiari II malformation. *Childs Nerv Syst*. 1985;1:312–318.
7. Stritzke AI, Dunham CP, Smyth JA, Steinbok P. Congenital stridor in the context of Chiari malformation type II: the etiological role of vernix caseosa granulomatous meningitis. *J Neurosurg Pediatr*. 2011;8:372–376.
8. Morley AR. Laryngeal stridor, Arnold-Chiari malformation and medullary haemorrhages. *Dev Med Child Neurol*. 1969;11:471–474.
9. Ocal E, Irwin B, Cochrane D, Singhal A, Steinbok P. Stridor at birth predicts poor outcome in neonates with myelomeningocele. *Childs Nerv Syst*. 2012;28:265–271.
10. Petersson RS, Wetjen NM, Thompson DM. Neurologic variant laryngomalacia associated with Chiari malformation and cervicomedullary compression: case reports. *Ann Otol Rhinol Laryngol*. 2011;120:99–103.
11. Cheng YS, Bhutta MF, Ramsden JD, Lennox P. Periodic botulinum toxin injections for paradoxical vocal fold motion in a child with cerebral palsy: a case study. *Int J Pediatr Otorhinolaryngol*. 2014;78:570–571.

12. Thevasagayam M, Rodger K, Cave D, Witmans M, El-Hakim H. Prevalence of laryngomalacia in children presenting with sleep-disordered breathing. *Laryngoscope.* 2010;120:1662–1666.
13. Adamczuk D, Krzemień G, Szmigielska A, et al. Congenital laryngeal stridor – an interdisciplinary problem. *Med Wieku Rozw.* 2013;17:174–178.
14. Gupta R, Williams A, Vetrivel M, Singh G. Stridor in children: is airway always the cause? *J Pediatr Neurosci.* 2014;9:270–272.
15. Singh D, Rath GP, Dash HH, Bithal PK. Anesthetic concerns and perioperative complications in repair of myelomeningocele: a retrospective review of 135 cases. *J Neurosurg Anesthesiol.* 2010;22:11–15.
16. Orme J, Kissack C, Becher JC. Stridor in asphyxiated neonates undergoing therapeutic hypothermia. *Pediatrics.* 2014;134:e261–e265.
17. Alshammari J, Monnier Y, Monnier P. Clinically silent subdural hemorrhage causes bilateral vocal fold paralysis in newborn infant. *Int J Pediatr Otorhinolaryngol.* 2012;76:1533–1534.
18. Forbes E, Patel N, Kasem K. Unilateral vocal cord paralysis associated with subdural haemorrhage in a newborn infant. *J Perinatol.* August 2010;30(8):563–565.
19. Fah KK, Tan HK. An unusual cause of stridor in a neonate. *J Laryngol Otol.* 1994;108:63–64.
20. Epstein SK, Ciubotaru RL. Independent effects of etiology of failure and time to reintubation on outcome for patients failing extubation. *Am J Respir Crit Care Med.* 1998;158:489–493.
21. Colice GL, Stukel TA, Dain B. Laryngeal complications of prolonged intubation. *Chest.* 1989;96:877–884.
22. Mackle T, Meaney J, Timon C. Tracheosophageal compression associated with substernal goiter. Correlation of symptoms with cross-sectional imaging findings. *J Laryngol Otol.* 2007;121:358–361.
23. Darmon JY, Rauss A, Dreyfuss D, et al. Evaluation of risk factors for laryngeal edema after tracheal extubation in adults and its prevention by desamethasone. *Anesthesiology.* 1992;77:245–251.
24. Kemper KJ, Benson MS, et al. Predictors of postextubation stridor in pediatric trauma patients. *Crit Care Med.* 1991;19:352–355.
25. Epstein SK, Ciubotaru RL, et al. Effect of failed extubation on the outcome of mechanical ventilation. *Chest.* 1997;1(12):186–192.
26. Torres A, Gatell JM, Aznar E, et al. Re-intubation increases the risk of nosocomial pneumonia in patients needing mechanical ventilation. *Am J Respir Crit Care Med.* 1995;152:137–141.
27. Demling RI-I, Read T, et al. Incidence and morbidity of extubation failure in surgical intensive care patients. *Crit Care Med.* 1988;16(6):573–577.
28. Miller RL, Cole RP. Association between reduced cuff leak volume and postextubation stridor. *Chest.* 1996;110:1035–1040.
29. Ding LW, Wang HC, Wu HD, Chang CJ, Yang PC. Laryngeal ultrasound: a useful method in predicting post-extubation stridor. A pilot study. *Eur Respir J.* 2006;27:384–389.
30. Mikaeili H, Yazdchi M, Tarzamni MK, Ansarin K, Ghasemzadeh M. Laryngeal ultrasonography versus cuff leak test in predicting postextubation stridor. *J Cardiovasc Thorac Res.* 2014;6:25–28.
31. MacDonnell SP, Timmins AC, Watson JD. Adrenaline administered via a nebulizer in adult patients with upper airway obstruction. *Anaesthesia.* 1995;50:35–36.
32. Fan T, Wang G, Mao B, et al. Prophylactic administration of parenteral steroids for preventing airway complications after extubation in adults: meta-analysis of randomised placebo controlled trials. *BMJ.* 2008;337:a1841.
33. Wang CL, Tsai YH, Huang CC, et al. The role of the cuff leak test in predicting the effects of corticosteroid treatment on postextubation stridor. *Chang Gung Med J.* 2007;30:53–61.
34. Sinha A, Jayashree M, Singhi S. Aerosolized L-epinephrine vs. budesonide for post extubation stridor: a randomized controlled trial. *Indian Pediatr.* 2010;47:317–322.

COMPLICATIONS RELATED TO FLUID AND ELECTROLYTE DISTURBANCES

Osmotic Demyelination Syndrome

Gyaninder P. Singh, Indu Kapoor

Department of Neuroanaesthesiology and Critical Care, All India Institute of Medical Sciences, New Delhi, India

Osmotic demyelination syndrome (ODS) refers to demyelination of white matter tracts traversing the pons (central pontine myelinolysis (CPM)) or in the extrapontine regions (extrapontine myelinolysis (EPM)).[1]

CPM is a noninflammatory, symmetric, demyelinating condition involving the central pons. EPM refers to demyelination, which occurs in the region outside the pons including midbrain, thalamus, basal ganglia, internal capsule, lateral geniculate bodies, cerebellum, and spinal cord. It is seen in approximately 10% of patients with CPM.

https://doi.org/10.1016/B978-0-12-804075-1.00027-4

CPM was first described in 1959 by Adams et al. in chronic alcoholics and malnourished individuals.[2] They observed that patients who were chronic alcoholics or undernourished developed spastic quadriplegia, pseudobulbar palsy, encephalopathy, or coma as a result of an acute, noninflammatory demyelinating lesion within the basis pontis. It was later recognized that lesions can occur even outside the pons, i.e., EPM. Though originally described in chronic alcoholics and malnourished patients, the condition is typically seen in the setting of rapid correction of hyponatremia.

Chronic alcoholism is the most common underlying condition seen in approximately 40% of patients who develop CPM.[1,3] Singh et al.[4] reported the incidence of CPM to be 29% during autopsy examination of liver transplant recipients. CPM is more commonly seen in females than males.

PATHOPHYSIOLOGY

The exact mechanism is still not well understood. According to one hypothesis, the central pons and other areas of EPM are the region of maximum admixture and apposition of gray and white matter.[3] In these regions of rich gray–white matter interface, a rapid change in osmotic forces (such as rapid correction of sodium following prolonged hyponatremia) causes osmotic endothelial damage, vasogenic edema, and release of myelinotoxic factors inducing demyelination of the adjacent white matter tracts. Histologically, demyelination in CPM is characterized by intramyelinitic splitting, vacuolization, and rupture of myelin sheaths presumably due to osmotic effects.[5] The lesion exhibits degeneration and loss of oligodendrocytes with relative sparing of neural cell bodies and axons. Therefore, the distribution of myelinolysis parallels the distribution of oligodendrocytes.

During hyponatremia, fall in serum osmolality leads to entry of water into the brain cells and causes edema. Various protective mechanisms prevent this from happening, which include a shift in interstitial sodium-rich fluid to CSF (within minutes), loss of inorganic ion (K^+, Cl^-) over a few hours, and loss of organic osmoles (myoinisotol, taurine, aspartate, glutamate, and glycine) from one to a few days, rendering the cell isotonic to extracellular fluid and maintaining cell volume. During correction of hyponatremia, the reverse happens and lost electrolytes are restored. Once the shift of inorganic ions has exhausted, the rate of rise in serum tonicity more than the rate of synthesis and/or transport of organic osmoles into the cell will cause the brain cell to shrink.[3] Oligodendrocytes are particularly susceptible to volume loss. In malnourished patients, impaired ability to regenerate organic osmoles makes them vulnerable to this condition.

TABLE 1 Common Conditions Associated with CPM and/or EPM[3]

1. Chronic alcoholism
2. Malnutrition
3. After surgery (hepatic transplant, pituitary surgery)
4. Chronic use of diuretics
5. Burns
6. Psychological polydipsia

ETIOLOGY

After the first description of CPM in alcoholics, a number of other illnesses have been recognized where this condition is reported. It is most commonly seen in the setting of osmotic changes, typically during rapid correction of hyponatremia. Risk factors for the development of CPM in hyponatremic patients include serum sodium <120 mEq/L for more than 48 h, aggressive IV fluid therapy with hypertonic saline solutions, and development of hypernatremia during treatment. CPM can also occur in patients with hypophosphatemia.[6]

Various conditions associated with CPM and EPM are given in Table 1. Myelinolysis has also been reported in patients with inadequate secretion of antidiuretic hormone, adrenal insufficiency,[7,8] Wilson's disease,[9] patients undergoing renal dialysis, eating disorders like anorexia and bulimia,[10,11] severe liver disease[12] and liver transplant,[13] pancreatic encephalopathy,[14] AIDS, lymphoma,[15] systemic lupus erythematous,[16] hematopoietic stem cell transplant patients,[17] hyperemesis gravidarum,[18,19] Marchiafava–Bignami disease, and hyperosmolar hyperglycemic state.[20]

SIGNS AND SYMPTOMS

The clinical presentation of CPM and EPM varies depending upon the regions of the brain involved. The initial symptoms of myelinolysis appear within 2–3 days following correction of hyponatremia. The symptoms include confusion, delirium, tremors,[21,22] seizures, dysphagia, dysarthria or mutism, diplopia, stiffness, weakness or paralysis of the limbs, sensory loss, and movement incoordination. Various signs such as oculomotor, abducens and facial nerve palsies, pyramidal tract lesions, spastic quadriparesis, pseudobulbar palsy, and Babinski sign may be present. The patient may develop "locked-in syndrome" (where the cognitive functions remain intact but all the voluntary muscles of the body are paralyzed except for those that control the eyes), coma, and death. These signs and symptoms result from rapid myelinolysis of the corticobulbar and corticospinal tracts in the basis pontis. EPM may lead to various movement disorders depending upon the site of lesion. Different presentations such as mutism, parkinsonism, dystonia, and catatonia have been described in the literature.[3,22] The patient may also develop "Uhtoff's syndrome" (where raised body temperature causes persistent dysarthria and oropharyngeal dysphagia) possibly due to the effect of increased temperature on nerve conduction.[23]

The clinical course of CPM is described as biphasic.[5,24] Initially, the patient has encephalopathy caused by hyponatremia, which improves transiently following rapid reversal of hyponatremia before developing the second phase of neurological syndrome caused by demyelination. The latter phase is characterized by spastic quadriparesis and pseudobulbar palsy and develops 2–3 days following correction or overcorrection of hyponatremia.

DIAGNOSIS

Early diagnosis of CPM requires a high degree of suspicion. CPM should be suspected if an alcoholic patient with hyponatremia subacutely develops pontine syndrome. The radiological findings lag behind and do not necessarily correlate with the clinical findings, limiting the utility of imaging in early diagnosis of CPM. Serial brain imaging is advocated as in the large proportion of cases, early scans may be normal[25] and the diagnosis of CPM is not ruled out in the setting of normal imaging. Magnetic resonance imaging (MRI) is the imaging technique of choice. Lesions are seen as hypointense on T1-weighted images (Figure 1(a)) and hyperintense on T2-weighted and FLAIR images (Figure 1(b) and (c)). A symmetrical, bat wing–shaped, partly confluent lesion in the center of pons giving a classic "trident-shaped" appearance is seen (Figure 1(c)). The lesions do not enhance on contrast. Diffusion weighed imaging (DWI) and diffusion tensor imaging are relatively new MRI techniques sensitive to the motion of water and might be capable of detecting early pathophysiological changes not detected on conventional MRI.[3,5,26] The lesion appears hyperintense on DWI. A computed tomography (CT) scan can detect lesion of CPM (seen as hypodense areas) but is less sensitive than an MRI. On a positron emission tomography scan, the affected areas show a high uptake initially followed by a subsequent low uptake.

Other investigations include serum electrolytes, cerebrospinal fluid (CSF) examination, and electrophysiological monitoring (electroencephalography (EEG), brain stem auditory–evoked potentials, and somatosensory-evoked potentials). CSF examination is usually normal but may sometimes demonstrate increased pressure, elevated proteins (myelin basic proteins), and cell counts (mononuclear macrophages). Abnormalities in EEG and evoked potentials aid in diagnosis of the condition and its location.

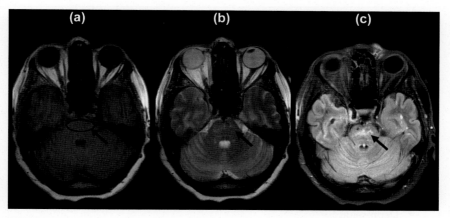

FIGURE 1   Axial MRI images through upper pons. T1-weighed MRI image (a) shows subtle hypointensity (encircled area marked by black arrow). T2-weighed MRI (b) and FLAIR (c) images shows symmetric hyperintensity (black arrows) in the pontine tegmentum.

DIFFERENTIAL DIAGNOSIS

Differential diagnosis includes multiple sclerosis, multifocal leukoencephalopathy, Binswanger's disease, pontine neoplasms (metastasis, gliomas), basilar artery thrombosis, and pontine infarct. The osmotic demyelination is noninflammatory, which distinguishes it from multiple sclerosis where marked perivascular inflammation is present. Preservation of neurons and axons in ODS lesions differentiate them from pontine infarcts.

PREVENTION AND TREATMENT

Prevention of the ODS is by avoiding the rapid correction of hyponatremia, which is the most frequent cause for its development. The rate of sodium correction should not exceed 0.5 mmol/L/h, and 24 h correction should not be greater than 10 mmol/L. Chronic alcoholics should receive vitamin supplementation and the nutritional status should be improved.

Once the CPM has occurred, the treatment is supportive only (such as prophylaxis against deep vein thrombosis, assisted ventilation in those with respiratory failure, prevention of aspiration and ventilator associated pneumonia, decubitus ulcers, and supplementation of vitamin B_1 in alcoholics). A number of therapeutic approaches have been tried but there is no specific therapy of choice. Various treatments that have been used include administration of steroids,[27] intravenous immunoglobins,[28–30] and thyrotropins with substantial improvement in the prognosis, but the results are from individual case reports or small case series and thus lack adequate level of evidence.

BOX 1

POSSIBLE COMPLICATIONS IN PATIENTS OF ODS

- Ventilator dependency
- Aspiration pneumonia
- Venous thrombosis
- Pulmonary embolism
- Contractures
- Muscle wasting
- Decubitus ulcers
- Urinary tract infections
- Depression

Patients of ODS are likely to receive extensive and prolonged physiotherapy and rehabilitation (such as physical, occupational, speech, and language therapy). Reinducing hyponatremia[31] and administration of organic osmolytes (myoinositol)[32] during the correction phase of hyponatremia are being explored as the potential treatment of this condition.

PROGNOSIS

In ODS, the prognosis remains guarded. The recovery varies from no improvement to substantial improvement, although the outcome may be frequently fatal. Both clinical features and radiological findings do not correlate with the outcome. Maximum recovery from CPM may require several months. Patients with extrapontine lesions may exhibit tremor and ataxia. In those patients who survive, the condition may develop various complications associated with severe central nervous system injury and reduced activity (Box 1).

CONCLUSION

In the past, ODS was primarily a postmortem diagnosis. However, the improved imaging techniques (CT and MRI) have facilitated the early diagnosis of the condition, which has led to better prognosis. Myelinolysis more commonly results following the treatment of chronic rather than acute hyponatremia and with a rapid rate of correction. Various animal and human studies suggest that correction of hyponatremia (of more than

48 h) should be done slowly and the rate of correction should not exceed more than 10 mmol/L/day. The overall prognosis is bleak. Those who survive usually suffer from disabilities ranging from minor tremors to spastic quadriparesis and locked-in syndrome.

References

1. Lampl C, Yazdi K. Central pontine myelinolysis. *Eur Neurol*. 2002;47:3–10.
2. Adams RD, Victor M, Mancall EL. Central pontine myelinolysis: a hitherto undescribed disease occurring in alcoholic and malnourished patients. *AMA Arch Neurol Psychiatry*. 1959;81:154–172.
3. Martin RJ. Central pontine and extrapontine myelinolysis: the osmotic demyelination syndromes. *J Neurol Neurosurg Psychiatry*. 2004;75(Suppl 3):iii22–iii28.
4. Singh N, Yu VL, Gayowski T. Central nervous system lesions in adult liver transplant recipients: clinical review with implications for management. *Med Baltimore*. 1994;73:110–118.
5. Ruzek KA, Campeau NG, Miller GM. Early diagnosis of central pontine myelinolysis with diffusion-weighted imaging. *Am J Neuroradiol*. 2004;25:210–213.
6. Turnbull J, Lumsden D, Siddiqui A, Lin JP, Lim M. Osmotic demyelination syndrome associated with hypophosphataemia: 2 cases and a review of literature. *Acta Paediatr*. 2013;102:164–168.
7. Imam YZ, Saqqur M, Alhail H, Deleu D. Extrapontine myelinolysis-induced parkinsonism in a patient with adrenal crisis. *Case Rep Neurol Med*. 2012;2012:327058.
8. Gujjar A, Al-Mamari A, Jacob PC, Jain R, Balkhair A, Al-Asmi A. Extrapontine myelinolysis as presenting manifestation of adrenal failure: a case report. *J Neurol Sci*. 2010;290: 169–171.
9. Yildirim T, Altinbaş A, Aydinli M, Ersoy O, Bayraktar Y. Is central pontine myelinolysis a sign of pre-symptomatic neurologic form of Wilson disease? *Turk J Gastroenterol*. 2012;23:419–420.
10. Ramirez N, Arranz B, Martín C, San L. Course and prognosis of a case of central pontine myelinolysis in eating behavior disorder. *Actas Esp Psiquiatr*. 2007;35:141–144. [Article in Spanish].
11. Amann B, Schäfer M, Sterr A, Arnold S, Grunze H. Central pontine myelinolysis in a patient with anorexia nervosa. *Int J Eat Disord*. 2001;30:462–466.
12. Chang Y, An DH, Xing Y, Qi X. Central pontine and extrapontine myelinolysis associated with acute hepatic dysfunction. *Neurol Sci*. 2012;33:673–676.
13. Al-Sarraf AJ, Haque M, Pudek M, Yoshida EM. Central pontine myelinolysis after orthotopic liver transplant-a rare complication. *Exp Clin Transplant*. 2010;8:321–324.
14. Hornik A, Rodriguez Porcel FJ, Agha C, et al. Central and extrapontine myelinolysis affecting the brain and spinal cord. An unusual presentation of pancreatic encephalopathy. *Front Neurol*. 2012;3:135.
15. Zhou AY, Barnes C, Razzaq R. Central pontine myelinolysis in a patient with non-Hodgkin lymphoma. *Br J Haematol*. 2013;161:156.
16. Tsai MH, Lu CS, Chen CJ, Tsai WP, Liou LB. Extrapontine myelinolysis in a patient with systemic lupus erythematosus: a case report. *J Formos Med Assoc*. 2002;101:505–508.
17. Lim KH, Kim S, Lee YS, et al. Central pontine myelinolysis in a patient with acute lymphoblastic leukemia after hematopoietic stem cell transplantation: a case report. *J Korean Med Sci*. 2008;23:324–327.
18. Tonelli J, Zurru MC, Castillo J, Casado P, Di Prizito C, Gutfraind E. Central pontine myelinolysis induced by hyperemesis gravidarum. *Med Buenos Aires*. 1999;59:176–178.
19. Sinn DI, Bachman D, Feng W. Simultaneous optic neuropathy and osmotic demyelinating syndrome in hyperemesis gravidarum. *Am J Med Sci*. 2014;347:88–90.

20. Rodríguez-Velver KV, Soto-Garcia AJ, Zapata-Rivera MA, Montes-Villarreal J, Villarreal-Pérez JZ, Rodríguez-Gutiérrez R. Osmotic demyelination syndrome as the initial manifestation of a hyperosmolar hyperglycemic state. *Case Rep Neurol Med*. 2014;2014:652523.
21. Sharma P, Sharma S, Panwar N, et al. Central pontine myelinolysis presenting with tremor in a child with Celiac disease. *J Child Neurol*. 2013;29:381–384.
22. Rizvi I, Ahmad M, Gupta A, Zaidi N. Isolated extra pontine myelinolysis presenting as acute onset parkinsonism. *BMJ Case Rep*. 2012;2012. pii: bcr2012007140.
23. Davis SL, Frohman TC, Crandall CG, et al. Modeling Uhthoff's phenomenon in MS patients with internuclear ophthalmoparesis. *Neurology*. 2008;70:1098–1106.
24. Laureno R, Karp BI. Myelinolysis after correction of hyponatremia. *Ann Intern Med*. 1997;126:57–62.
25. Graff-Radford J, Fugate JE, Kaufmann TJ, Mandrekar JN, Rabinstein AA. Clinical and radiologic correlations of central pontine myelinolysis syndrome. *Mayo Clin Proc*. 2011;86:1063–1067.
26. Nair SR, Ramli NM, Rahmat K, Mei-Ling ST. Central pontine and extrapontine myelinolysis: Diffusion weighted imaging and diffusion tensor imaging on follow-up. *Neurol India*. 2012;60:426–428.
27. Sakamoto E, Hagiwara D, Morishita Y, Tsukiyama K, Kondo K, Yamamoto M. Complete recovery of central pontine myelinolysis by high dose pulse therapy with methylprednisolone. *Nihon Naika Gakkai Zasshi*. 2007;96:2291–2293. [Article in Japanese].
28. Escribano-Gascón AB, Casanova-Peño LI, Bartolomé-Puras M, Porta-Etessam J. Efficacy of intravenous immunoglobulins in central pontine myelinolysis. *Neurologia*. 2008;23:392–394. [Article in Spanish].
29. Finsterer J, Engelmayer E, Trnka E, Stiskal M. Immunoglobulins are effective in pontine myelinolysis. *Clin Neuropharmacol*. 2000;23:110–113.
30. Deleu D, Salim K, Mesraoua B, El Siddig A, Al Hail H, Hanssens Y. "Man-in-the-barrel" syndrome as delayed manifestation of extrapontine and central pontine myelinolysis: beneficial effect of intravenous immunoglobulin. *J Neurol Sci*. 2005;237:103–106.
31. Oya S, Tsutsumi K, Ueki K, Kirino T. Reinduction of hyponatraemia to treat central pontinemyelinolysis. *Neurology*. 2001;57:1931–1932.
32. Silver SM, Schroeder BM, Sterns RH, Rojiani AM. Myoinositol administration improves survival and reduces myelinolysis after rapid correction of chronic hyponatremia in rats. *J Neuropathol Exp Neurol*. 2006;65:37–44.

Cerebral Salt Wasting

Indu Kapoor, Gyaninder P. Singh

Department of Neuroanaesthesiology and Critical Care, All India Institute
of Medical Sciences, New Delhi, India

DEFINITION

Cerebral salt wasting (CSW) is a condition characterized by renal loss of sodium leading to hyponatremia and concomitant decrease in extracellular fluid volume due to an intracranial disease.[1]

CSW was first described in 1950 by Peters et al.[2] They reported three patients with intracranial disorder exhibiting renal salt wasting. In patients with intracranial disorders, hyponatremia is frequently attributed to syndrome of inappropriate hormone secretion (SIADH). However, CSW is another important entity to consider in such patients. As both the conditions have many similar clinical and laboratory findings, it is important to differentiate between the two conditions. This is crucial because the management of each is fundamentally different,[3] and improper treatment may significantly increase the morbidity and mortality.[3,4]

In clinical practice, hyponatremia (serum Na+ concentration <136 mEq/L) is the commonest electrolyte abnormality encountered.[5] The incidence of mild hyponatremia (serum Na+ 130–135 mEq/L) is estimated to be approximately 30%[6] and moderate to severe hyponatremia is observed in 7%[7,8] of hospitalized patients. There are varied causes of hyponatremia such as hormone disorders, medications, volume status of the patient, etc., and thus diagnosis of exact etiology is important for its management.

ETIOLOGY

CSW chiefly occurs in patients with subarachnoid hemorrhage (SAH).[9] Other conditions where it has been reported to occur include head injury, brain tumors, brain infarction, intracranial hemorrhage, arteriovenous malformations, meningitis, central nervous system derangements, and intracranial surgeries.[9–20] In a study by Wijdicks et al.,[21] approximately 67% of patients with hyponatremia after SAH (rupture of intracranial aneurysm) had CSW as the etiology for hyponatremia. However, Sherlock et al.[22] found CSW as the cause of hyponatremia in only 6.5% of patients who presented with spontaneous SAH and hyponatremia. Vespa[11] reported CSW in 5–10% of patients with traumatic brain injury. The CSW syndrome can also be associated with status epilepticus.[23] Hence, hydration status and electrolytes should be monitored closely in these patients.

PATHOPHYSIOLOGY

Though a clear association between neurological disorders and CSW exist, the precise mechanism underlying this is not well understood. Maintenance of body Na+ and water homeostasis is a vital physiological process that is regulated by close interaction between the autonomic nervous system, humoral factors (hormones), and kidneys.[3] Any disruption of this system may lead to Na+ and water dysregulation. Interference of the sympathetic outflow to the kidneys and high levels of circulating natriuretic factors are postulated as the cause of CSW syndrome.[3] Natriuretic peptides (NPs; discovered in early 1980s)[3] are molecules that prevent excess water and salt retention. NPs identified as associated with

CSW are atrial natriuretic peptide, brain natriuretic peptide (BNP), C-type natriuretic peptide and dendroaspis natriuretic peptide Endogenous peptide adrenomedullin has also been proposed as a mediator of CSW.[3] It is found in human brain tissue (hypothalamus)[24,25] and is a potent vasodilator[26] with natriuretic and diuretic properties.[3] However, BNP remains the primary suspect for the development of CSW.

All NPs cause relaxation of vascular smooth muscle by inhibiting sympathetic vascular tone,[3,27] leading to vasodilatation. Dilatation of renal afferent tubules causes increased Na^+ and water filtration through the glomerulus. Also, NPs have direct renal natriuretic and diuretic effects by antagonizing the effect of angiotensin and vasopressin on the proximal convoluted tubule and the collecting duct, respectively.[28,29]

Several hypotheses to explain the rise of serum concentration of NPs during intracranial insult have been proposed: (1) direct release of BNP into circulation, due to damage to cortical and subcortical areas where BNP exists[2]; (2) generation and release of NPs from the hypothalamus in conditions such as SAH to protect against elevated intracranial pressure[30]; (3) surges in sympathetic outflow in response to intracranial injury[31] may cause catecholamine-induced myocardial strain, thereby causing release of NPs from the atrial myocardium[32–34]; and (4) hypervolemic therapy (frequently administered after SAH to prevent vasospasm) causing myocardial stretch and release of NPs have also been speculated by some authors.[35]

SIGNS AND SYMPTOMS

Signs and symptoms of CSW are those of hyponatremia (see Chapter 30 on SIADH) and of hypovolemia and diminished extracellular volume (such as tachycardia, hypotension, lassitude, increased thirst, muscle cramps, weight loss, absence of jugular venous distension, orthostatic hypotension, prolonged capillary refill time, diminished skin turgor, or dry mucous membranes). However, the accurate determination of volume status is difficult in routine clinical practice[3] and thus the differentiation between hypovolemic, euvolemic, and hypervolemic hyponatremia is not consistently possible.

DIAGNOSIS

Obtaining a meticulous history, physical examination, and laboratory investigation often helps in arriving at a correct diagnosis. CSW is a disorder of sodium and water regulation that occurs as a result of cerebral disorder in the presence of normal renal function.[3] The major features of CSW syndrome are hypovolemia, hyponatremia, serum hypoosmolality, and elevated urine osmolality (increased urinary Na^+). The urine is inappropriately concentrated for the degree of serum hypoosmolality as the sodium excretion is disproportionately higher than that of water. The daily fluid intake, output record, and weight changes are helpful in determining the volume status of the patients. Measurement of central venous pressure (CVP) provides information about the intravascular volume status and also helps in precise management of the fluid. Awareness of CSW is important for recognition of the changes mentioned above early in their course so that timely therapeutic measures and treatment can be initiated.[36]

DIFFERENTIAL DIAGNOSIS

Differentiating CSW from other causes of hyponatremia, particularly SIADH, is important. CSW and SIADH have many identical clinical and laboratory findings and occur in similar intracranial disorders.[4,37] Determination of volume status of the patient is the key to differentiation between these two conditions; however, in clinical practice, determination of volume status is difficult. Differentiating features between CSW and SIADH are given in Table 1.

TREATMENT

CSW is characterized by hypovolemic hyponatremia caused by diuresis and natriuresis (i.e., renal loss of sodium and water). Thus, replacement of sodium and water remains the mainstay of treatment in these patients. Initial management strategy is intravenous administration of normal saline (0.9%) at 100–125 mL/h to restore intravascular volume. Oral salt supplementation may be considered in stable patients. In case of severe hyponatremia (i.e., serum Na^+ concentration <125 mEq/L) or if large volumes of intravenous fluid are required to maintain euvolemia, infusion of hypertonic saline may be necessary. Normally, 1.5% NaCl solution at a rate of 50–150 mL/h titrated to achieve a normal to slightly positive fluid balance may be administered.[3] Occasionally, 3% hypertonic saline infusion at a rate of 25–50 mL/h may be required in symptomatic patients with serum Na <120 mEq/L. However, rapid correction of hyponatremia may cause osmotic demyelination and thus should be avoided (see Chapter 30 SIADH). In general, the rate of correction of serum Na^+ concentration should not exceed 0.5 mEq/L/h, and the end point of correction should be around 130 mEq/L (rather than complete correction). Drug therapy includes the use of hormone mineralocorticoid (fludrocortisone). Mineralocorticoid

TABLE 1   Differentiating Features between CSW and SIADH

Clinical parameters	CSW	SIADH
Heart rate	Normal or increased	Normal
Urine output	Normal or increased	Decreased
CVP	Decreased (<6 cm of H_2O)	Normal or slightly increased
Wedge pressure	Decreased (<8 cm of H_2O)	Normal or slightly increased
Body weight	Decreased	Normal or slightly increased
Fluid balance	Negative	Neutral or slightly positive
Extracellular fluid volume	Decreased	Normal or increased
Laboratory variables		
Hematological		
Hematocrit	Increased	Normal
Sodium balance	Negative	Neutral or increased
Serum osmolality	Increased or normal	Decreased
Serum Na^+ concentration	Decreased	Decreased
Serum K^+ concentration	Increased or normal	Decreased or normal
Serum albumin	Increased	Normal
Serum bicarbonate	Increased	Normal or increased
Serum uric acid	Normal or decreased	Decreased
Blood urea nitrogen (BUN)	Increased	Normal or increased
Serum [BUN]:[creatinine] ratio	Increased	Normal
Urinary		
Urine osmolality	Increased (>100 mOsm/kg)	Increased (>100 mOsm/kg)
Urinary Na^+ concentration	Increased (>40 mmol/L)	Increased (>40 mmol/L)
Fractional excretion of uric acid (after correction of hyponatremia)	Increased	Normal

enhances reabsorption of sodium and water from the renal tubules, thereby causing correction of hyponatremia and hypovolemia. When used in SAH patients, renal salt excretion was reduced, and sodium balance was achieved more frequently.[38,39] A dose of 0.1–0.2 mg orally twice daily may be administered until normal serum Na^+ concentration and intravascular

---

BOX 1   MANAGEMENT OF CSW

- Administration of isotonic saline (0.9% NaCl) to achieve positive fluid balance.
- Monitoring of fluid intake and output, volume status, and serum Na$^+$ concentration.
- Intravenous infusion of hypertonic saline (1.5% or 3%) in severe and symptomatic hyponatremia. (Avoid rapid correction to prevent osmotic myelinolysis.)
- Fludrocortisone (mineralocorticoid) in the dose of 0.1–0.2 mg orally twice a day may be used (enhances renal reabsorption of Na and water).
- Oral salt supplementation as an adjuvant therapy.
- Treatment of the underlying intracranial pathology.

---

volume is restored. Adverse effects of fludrocortisone are hypokalemia (73%),[39] fluid retention, pulmonary edema, and hypertension.[3,39]

PREVENTION

CSW, which was once thought to be rare, is not uncommon in patients with certain intracranial disorders. However, the incidence of CSW is significantly high in children with an acute central nervous system disorder compared to SIADH.[40] Thus it is essential to consider CSW in addition of SIADH in patients who present with hyponatremia and intracranial disorder, as both have very similar biochemical profiles and clinical presentations but different management strategies. Though the condition cannot be prevented, early and correct diagnosis is important to obtain a good outcome and decrease morbidity and mortality (Box 1).

References

1. Harrigan MR. Cerebral salt wasting syndrome: a review. *Neurosurgery*. 1996;38:152–160.
2. Peters JP, Welt LG, Sims EA, Orloff J, Needham J. A salt-wasting syndrome associated with cerebral disease. *Trans Assoc Am Physicians*. 1950;63:57–64.
3. Yee AH, Burns JD, Wijdicks EFM. Cerebral salt wasting: pathophysiology, diagnosis, and treatment. *Neurosurg Clin N Am*. 2010;21:339–352.
4. Momi M, Tang CM, Abcar AC, Kuju bu DA, Sim JJ. Hyponatremia—what is cerebral salt wasting? *Perm J*. 2010;14:62–65.
5. Thompson C, Hoorn EJ. Hyponatremia: an overview of frequency, clinical presentation and complications. *Best Pract Res Clin Endocrinol Metab*. 2012;26(suppl 1):S1–S6.
6. Upadhyay A, Jaber BL, Madias NE. Epidemiology of hyponatremia. *Semin Nephrol*. 2009;29:227–238.

7. Ellison DH, Berl T. Clinical practice. The syndrome of inappropriate antidiuresis. *N Engl J Med*. 2007;356:2064–2072.
8. Hoorn EJ, Lindemans J, Zietse R. Development of severe hyponatraemia in hospitalized patients: treatment-related risk factors and inadequate management. *Nephrol Dial Transplant*. 2006;21:70–76.
9. Kruse JA. An endocrinology consult. In: Torbey MT, ed. *Neurocritical Care*. New York, USA: Cambridge University Press; 2010:397–409.
10. Lu DC, Binder DK, Chien B, et al. Cerebral salt wasting and elevated brain natriuretic peptide levels after traumatic brain injury: 2 case reports. *Surg Neurol*. 2008;69:226–229.
11. Vespa P. Cerebral salt wasting after traumatic brain injury: an important critical care treatment issue. *Surg Neurol*. 2008;69:230–232.
12. Jimenez R, Casado-Flores J, Nieto M, et al. Cerebral salt wasting syndrome in children with acute central nervous system injury. *Pediatr Neurol*. 2006;35:261–263.
13. Oruckaptan HH, Ozisik P, Akalan N. Prolonged cerebral salt wasting syndrome associated with the intraventricular dissemination of brain tumors: report of two cases and review of the literature. *Pediatr Neurosurg*. 2000;33:16–20.
14. Kim JH, Kang JK, Lee SA. Hydrocephalus and hyponatremia as the presenting manifestations of primary CNS lymphoma. *Eur Neurol*. 2006;55:39–41.
15. Huang SM, Chen CC, Chiu PC, et al. Tuberculous meningitis complicated with hydrocephalus and cerebral salt wasting syndrome in a three-year old boy. *Pediatr Infect Dis J*. 2004;23:884–886.
16. Brookes MJ, Gould TH. Cerebral salt wasting syndrome in meningoencephalitis: a case report. *J Neurol Neurosurg Psychiatr*. 2003;74:277.
17. Ti LK, Kang SC, Cheong KF. Acute hyponatraemia secondary to cerebral salt wasting syndrome in a patient with tuberculous meningitis. *Anaesth Intensive Care*. 1998;26:420–423.
18. Papadimitriou DT, Spiteri A, Pagnier A, et al. Mineralocorticoid deficiency in postoperative cerebral salt wasting. *J Pediatr Endocrinol Metab*. 2007;20:1145–1150.
19. Roca-Ribas F, Ninno JE, Gasperin A, et al. Cerebral salt wasting syndrome as a postoperative complication after surgical resection of acoustic neuroma. *Otol Neurotol*. 2002;23:992–995.
20. Poon WS, Lolin YI, Yeung TF, et al. Water and sodium disorders following surgical excision of pituitary region tumours. *Acta Neurochir (Wien)*. 1996;138:921–927.
21. Wijdicks EF, Vermeulen M, ten Haaf JA, et al. Volume depletion and natriuresis in patients with a ruptured intracranial aneurysm. *Ann Neurol*. 1985;18:211–216.
22. Sherlock M, O'Sullivan E, Agha A, et al. The incidence and pathophysiology of hyponatraemia after subarachnoid haemorrhage. *Clin Endocrinol (Oxf)*. 2006;64:250–254.
23. Çelik T, Tolunay O, Tolunay I, Çelik Ü. Cerebral salt wasting in status epilepticus: two cases and review of the literature. *Pediatr Neurol*. 2014;50:397–399.
24. Satoh F, Takahashi K, Murakami O, et al. Adrenomedullin in human brain, adrenal glands and tumor tissues of pheochromocytoma, ganglioneuroblastoma and neuroblastoma. *J Clin Endocrinol Metab*. 1995;80:1750–1752.
25. Satoh F, Takahashi K, Murakami O, et al. Immuno-cytochemical localization of adrenomedullin-like immunoreactivity in the human hypothalamus and the adrenal gland. *Neurosci Lett*. 1996;203:207–210.
26. Lang MG, Paterno R, Faraci FM, et al. Mechanisms of adrenomedullin-induced dilation of cerebral arterioles. *Stroke*. 1997;28:181–185.
27. Schultz HD, Steele MK, Gardner DG. Central administration of atrial peptide decreases sympathetic outflow in rats. *Am J Physiol*. 1990;258:R1250–R1256.
28. Harris PJ, Thomas D, Morgan TO. Atrial natriuretic peptide inhibits angiotensin-stimulated proximal tubular sodium and water reabsorption. *Nature*. 1987;326:697–698.
29. Dillingham MA, Anderson RJ. Inhibition of vasopressin action by atrial natriuretic factor. *Science*. 1986;231:1572–1573.

30. Berendes E, Walter M, Cullen P, et al. Secretion of brain natriuretic peptide in patients with aneurismal subarachnoid haemorrhage. *Lancet.* 1997;349:245–249.
31. Samuels MA. The brain–heart connection. *Circulation.* 2007;116:77–84.
32. Tomida M, Muraki M, Uemura K, et al. Plasma concentrations of brain natriuretic peptide in patients with subarachnoid hemorrhage. *Stroke.* 1998;29:1584–1587.
33. Espiner EA, Leikis R, Ferch RD, et al. The neurocardio-endocrine response to acute subarachnoid haemorrhage. *Clin Endocrinol (Oxf).* 2002;56:629–635.
34. Rosenfeld JV, Barnett GH, Sila CA, et al. The effect of subarachnoid hemorrhage on blood and CSF atrial natriuretic factor. *J Neurosurg.* 1989;71:32–37.
35. Inoha S, Inamura T, Nakamizo A, et al. Fluid loading in rats increases serum brain natriuretic peptide concentration. *Neurol Res.* 2001;23:93–95.
36. Bajwa SJ, Haldar R. Endocrinological disorders affecting neurosurgical patients: an intensivists perspective. *Indian J Endocrinol Metab.* 2014;18:778–783.
37. Palmer BF. Hyponatremia in patients with central nervous system disease: SIADH versus CSW. *Trends Endocrinol Metab.* 2003;14:182–187.
38. Hasan D, Lindsay KW, Wijdicks EF, et al. Effect of fludrocortisone acetate in patients with subarachnoid hemorrhage. *Stroke.* 1989;20:1156–1161.
39. Mori T, Katayama Y, Kawamata T, Hirayama T. Improved efficiency of hypervolemic therapy with inhibition of natriuresis by fludrocortisone in patients with aneurysmal subarachnoid hemorrhage. *J Neurosurg.* 1999;91:947–952.
40. Sorkhi H, Salehi Omran MR, Barari Savadkoohi R, Baghdadi F, Nakhjavani N, Bijani A. CSWS versus SIADH as the probable causes of hyponatremia in children with acute CNS disorders. *Iran J Child Neurol.* 2013;7:34–39.

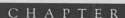

CHAPTER

29

Diabetes Insipidus

Gyaninder P. Singh, Indu Kapoor

Department of Neuroanaesthesiology and Critical Care, All India Institute of Medical Sciences, New Delhi, India

OUTLINE

DEFINITION

Diabetes insipidus (DI) is a heterogeneous condition characterized by polyuria and polydipsia caused either due to a lack of secretion of vasopressin (antidiuretic hormone) from posterior pituitary, its physiological suppression following excessive water intake, kidney resistance to its action, or its increased degradation.[1]

DI is a rare condition, with a reported prevalence of 1 in 25,000.[2] The impaired water conservation in DI leads to hypernatremia without apparent volume deficits.[3,4] The underlying abnormality is decreased action of vasopressin on the kidneys, either due to a low level of the hormone or refractoriness of the kidneys to a normal level of hormone.

CLASSIFICATION

DI is broadly classified into two types: neurogenic DI (also known as neurohypophyseal, hypothalamic, cranial, or central), which is due to inadequate synthesis and release of vasopressin from the hypothalamic–pituitary axis (neurohypophyseal axis); and nephrogenic or renal DI, due to inadequate responses of the kidneys to adequate levels of circulating vasopressin.

Two other rare forms of the DI are recognized viz. dipsogenic DI and gestational DI.

Dipsogenic DI (or primary polydipsia) occurs due to excessive fluid intake, causing suppression of vasopressin (low circulating levels of vasopressin) and inducing polyuria.

Gestational DI occurs due to the actions of placental vasopressinase, which causes accelerated degradation of vasopressin during pregnancy, thereby leading to a decreased level of circulating vasopressin.

PHYSIOLOGY OF WATER REGULATION

Water balance in the human body is principally attained by three interrelated mechanisms, i.e., thirst, vasopressin, and renal function. Under normal conditions, body–water balance is maintained by regulating renal water excretion and thirst so as to confine plasma osmolality within the narrow range of 282–295 mmol/kg.[5] Synthesis and release of vasopressin is precisely controlled by serum osmolality. Increases in serum osmolality stimulates the release of vasopressin, and vice versa. The vasopressin acts on renal collecting ducts (V_2 receptors) and activates adenyl cyclase, increasing intracellular cAMP. This stimulates protein kinase A, which causes phosphorylation of aquaporin 2 (AQP2) and their insertion into the cell membrane. The insertion of AQP2 (i.e., water channel protein) renders the collecting duct permeable to water and allows free passage of water from the lumen of nephrons into the cells of the collecting duct along the osmotic gradient. Further passage of water from within the cell to renal interstitium and circulation is mediated by aquaporin 3 and aquaporin 4, present in the basolateral membrane.[2,5]

Similar to secretion of vasopressin, the sensation of thirst is also under the fine control of serum osmolality.[6] When there is a large amount of water loss from the body, plasma osmolality may rise above 300 mmol/kg.

In such situations, the increased plasma concentration of vasopressin (plasma concentration >4 pmol/L) will not be able to conserve more renal water, and a thirst sensation leading to ingestion of water restores the water balance.

ETIOLOGY

Numerous causes result in partial or complete impairment of urinary concentrating ability leading to DI. Neurogenic or central DI may be caused by destruction or degeneration of neurons in the supraoptic and paraventricular nuclei of hypothalamus by tumors, trauma, infection, surgery, anesthetic agents,[7] inflammatory or autoimmune disease, granulomatous disease, and congenital cranial malformations. It may also be caused by inherited genetic defects leading to impaired vasopressin synthesis. DI is said to occur when more than 80% of the vasopressin-secreting neurons are destroyed.[2] Causes for renal or nephrogenic DI includes various renal disorders, electrolyte disturbances, drugs, or mutations of vasopressin receptors in the kidneys. Excessive thirst and fluid intake due to any cause may lead to dipsogenic DI. Few patients may have a lowered osmotic threshold for the onset of the thirst sensation but normal osmoregulation of vasopressin secretion.[5] Various causes of central, nephrogenic, and dipsogenic DI are given in Table 1. Incidences of central DI during pregnancy are more than in the postpartum period, likely favored by some conditions occurring in pregnancy. The monitoring of vasopressin–cell antibodies (AVPcAb) in pregnant patients with an autoimmune disease and posterior pituitary function during pregnancy may allow an early diagnosis and treatment.[8]

SIGNS AND SYMPTOMS

The primary symptoms of DI are persistent polyuria and polydipsia. This may be accompanied by severe dehydration, vomiting, constipation, fever, irritability, sleep disturbances, nocturia, bed wetting, failure to thrive, and growth retardation in children. Some mental retardation has also been reported, probably due to unrecognized repeated dehydration.[2] Signs and symptoms of the underlying causes may be present in a few patients, e.g., headache, visual defects, growth retardation, etc. in cases of intracranial tumors leading to central DI. In Wolfram syndrome, the first symptom to appear is diabetes mellitus (median age of 6 years), followed by optic atrophy (median age of 11 years), while polyuria and/or enuresis usually appear during the second or third decade of life.[2,9]

TABLE 1   Causes of Diabetes Insipidus

1. Causes of neurogenic or central DI:
  a. Injury to the central nervous system
- Neoplasms (craniopharyngeoma, pineal gland tumors, germinoma, suprasellar tumors, optic glioma, pituitary adenoma/apoplexy, leukemia, lymphoma, brain metastases and, rarely, colloid cyst)
- Trauma (head injury)
- Brain surgery (hypothalamic or pituitary surgeries)
- Hypoxic or ischemic brain damage (cardiac arrest, carbon monoxide poisoning)
- Radiation to brain
- CNS infections (encephalitis, meningitis, toxoplasmosis, congenital CMV, Guillain-Barre syndrome)
- Granulomatous infiltration (sarcoidosis, tuberculosis, Langerhans cell histiocytosis, Wegener's granulomatosis)
- Autoimmune (lymphocytic infundibulohypophysitis)
- Cerebrovascular disease (aneurysm, brain infarction, intracranial hemorrhage, Sheehan's syndrome, damage to posterior pituitary vascular system due to congenital malformations (i.e., poor development), or local vasculitis affecting posterior pituitary blood supply)
- Brain death (hypothalamic production of vasopressin ceases)

  b. Familial disease
    Wolfram syndrome or DIDMOAD syndrome (diabetes insipidus, diabetes mellitus, optic atrophy, and deafness)
    Familial neurohypophyseal DI

  c. Cerebral malformations
    Septo-optic dysplasia
    Laurence-Moon-Beidl syndrome

  d. Drugs induced (inhibit vasopressin release)
    Phenytoin
    Ethanol

  e. Idiopathic

2. Causes of nephrogenic DI
  a. Familial
    V_2 receptor gene mutation (X-linked recessive inheritance)
    AQP2 gene mutation (autosomal recessive inheritance)

  b. Renal disease
    Chronic renal failure, renal medullary sponge disease, pyelonephritis, polycystic kidney disease, obstructive uropathy, renal amyloidosis, sarcoidosis, Sjogren's syndrome, renal transplantation

  c. Electrolyte disturbance
    Hypercalcemia, Hypokalemia

  d. Drugs
    Lithium, amphotericin B, demeclocycline, gentamicin, ofloxacin, orlistat, vinblastine, loop diuretics, methoxyflurane, cidofovir, ifosfamide, etc.

  e. Others
    Multiple myeloma, sickle cell disease, diabetes mellitus (osmotic diuresis)

3. Causes of dipsogenic DI
  a. Compulsive or habitual excessive fluid intake
  b. Psychiatric disorder
  c. Hypothalamic lesion
  d. Drugs (lithium, carbamazepine)
  e. Lowered osmotic threshold for thirst

VII. COMPLICATIONS RELATED TO FLUID AND ELECTROLYTE DISTURBANCES

DIAGNOSIS

A meticulous history and examination along with laboratory parameters is required for the diagnosis of DI, differentiating it from other causes of polyuria. A 24 h, urine volume should be documented to confirm polyuria. Polyuria is defined as the passage of large volumes of dilute urine, in excess of $2 L/m^2/day$ or approximately $40 mL/kg/day$ in older children and adults.[5] Other investigations which assist in correct diagnosis include serum electrolyte, plasma and urine osmolality, and renal function tests. Measurement of blood glucose, serum Ca^{2+}, and K^+ levels helps to exclude the common causes of nephrogenic DI.

The diagnostic approach to determine the pathogenesis of DI is the fluid deprivation test coupled with the renal response to exogenous vasopressin. The ability to secrete vasopressin from posterior pituitary can be established through water deprivation tests, and the renal response to vasopressin can be tested by desmopressin (DDAVP) trial tests.[5] After confirming the pathogenic mechanism of DI, the underlying cause for it should be searched. Magnetic imaging of the hypothalamic, pituitary, and surrounding structure is performed to rule out any intracranial mass. Genetic studies help to identify the familial causes (abnormality in the vasopressin molecule).

Following pituitary surgery or excision of craniopharyngiomas, injury to posterior pituitary or pituitary stalk causes central DI in the postoperative period.[10] The various pattern of DI[10] seen are: (1) transient DI (polyuria and polydipsia lasting for 12–36 h); (2) prolonged DI (symptoms may last for weeks to months or sometimes permanently); or (3) triphasic response.[11] In triphasic response, the initial phase of DI (polyuria and polydipsia) lasts for 4–5 days due to reduced level of vasopressin. This is followed by the second phase of oliguria (for the next 4–5 days) due to liberation of vasopressin as a result of vasopressin-secreting neurons degenerating. The third and final phase is again of polyuria (DI) due to deficiency of vasopressin for either a transient or a prolonged period. Diagnosis of DI is usually made a few hours after surgery, although the abnormalities of vasopressin and fluid balance often begin intraoperatively.[12]

TREATMENT

Treatment depends on the mechanism causing the disorder. For the neurogenic or central DI, the drug of choice is desmopressin. It is the synthetic analog of the hormone arginine vasopressin. The drug may be administered orally, intranasally, or parenterally. The daily oral dose is 100–1000 μg in three divided doses. For parenteral preparations, the dose is 0.1–1 µg given intravenously. Intranasal preparations are given in the dose of 2–40 µg.[5] A low dose should be started initially and further titrated according to the response. A potential side effect of the drug is dilutional hyponatremia if the desmopressin is administered in excess for a prolonged period. However, it has been found that the incidence of hyponatremia is significantly less with oral disintegrating tablets than intranasal desmopressin.[13] Daily record of weight should be used as an index for fluid balance along with measurements of serum electrolytes, particularly on the initial phase of treatment. Treatment of the underlying cause of DI may sometimes cure the condition.

Nephrogenic DI may be treated by addressing the underlying pathology. Withdrawal of the culprit drug or correction of metabolic disturbances usually reverses the condition. Familial (genetic) form of nephrogenic DI is difficult to treat. Restriction of salt intake along with administration of diuretic thiazide may help reduce the urinary output. Thiazide diuretics act by enhancing excretion of Na^+ at the expense of water and reducing the glomerular filtration rate.[5] Prostaglandin synthetase inhibitor indomethacin (1.5–3.0 mg/kg) may be administered alone or in combination with thiazide and desmopressin to reduce urine output. However, adequate fluid intake to quench the thirst should be taken. Statins also have a therapeutic effect on nephrogenic DI. It increases water reabsorption by the kidneys, thus opening up a new avenue in treating patients with nephrogenic DI.[14]

In case of compulsive or habitual water intake leading to dipsogenic DI (primary polydipsia), fluid intake should be reduced. Treatment of associated psychological or psychiatric illness helps in treating the condition.

References

1. Robertson GL. Diabetes insipidus. *Endocrinol Metab Clin North Am*. 1995;24:549–572.
2. Di Iorgi N, Napoli F, Allegri AE, et al. Diabetes insipidus–diagnosis and management. *Horm Res Paediatr*. 2012;77:69–84.
3. Makaryus AN, McFarlane SI. Diabetes insipidus: diagnosis and treatment of complex disease. *Cleve Clin J Med*. 2006;73:65–71.
4. Blevins Jr LS, Wand GS. Diabetes insipidus. *Crit Care Med*. 1992;20:69–79.
5. Baylis PH, Cheetham T. Diabetes insipidus. *Arch Dis Child*. 1998;79:84–89.
6. Thompson CJ, Bland J, Burd J, Baylis PH. The osmotic thresholds for thirst and vasopressin release are similar in healthy man. *Clin Sci*. 1986;71:651–656.
7. Soo J, Gray J, Manecke G. Propofol and diabetes insipidus. *J Clin Anesth*. 2014;26:679–683.
8. Bellastella G, Bizzarro A, Aitella E, et al. Pregnancy may favour the development of severe autoimmune central diabetes insipidus in women with vasopressin-cell antibodies: description of two cases. *Eur J Endocrinol*. 2015;172:K11–17.
9. Barrett TG, Bundey SE, Macleod AF. Neurodegeneration and diabetes: UK nationwide study of Wolfram (DIDMOAD) syndrome. *Lancet*. 1995;346:1458–1463.
10. Neurocritical care. In: Greenberg MS, ed. *Handbook of Neurosurgery*. New York, USA: Thieme publishers; 2010:7–30.

11. Finken MJ, Zwaveling-Soonawala N, Walenkamp MJ, Vulsma T, van Trotsenburg AS. Rotteveel J. Frequent occurrence of the triphasic response (diabetes insipidus/hyponatremia/diabetes insipidus) after surgery for craniopharyngioma in childhood. *Horm Res Paediatr*. 2011;76:22–26.
12. Ghirardello S, Hopper N, Albanese A, Maghnie M. Diabetes insipidus in craniopharyngioma: postoperative management of water and electrolyte disorders. *J Pediatr Endocrinol Metab*. 2006;19(suppl 1):413–421.
13. Kataoka Y, Nishida S, Hirakawa A, Oiso Y, Arima H. Comparison of incidence of hyponatremia between intranasal and oral desmopressin in patients with central diabetes insipidus. *Endocr J*. 2015;62:195–200.
14. Bonfrate L, Procino G, Wang DQ, Svelto M, Portincasa P. A novel therapeutic effect of statins on nephrogenic diabetes insipidus. *J Cell Mol Med*. 2015;19:265–282.

VII. COMPLICATIONS RELATED TO FLUID AND ELECTROLYTE DISTURBANCES

Syndrome of Inappropriate Antidiuretic Hormone Secretion (SIADH)

Indu Kapoor, Gyaninder P. Singh

Department of Neuroanaesthesiology and Critical Care, All India Institute of Medical Sciences, New Delhi, India

http://dx.doi.org/10.1016/B978-0-12-804075-1.00030-4

DEFINITION

Syndrome of inappropriate antidiuretic hormone secretion (SIADH) is caused by excessive or inappropriate secretion or action of antidiuretic hormone (ADH), resulting in:

- Dilutional hyponatremia without clinically apparent hypervolemia (also known as euvolemic)
- Reduced plasma osmolality
- Impaired water excretion with decreased volumes of urine that is inappropriately concentrated for the prevailing plasma osmolality and volume status.[1]

Schwartz first described SIADH in 1957 (also known as Schwartz–Bartter syndrome).[2] SIADH is uncommon in the general population and is mainly seen in hospitalized patients. Both genders are equally affected. Risk factors for SIADH are neoplasms, central nervous system (CNS) disorders, pulmonary disease, and some medications; elderly patients are also at a high risk for SIADH.

ETIOLOGY

ADH, or arginine vasopressin (AVP), is secreted from the posterior pituitary in response to hypovolemia or hyperosmolality.[3] Physiological action of ADH is to cause water reabsorption from renal tubules, causing concentration of urine. In SIADH, secretion of ADH is unregulated and is secreted despite serum hypotonicity.[4,5] This leads to retention of water by the kidneys and hypotonic euvolemic hyponatremia. SIADH is the most common cause of euvolemic hyponatremia.[5,6]

Mechanisms of increased production of ADH include:

1. Increased production of ADH from posterior pituitary
2. Ectopic production of ADH from primary or metastatic tumor
3. Exogenous administration of ADH or its analog (e.g., desmopressin, high-dose oxytocin, chlorpropamide, carbamazepine, vincristine, etc.)

Various conditions that may produce SIADH are given in Table 1. The most common cause of hyponatremia after acute nontraumatic aneurysmal subarachnoid hemorrhage is SIADH followed by glucocorticoid insufficiency and cerebral salt wasting syndrome (CSWS).[7]

SIGNS AND SYMPTOMS

Signs and symptoms of SIADH develop because of hyponatremia and possibly because of water overload. Patients with mild to moderate

TABLE 1   Etiologies of SIADH

1. **Neoplasm:** Various tumors that can secrete ADH ectopically such as:
    a. Carcinomas
        - Small-cell carcinoma of the lung (most common neoplastic cause of SIADH)
        - Duodenum, pancreas, ovary, prostrate, urinary bladder, ureter
        - Head and neck
    b. Other neoplasms
        - Thymoma, mesothelioma, bronchial adenoma, carcinoid, gangliocytoma, lymphomas, Ewing's sarcoma
2. **Neurological disorders:**
    a. CNS disorders
        - Head trauma
        - Postcraniotomy following pituitary surgery, craniopharyngiomas, hypothalamic tumors
        - Brain tumors
        - Stroke (cerebrovascular occlusion, intracranial hemorrhage)
        - Cavernous sinus thrombosis
        - Infection: Meningitis (bacterial, tubercular, or viral), encephalitis, brain abscess, AIDS
        - Hydrocephalus
        - Neurosarcoidosis, multiple sclerosis, amyotrophic lateral sclerosis
        - Psychosis, delirium tremens
        - Congenital malformations: Agenesis of corpus callosum, cleft lip/palate with or without recognized CNS abnormality
    b. Peripheral nervous system disease
        - Guillain–Barré syndrome
        - Peripheral neuropathy
3. **Pulmonary/Thoracic disorder:**
    a. Infection: Pneumonia (bacterial or viral), lung abscess, tuberculosis, AIDS-related lung infections
    b. Cavitation (tuberculosis, aspergillosis)
    c. Chronic obstructive pulmonary disease, asthma
    d. Pneumothorax, pulmonary embolism, atelectasis
    e. Positive-pressure ventilation
4. **Drugs**
    a. Vasopressin or desmopressin, chlorpropamide, high-dose oxytocin, vincristine, carbamazepine, nicotine, phenothiazines, cyclophosphamide, tricyclic antidepressants, monoamine oxidase inhibitors, serotonin reuptake inhibitors, opioids, NSAIDs, theophylline, bromocriptine, clofibrate
5. **Miscellaneous**
    a. Anemia, stress, severe pain, nausea, endurance exercise combined with solute-free water intake
    b. Major surgery, general anesthesia, postoperative pain
    c. Acute intermittent porphyria
    d. Idiopathic

hyponatremia that develops slowly may be asymptomatic. Various signs and symptoms that may be present in patients of SIADH include malaise, apathy, lethargy, headache, dysgeusia, personality changes, confusion, agitation, ataxia, muscle weakness, myoclonus, anorexia, nausea, vomiting, hyporeflexia, seizures, stupor, coma, respiratory arrest, and death.

VII. COMPLICATIONS RELATED TO FLUID AND ELECTROLYTE DISTURBANCES

DIAGNOSIS

Diagnosis of SIADH is made on history, clinical examination, and laboratory investigations. Diagnosis requires exclusion of other causes of hyponatremia. Criteria for the diagnosis of SIADH includes:

1. Lack of evidence for volume overload (e.g., edema)
2. Hyponatremia
3. Hypotonicity (plasma osmolality <270 mOsmol/kg)
4. Inappropriately concentrated urine (urine osmolality >100 mOsmol/kg H_2O)
5. Urine sodium level >30 mEq/L
6. Sodium corrects with fluid restriction but not with 0.9% (normal) saline infusion
7. Normal renal, thyroid, and adrenal function.

DIFFERENTIAL DIAGNOSIS

- CSWS: It is characterized by hypovolemic hyponatremia compared to euvolemic hyponatremia in SIADH.
- Psychogenic polydipsia: It is characterized by euvolemic hyponatremia but can be distinguished from the SIADH on the basis of urine sodium and urine osmolality. In psychogenic polydipsia, the urine Na^+ is <10 mEq/L and urine osmolality is <100 mOsmol/kg compared to SIADH (>20 mEq/L and >100 mOsmol/kg, respectively).
- Inappropriate antidiuresis of nephrogenic origin (or nephrogenic syndrome of inappropriate antidiuresis): The clinical and laboratory features are consistent with SIADH but undetectable as levels of ADH. This may be due to gain of function mutations in the *AVPR2* gene (X-linked gene) on chromosome Xq28, which encodes the vasopressin V2 receptor.[8]

TREATMENT

In most cases, SIADH is an acute, self-limiting disorder that remits over several days to weeks.[1] However, during this period, correction of salt and water imbalances is usually essential. In most patients, fluid restriction is the treatment of choice. In case of severe hyponatremia (serum Na^+ <125 mmol/L), hypertonic saline (3%) infusion is used to correct the hyponatremia. The rate of correction of serum Na^+ should be 0.5–1 mmol/L/h with frequent monitoring of serum Na^+. The total serum sodium correction should not exceed 12 mmol/L over 24 h, and infusion should be stopped once the serum Na$^+$ reaches 130 mmol/L.[9] Rapid correction of hyponatremia is avoided to prevent central pontine myelinolysis. In patients where some underlying causes, such as tumor, drug, or disease is present, SIADH can be managed by eliminating the underlying disorder.

Close monitoring is required in patients who develop symptomatic hyponatremia and during correction of hyponatremia. Total fluid intake, urine output, and serum sodium levels should be measured. During correction of hyponatremia using hypertonic saline, serum Na$^+$ should be regularly measured every 2 h to monitor the speed of correction.

Medical therapy is indicated for refractory cases. Drugs used are given in Table 2. Vasopressin receptor antagonists (vaptans) are the armamentarium in this class that offers the targeted approach to the treatment of hyponatremia due to SIADH.[10] Conivaptan is Food and Drug Administration–approved for the treatment of euvolemic and hypervolemic hyponatremia in adults; however, the data related to its use in the pediatric population are extremely limited.[11]

Urea has been suggested for the management of hyponatremia linked to SIADH. A systemic review was performed, and the end result showed

TABLE 2 Drug Therapy for Treatment of SIADH

Drug	Action	Dose	Adverse effects
Demeclocycline	Inhibits action of ADH in the kidney	150–300 mg orally; Three times a day or Four times a day	Phototoxicity, azotemia
Fludrocortisone	Increases retention of Na$^+$ Possibly inhibits thirst	0.05–0.2 mg orally; Two times a day	Hypokalemia, hypertension
Conivaptan (combined V1a/V2 ADH receptor antagonist)	Block the antidiuretic effect of ADH Produces an increase in urinary free-water excretion	Administered only intravenously Loading dose 20 mg followed by infusion of 20–40 mg/24 h Maximum duration of treatment: 4 days	Thirst, central pontine myelinolysis, nausea, dry mouth, polyuria, fever, orthostatic hypotension, hypokalemia, inflammation of the infusion site
Tolvaptan (selective V2 ADH receptor antagonist)	Block the antidiuretic effect of ADH Produces an increase in urinary free-water excretion	15 mg once daily orally; may be increased to 30–60 mg qid	Thirst, central pontine myelinolysis, nausea, dry mouth, polyuria
Lithium carbonate	Inhibits ADH action in the kidney		

no evidence to support the efficacy of urea for the treatment of hyponatremia following SIADH.[12]

COMPLICATIONS OF SIADH

Complications during SIADH may develop due to hyponatremia or its correction. The complication depends on the rapidity of onset and the absolute decrease in serum Na^+ concentration. Hyponatremia promotes cerebral edema leading to encephalopathy. Hyponatremic encephalopathy carries a poor prognosis, especially in females.[13] Rapid and severe decrease in serum sodium may cause seizure, obtundation, coma, or death. Similarly, if the hyponatremia has been present for more than 24–48 h, the rapid correction of hyponatremia may cause central pontine myelinolysis, an acute and potentially fatal neurological complication caused due to osmotic demyelination of neurons. It is characterized by quadriparesis, ataxia, and abnormal extraocular movements.

PROGNOSIS AND PREVENTION

Prognosis of the condition depends on the severity and rate of development of hyponatremia and the underlying cause. Severe hyponatremia in SIADH, however, carries a high mortality rate.[14] There are no preventive strategies, but prompt treatment of the condition may improve the outcome.

References

1. Ellison DH, Berl T. The syndrome of inappropriate antidiuresis. *N Engl J Med*. 2007;356:2064–2072.
2. Schwartz WB, Bennett W, Curelop S, Bartter FC. A syndrome of renal sodium loss and hyponatremia probably resulting from inappropriate secretion of antidiuretic hormone. *Am J Med*. 1957;23:529–542.
3. Kruse JA. An endocrinology consult. In: Torbey, MT, ed. Neurocritical Care. 1st ed. New York, USA: Cambridge University Press; 2010: 397–409 [Chapter 29].
4. Bartter FC, Schwartz WB. The syndrome of inappropriate secretion of antidiuretic hormone. *Am J Med*. 1967;42:790–806.
5. Thompson C, Hoorn EJ. Hyponatremia: an overview of frequency, clinical presentation and complications. *Best Pract Res Clin Endocrinol Metab*. 2012;26(suppl 1):S1–S6.
6. Baylis PH. The syndrome of inappropriate antidiuretic hormone secretion. *Int J Biochem Cell Biol*. 2003;35:1495–1499.
7. Hannon MJ, Behan LA, O'Brien MM, Tormey W, Ball SG, Javadpour M, et al. Hyponatremia following mild/moderate subarachnoid hemorrhage is due to SIAD and glucocorticoid deficiency and not cerebral salt wasting. *J Clin Endocrinol Metab*. 2014;99:291–298.
8. Feldman BJ, Rosenthal SM, Vargas GA, et al. Nephrogenic syndrome of inappropriate antidiuresis. *N Engl J Med*. 2005;352:1884–1890.

9. Zietse R, van der Lubbe N, Hoorn EJ. Current and future treatment options in SIADH. *NDT Plus*. 2009;2(suppl 3):iii12–iii19.

10. Sherlock M, Thompson CJ. The syndrome of inappropriate antidiuretic hormone: current and future management options. *Eur J Endocrinol*. 2010;162:13–18.

11. Peters S, Kuhn R, Gardner B, Bernard P. Use of conivaptan for refractory syndrome of inappropriate secretion of antidiuretic hormone in a pediatric patient. *Pediatr Emerg Care*. 2013;29:230–232.

12. de Solà-Morales O, Riera M. Urea for management of the syndrome of inappropriate secretion of ADH: a systematic review. *Endocrinol Nutr*. November 2014;61(9):486–492. http://dx.doi.org/10.1016/j.endonu.2014.04.006. Epub June 19, 2014.

13. Arieff A. Influence of hypoxia and sex on hyponatremic encephalopathy. *Am J Med*. 2006;119:559–564.

14. Basu A, Ryder RE. The syndrome of inappropriate antidiuresis is associated with excess long-term mortality: a retrospective cohort analyses. *J Clin Pathol*. 2014;67:802–806.

POSTOPERATIVE PAIN

Pain Following Spinal Surgery

Zulfiqar Ali¹, Hemanshu Prabhakar²

¹Division of Neuroanesthesiology, Department of Anesthesiology, SKIMS,
Srinagar, Jammu and Kashmir, India; ²Department of Neuroanaesthesiology and
Critical Care, All India Institute of Medical Sciences, New Delhi, India

After a spinal surgery, acute pain is mainly generated from the skin, muscle, vertebrae, intervertebral discs, and facet joints. Following a spine surgery, most of the patients may have moderate to severe pain for the initial 3–4 days. The intensity of pain generated depends on the number of levels operated.[1] There seems to be no difference in the severity of pain, according to the region of the surgery, between cervical, thoracic, and lumbar spine surgeries.[2,3] Minimally invasive neurosurgical techniques are associated with minimum postoperative pain.[4]

TABLE 1   Pain Sensitive Tissues in the Spine

Skin, subcutaneous tissue, and adipose tissue
Paravertebral muscles
Capsules of facet and sacroiliac joints
Ligaments: longitudinal, interspinous, sacroiliac
Periosteum
Dura mater and epidural fibroadipose tissue
Nerve root sleeves

Pain management after surgery of the spine should be effective with minimum side effects. It should promote early rehabilitation and reduce postoperative morbidity. Several strategies have been used after spine surgery; however, there is a lack of systematic documentation with no known single strategy that has emerged as a "gold standard."[5]

PATHOPHYSIOLOGY

The spine has an adjacent, complex network of bones, joints, muscles, and ligaments, with multilevel crossovers in nerve supply. The causes of acute postoperative pain are the injury to the vertebral column, surrounding muscle, tendons, ligaments, fasciae, dura, nerve root sleeves, facet joint capsules, or a combination of these structures (Table 1).

The pain from these structures is transmitted from various nociceptors and mechanoreceptors via the posterior rami of spinal nerves to the sympathetic and parasympathetic nervous system. When compared to chronic spinal pain, which is mostly referred, the acute postoperative pain is mainly localized to the surgical site.[3]

TREATMENT MODALITIES FOR ACUTE POSTOPERATIVE SPINAL PAIN

Nonsteroidal Antiinflammatory Drugs

Nonsteroidal antiinflammatory drugs (NSAIDs) block the inflammatory mediators by acting on the cyclooxygenase (COX) enzyme, reducing the postoperative pain, and facilitating an early ambulation. Jirarattanaphochai and Jung conducted a metaanalysis comprising of 17 studies and found that patients receiving a combination of NSAIDs and opioids had lower pain scores than the group receiving opioids alone.[6] NSAIDs may be administered either orally (diclofenac sodium, ibuprofen, mefenamic acid) or intravenously (diclofenac or ketorolac). It has been found that ketorolac, when used with parenteral narcotics, is more effective than parenteral narcotics alone for postoperative pain following lumbar disc surgery. This combination has been found to contribute to an early discharge from the hospital after lumbar disc surgery.[7] NSAIDs are mainly helpful for the initial three days after surgery. In addition to causing platelet dysfunction, risk of hemorrhage, gastric ulceration, and renal toxicity, there are concerns that NSAIDs may affect the bone metabolism and osteoblastic proliferation. Reuben et al.[8] found that short-term perioperative administration of celecoxib, rofecoxib, or low-dose ketorolac (< or = 110 mg/day) had no significant deleterious effect on skeletal nonunion. In contrast, higher doses of ketorolac (120–240 mg/day), a history of smoking, and two-level vertebral fusions were found to significantly increase the incidence of nonunion following the spinal fusion surgery. Li et al.[9] did a metaanalysis comprising of five retrospective studies with 1,403 participants. The authors found that short-time (<14 days) exposure to normal-dose NSAIDs (ketorolac, diclofenac sodium, celecoxib, or rofecoxib) were safe after spinal fusion, whereas short-time (<14 days) exposure to high-dose ketorolac increased the risk of nonunion. Therefore, the effect of perioperative NSAIDs on spinal fusion might be dose-dependent. NSAIDs should be used cautiously in renal, coronary, and cerebrovascular diseases.

Paracetamol (acetaminophen) has emerged as an effective and safe drug for the treatment of postoperative pain. Acetaminophen has analgesic and antipyretic effects, but unlike NSAIDs, it has weak peripheral antiinflammatory effects.[10] It has minimal effect on the platelet function, making it useful during the intraoperative and postoperative periods.[11] The analgesic mechanism of acetaminophen is not understood properly. It is believed to have a central action by acting as an inhibitor of the prostaglandins via the COX pathway.[12,13] Acetaminophen rapidly enters the central nervous system (CNS), producing profound analgesia.[14,15] In vitro, acetaminophen demonstrated a 4.4 times receptor selectiveness to COX-2 compared with COX-1.[16] It is known to act as a nitric oxide pathway inhibitor through substance P or N-methyl-D-aspartate (NMDA)[17,18] and strengthens the descending serotonergic inhibitory pathways.[19] Active metabolites of acetaminophen have shown to affect the cannabinoid receptors.[20] After intravenous administration of acetaminophen, a rapid and high plasma concentration is achieved within 5 min.[21] Peak plasma concentration occurs within 15 min after administration.[22] The dose of intravenous acetaminophen in adolescents and adults is 1 g every 4–6 h, with a maximum daily dose of 4 g. In children more than 2 years, and adults weighing less than 50 kg, 15 mg/kg should be administered at the same interval. Children and infants less than 2 years of age should receive no more than 10 mg/kg, and neonates and premature infants 7.5 mg/kg. The elimination half-life is 2–3 h, and the duration of analgesic effect is approximately 4–6 h. This may be prolonged in infants, neonates, and patients with renal impairment.[23,24]

Corticosteroids

Aminmansour et al.[25] found that the administration of 40 mg dexamethasone effectively reduces the postoperative radicular leg pain and narcotics usage in patients operated on for single-level herniated lumbar disc. A systemic review was published in 2014 by Jamjoom et al.[26] to review the literature aimed at examining the efficacy of the use of intraoperative epidural steroids in lumbar disc surgery. Steroids may reduce the inflammation, inhibit phospholipase A2, and decrease substance P levels at the dorsal root ganglion.[27] Sixteen trials published from 1990 to 2012[26] showed strong evidence favoring the use of epidural steroids to reduce pain in the early postoperative stage (0–2 weeks). They found, however, that steroids are ineffective in reducing pain in the late stage (more than 2 months to 1 year) or in reducing the duration of hospital stay. Their effectiveness in reducing pain in the intermediate stage (more than 2 weeks to 2 months) was found to be limited. The authors, however, concluded that the heterogeneity between the trials made it difficult to make undisputed conclusions. Before any valid conclusions can be made, there is a need for a large multicenter trial.

Ketamine

Ketamine is an NMDA receptor antagonist that has been shown to be useful in the reduction of acute postoperative pain and analgesic consumption in a variety of surgical interventions. It is believed to reduce or reverse opioid tolerance in patients who are chronic opioid users. Loftus et al.[28] observed that intraoperative ketamine (0.5 mg/kg on induction of anesthesia, and a continuous infusion at 10 μg/kg/min) reduced the opiate consumption in the 48-h postoperative period in opiate-dependent patients with chronic pain. Abrishamkar et al.[29] found that ketamine could be a good alternative analgesic after fusion of lumbar spondylolisthesis. In comparison with morphine, it was found that ketamine was more efficient in pain reduction during the first 24 h (p < 0.001). Contradictory findings were observed by Subramaniam et al.,[30] who found out that the addition of low-dose ketamine infusion (2 μg/kg/min) regimen did not improve postoperative analgesia.

Another trial (https://clinicaltrials.gov/ct2/show/NCT02085577) is underway at the Department of Anesthesiology, Glostrup Hospital, Denmark, to address this issue. The data compilation will be completed by December 2016. This study may clarify some of the controversies on this issue.

Gabapentin

Turan et al.[31] studied the effects on gabapentin in patients undergoing spinal surgery. 1,200 mg of gabapentin 1 h before surgery was administered orally in a randomized fashion to 25 patients, and the results were compared with the placebo group. It was found that preoperative oral gabapentin decreased pain scores and postoperative morphine consumption in the early postoperative period. There was a decrease in morphine-associated side effects like vomiting and urinary retention, which were significantly ($P < 0.05$) higher in the placebo group. Similar results were observed with lower doses of gabapentin administered orally 2 h before surgery.[32] In pediatric patients, gabapentin administered at a dose of 5 mg/kg was found to reduce the amount of morphine used for postoperative pain in children undergoing surgery for spinal fusion. However, there was no reduction in the overall opioid-related side effects.[33]

Intravenous Patient-Controlled Analgesia

In Intravenous patient-controlled analgesia (PCA) therapy, the patients titrate their own need for analgesics to relieve the acute postoperative pain. An ideal drug for PCA should be highly efficacious, with a rapid onset of action and a moderate duration of action. It should not accumulate with repeated administrations and must have a large therapeutic window. Morphine, in the dose of 1–1.5 mg with a lock-out period of 5–10 min, is a commonly used drug for PCA.

Intrathecal Drug Administration

Administration of local anesthetics via intrathecal route for management of acute postspinal surgery pain is not popular as it may cause a motor and sensory block that hampers an adequate neurological assessment. Intrathecal morphine (0.4 mgs)[34] and fentanyl (15 µg)[35] have been evaluated for the control of postspinal surgery pain. It was seen that PCA requirements were significantly lower in the morphine group throughout the observed 20-h period after surgery. However, patients in the morphine group experienced mild respiratory depression 4 h after surgery, which did not require any intervention.[34] Chan et al.[35] found that the patients who received fentanyl demonstrated a significant decrease in their mean pain visual analog scale (VAS), an increase in the time to first PCA bolus, and a 41% reduction in the total PCA morphine received. No patients had respiratory compromise requiring treatment.

Epidural Drug Administration

Epidural catheters for postoperative pain relief are usually placed intraoperatively by the operating surgeon under direct vision. With epidural drug administration, there is an advantage of analgesia for a prolonged period with decreased incidences of respiratory and thromboembolic events. Local anesthetics commonly used are bupivacaine and ropivacaine. They should be used judiciously as they may interfere with the neurological assessment and may lead to hypotension. Among the local anesthetics, ropivacaine is the choice of agent due to its better safety profile and selectivity toward sensory blockade.

After epidural administration, variable quantities (depending on the opioid used) of the drug diffuse across the dura and arachnoid mater into the subarachnoid space to bind opioid receptors in the dorsal horn of the spinal cord. The lipid solubility of the drug determines the rate of diffusion and the onset and duration of analgesia. Lipophilic opioids such as fentanyl and sufentanil diffuse rapidly across the dura into the cerebrospinal fluid (CSF) compared to hydrophilic opioids such as morphine. Lipophilic opioids produce rapid onset of analgesia, which is of a short duration. After epidural delivery, CSF opioid levels peak at 6 min for sufentanil, 20 min for fentanyl, and 1–4 h for morphine. The epidural space is extremely vascular and there is extensive absorption of opioids via the epidural venous plexus into the systemic circulation. Systemic opioids reach the CNS and bind receptors in areas of the brain that modulate pain perception and response.

Guilfoyle et al.[36] observed the effects of 100-μg bolus of fentanyl administered via an epidural catheter inserted 10 cm rostral to the operated level in patients undergoing a lumbar canal decompression. The authors found that the VAS score in the recovery area was significantly lower in patients treated with fentanyl when compared with the control group. However, the patients who received fentanyl required temporary urethral catheterization more frequently when compared with the control group.

Other studies[37,38] have shown that the intravenous PCA and epidural PCA are equally effective in controlling the pain in patients undergoing spine surgery. However, a greater incidence of side effects is seen in the patients in whom the drugs are administered epidurally.[38] The epidural administration of opioids should be monitored carefully for inadvertent respiratory depression due to the diffusion of opioids in the CSF.

Alpha 2 Adrenoreceptor Antagonists

Both clonidine and dexmedetomidine potentiate the actions of local anesthetics and opioids providing better analgesia in postspinal surgery. Both epidural clonidine and subcutaneous incisional bupivacaine,[39] added to spinal anesthesia for lumbar spine surgery, have been found to improve pain relief and reduce the need for postoperative opioids. Ekatodramis et al.[40]

found that when a double epidural catheter (one cranial, one caudal to the surgical field) was inserted by the surgeon at the end of the surgery and a combination of three drugs (bupivacaine, fentanyl, and clonidine) was used, a complete analgesia (VAS=0) was obtained at rest in all patients. During mobilization and physiotherapy, four patients (17%) had a VAS of 30. Farmery et al. found that use of epidural clonidine reduced the demand for morphine in the initial 36 h with an associated reduction in the incidence of nausea.[41]

Dexmedetomidine is a better neuraxial adjuvant compared with clonidine for providing early onset and prolonged postoperative analgesia and stable cardiorespiratory parameters. Saravana et al. found that those patients who received 20 mL of 0.2% ropivacaine and 1 μg/kg of dexmedetomidine had early onset, early peak effect, prolonged duration, and stable cardiorespiratory parameters when compared with those patients who received 20 mL of 0.2% ropivacaine and 2 μg/kg of clonidine through the epidural catheter.[42] Similarly, dexmedetomidine has displayed superior efficacy in alleviating pain after posterior lumbar interbody fusion for 48 h.[43] Rapid and predictable recovery with dexmedetomidine allows for early neurological assessment that is important following spinal surgeries.

Newer Modalities

One of the limitations of local anesthetics in the postoperative setting is its relatively short duration of action. Multivesicular liposomes containing bupivacaine have been increasingly utilized for their increased duration of action. Compared with bupivacaine hydrochloride, local infiltration of liposomal bupivacaine has shown to have an increase in duration of action. Preliminary clinical trials suggest that liposomal bupivacaine has predictable pharmacokinetics, a similar side effect profile compared with bupivacaine hydrochloride, and is effective in providing increased postoperative pain control.[44] Though liposomal bupivacaine has been compared with placebo in two multicenter trials[45] in patients undergoing soft-tissue surgery and orthopedic surgeries, its application in spinal surgeries has not been studied so far.

Extended-release epidural morphine (EREM) has been developed and is believed to provide effective postoperative analgesia for 48 h following injection. It is administered as a single bolus into the lumbar epidural space and is indicated for lower abdominal and lower extremity surgery associated with moderate to severe pain.[46] While its efficacy has been well documented in randomized controlled trials, the safety and clinically appropriate dosing are less well defined. Epidural morphine 15 mg or greater was associated with a trend toward an increased incidence of hypoventilation, pruritus, and vomiting when compared with placebo. A multimodal analgesic regime is recommended to permit the use of lower EREM doses, thus reducing the risk for adverse effects including respiratory depression.

Vineyard JC et al. compared the analgesic effects of extended release epidural morphine formulation (DepoDur) with preservative-free morphine sulfate injection (Duramorph) for pain control after lumbar spine surgery.[47] The authors found that there were no significant differences between the two groups in postoperative pain VAS scores. Patients receiving DepoDur were less likely to receive naloxone and oxygen supplementation or experience nausea or fever; however, they had higher incidences of hypotension.

CONCLUSION

In a prospective cohort study comparing 179 surgical procedures, the spinal surgeries were among the first 6 procedures in terms of the intensity of postoperative pain.[48] Hence, adequate postoperative pain management is needed to improve the functional outcome after surgery. An adequate pain control will lead to early ambulation and shorter hospital stays with a decreased incidence of respiratory complications and venous thrombosis. There is no single drug that may be the "gold standard" for pain control following spinal surgery.

Devin and McGirt[49] did a comprehensive literature review to determine grades of recommendation for commonly used agents in multimodal pain management and tried to provide a best practice guideline for patients undergoing spinal surgery. The authors found a good (Grade A) evidence for gabapentinoids, acetaminophen, neuraxial blockade, and extended-release local anesthetics in reducing postoperative pain and narcotic requirements. There was fair (Grade B) evidence that preemptive analgesia and NSAIDs result in reduced postoperative pain. There was insufficient and conflicting evidence that muscle relaxants and ketamine provide a significant reduction in postoperative pain or narcotic usage. They found fair (Grade B) evidence that short-term use of NSAIDs results in no long-term reduction in bone healing or fusion rates. Evidence (49) shows that multimodal pain management protocols allow for improved pain control with less reliance on opioids. Table 2 summarizes the commonly used drugs along with their doses in the postoperative period for management of postspinal surgery pain. There is quality evidence to support many of the common agents utilized in multimodal therapy; however, there is a lack of evidence regarding optimal postoperative protocols or pathways. The development of such protocols could be an area for future research.

TABLE 2 Commonly Used Drugs Along With Their Doses in the Postoperative
Period for Management of Postspinal Surgery Pain

Drug	Dose	Remarks
1. Paracetamol	IV 1. Adults 1 g every 4–6 h, maximum daily dose of 4 g 2. In children of 2 years, and adolescents, and adults weighing less than 50 kg, 15 mg/kg. 3. Children and infants less than 2 years of age not more than 10 mg/kg, and neonates and premature infants 7.5 mg/kg	Dose reduction if weight <50 kg and/or risk factors for hepatic impairment
2. NSAIDs	1. First line: Ibuprofen 400 PO mg qds 2. Second line: Naproxen 500 PO mg bd or diclofenac 50 PO mg tds	
3. Gabapentin	1. 600 mg PO 2 h preoperatively and then 300 mg PO tds while an inpatient	Modify dose in renal impairment eGFR <50 mL/min
4. Opioids minor procedures, e.g., lumbar discectomy/ ACDF	Regimen I 1. Oral morphine 10–20 mg qds + 10 mg q2h prn 2. Oxycodone 5–10 mg qds + 5 mg q2h prn Regimen II Modified release regimen: 1. Morphine sulfate capsules 20–30 mg bd + oral morphine 10 mg q2h prn 2. Oxycodone capsules 10–15 mg bd + oxycodone 5–10 mg q2h prn	Morphine first-line unless contraindicated or previous side effects Prescriptions should include a stop date and all opioids should be reviewed on discharge
Major procedures	Morphine IV PCA 1 mg bolus 5 min lockout, no background Oxycodone IV PCA 1 mg bolus 5 min lockout, no background	Dosing modification is required for opioid-tolerant patients Consider ketamine
4a. PCA analgesic failure	1. In case of analgesic failure oral morphine PO 10–20 mg stat	Consider stopping PCA and transferring to oral analgesia
5. Ketamine	For patients >50 kg if no contraindications: Prepare a ketamine 2 mg/mL infusion (ketamine 100 mg made up to 50 mL with 0.9% saline). Typical starting dose 0.1 mg/kg/h Dose range: Ketamine 2–8 mg/h This may be preceded by a bolus: 0.25–0.5 mg/kg	Precautions: Elderly patients, ischemic heart disease, hypertension, raised intracranial pressure, head trauma, acute porphyria, and any condition where elevation of blood pressure is hazardous. In case of hallucinations, consider diazepam 0.5–1 mg prn

Continued

VIII. POSTOPERATIVE PAIN

TABLE 2   Commonly Used Drugs Along With Their Doses in the Postoperative Period for Management of Postspinal Surgery Pain—cont'd

Drug	Dose	Remarks
5a. Oral ketamine: Patient discharged toward/ neurosurgical postoperative unit	Dose: Ketamine PO 10–20 mg qds PO increasing in 10 mg increments up to a maximum 50 mg qds	
5b. Opioid-dependent patients	Patients receiving morphine intravenous equivalent 0.5 mg/h preoperatively may benefit from: Ketamine bolus 0.5 mg/kg followed by 10 mcg/kg/min throughout the operation	For opioid-dependent patients, the baseline opioid should be maintained or replaced

References

1. Sharma S, Balireddy RK, Vorenkamp KE, et al. Beyond opioid patient-controlled analgesia: a systematic review of analgesia after major spine surgery. *Reg Anesth Pain Med.* 2012;37:79–98.
2. Bernard JM, Surbled M, Lagarde D, Trennec A. Analgesia after surgery of the spine in adults and adolescents. *Cah Anesthesiol.* 1995;43:557–564.
3. Klimek M, Ubben JF, Ammann J, Borner U, Klein J, Verbrugge SJ. Pain in neurosurgically treated patients: a prospective observational study. *J Neurosurg.* 2006;104:350–359.
4. Oskouian RJ, Johnson JP. Endoscopic thoracic microdiscectomy. *J Neurosurg Spine.* 2005;3:459–464.
5. Borgeat A, Blumenthal S. Postoperative pain management following scoliosis surgery. *Curr Opin Aneasthesiol.* 2008;21:313–316.
6. Jirarattanaphochai K, Jung S. Nonsteroidal antiinflammatory drugs for postoperative pain management after lumbar spine surgery: a meta-analysis of randomized controlled trials. *J Neurosurg Spine.* 2008;9:22–31.
7. Le Roux PD, Samudrala S. Postoperative pain after lumbar disc surgery: a comparison between parenteral ketorolac and narcotics. *Acta Neurochir (Wien).* 1999;141:261–267.
8. Reuben SS, Ablett D, Kaye R. High dose nonsteroidal anti-inflammatory drugs compromise spinal fusion. *Can J Anaesth.* 2005;52:506–512.
9. Li Q, Zhang Z, Cai Z. High-dose ketorolac affects adult spinal fusion: a meta-analysis of the effect of perioperative nonsteroidal anti-inflammatory drugs on spinal fusion. *Spine (Phila Pa 1976).* 2011;36:E461–E468.
10. Niemi TT, Backman JT, Syrjälä MT, Viinikka LU, Rosenberg PH. Platelet dysfunction after intravenous ketorolac or propacetamol. *Acta Anaesthesiol Scand.* 2000;44:69–74.
11. Cattabriga I, Pacini D, Lamazza G, et al. Intravenous paracetamol as adjunctive treatment for postoperative pain after cardiac surgery: a double blind randomized controlled trial. *Eur J Cardiothorac Surg.* 2007;32:527–531.
12. Smith HS. Perioperative intravenous acetaminophen and NSAIDs. *Pain Med.* 2011;12:961–981.

13. Boutaud O, Aronoff DM, Richardson JH, Marnett LJ, Oates JA. Determinants of the cellular specificity of acetaminophen as an inhibitor of prostaglandin H(2) synthases. *Proc Natl Acad Sci USA*. 2002;99:7130–7135.
14. Smith HS. Potential analgesic mechanisms of acetaminophen. *Pain Physician*. 2009;12: 269–280.
15. Kumpulainen E, Kokki H, Halonen T, Heikkinen M, Savolainen J, Laisalmi M. Paracetamol (acetaminophen) penetrates readily into the cerebrospinal fluid of children after intravenous administration. *Pediatrics*. 2007;119:766–771.
16. Hinz B, Cheremina O, Brune K. Acetaminophen (paracetamol) is a selective cyclooxygenase-2 inhibitor in man. *FASEB J*. 2008;22:383–390.
17. Björkman R, Hallman KM, Hedner J, Hedner T, Henning M. Acetaminophen blocks spinal hyperalgesia induced by NMDA and substance P. *Pain*. 1994;57:259–264.
18. Bujalska M. Effect of nitric oxide synthase inhibition on antinociceptive action of different doses of acetaminophen. *Pol J Pharmacol*. 2004;56:605–610.
19. Pickering G, Esteve V, Loriot MA, Eschalier A, Dubray C. Acetaminophen reinforces descending inhibitory pain pathways. *Clin Pharmacol Ther*. 2008;84:47–51.
20. Ottani A, Leone S, Sandrini M, Ferrari A, Bertolini A. The analgesic activity of paracetamol is prevented by the blockade of cannabinoid CB1 receptors. *Eur J Pharmacol*. 2006;531:280–281.
21. Moller PL, Sindet-Pedersen S, Petersen CT, Juhl GI, Dillenschneider A, Skoglund LA. Onset of acetaminophen analgesia: comparison of oral and intravenous routes after third molar surgery. *Br J Anaesth*. 2005;94:642–648.
22. Holmer Pettersson P, Owall A, Jakobsson J. Early bioavailability of paracetamol after oral or intravenous administration. *Acta Anaesthesiol Scand*. 2004;48:867–870.
23. Palmer GM, Atkins M, Anderson BJ, et al. I.V. acetaminophen pharmacokinetics in neonates after multiple doses. *Br J Anaesth*. 2008;101:523–530.
24. Duggan ST, Scott LJ. Intravenous paracetamol (acetaminophen). *Drugs*. 2009;69:101–113.
25. Aminmansour B, Khalili HA, Ahmadi J, Nourian M. Effect of high-dose intravenous dexamethasone on postlumbar discectomy pain. *Spine (Phila Pa 1976)*. 2006;31:2415–2417.
26. Jamjoom BA, Jamjoom AB. Efficacy of intraoperative epidural steroids in lumbar discectomy: a systematic review. *BMC Musculoskelet Disord*. 2014;5(15):146.
27. Wong HK, Tan KJ. Effects of corticosteroids on nerve root recovery after spinal nerve root compression. *Clin Orthop Relat Res*. 2002;403:248–252.
28. Loftus RW, Yeager MP, Clark JA, et al. Intraoperative ketamine reduces perioperative opiate consumption in opiate-dependent patients with chronic back pain undergoing back surgery. *Anesthesiology*. 2010;113:639–646.
29. Abrishamkar S, Eshraghi N, Feizi A, Talakoub R, Rafiei A, Rahmani P. Analgesic effects of ketamine infusion on postoperative pain after fusion and instrumentation of the lumbar spine: a prospective randomized clinical trial. *Med Arh*. 2012;66:107–110.
30. Subramaniam K, Akhouri V, Glazer PA, et al. Intra- and postoperative very low dose intravenous ketamine infusion does not increase pain relief after major spine surgery in patients with preoperative narcotic analgesic intake. *Pain Med*. 2011;12:1276–1283.
31. Turan A, Karamanlioğlu B, Memiş D, et al. Analgesic effects of gabapentin after spinal surgery. *Anesthesiology*. April 2004;100(4):935–938.
32. Pandey CK, Sahay S, Gupta D, et al. Preemptive gabepentine decreases postoperative pain after lumbar discectomy. *Can J Anaesth*. 2004;51:986–989.
33. Rusy LM, Hainsworth KR, Nelson TJ, et al. Gabapentine use in pediatric spinal fusion patients: a randomized double-blind, control trial. *Anesth Analg*. 2010;110: 1393–1398.
34. Ziegeler S, Fritsch E, Bauer C, et al. Therapeutic effect of intrathecal morphine after posterior lumbar interbody fusion surgery: a prospective, double-blind, randomized study. *Spine (Phila Pa 1976)*. 2008;33:2379–2386.

35. Chan JH, Heilpern GN, Packham I, Trehan RK, Marsh GD, Knibb AA. A prospective randomized double-blind trial of the use of intrathecal fentanyl in patients undergoing lumbar spinal surgery. *Spine (Phila Pa 1976)*. 2006;31:2529–2533.

36. Guilfoyle MR, Mannion RJ, Mitchell P, Thomson S. Epidural fentanyl for postoperative analgesia after lumbar canal decompression: a randomized controlled trial. *Spine J.* 2012;12:646–651.

37. O'Hara Jr JF, Cywinski JB, Tetzlaff JE, Xu M, Gurd AR, Andrish JT. The effect of epidural vs intravenous analgesia for posterior spinal fusion surgery. *Paediatr Anaesth.* 2004;14:1009–1015.

38. Fisher CG, Belanger L, Gofton EG, et al. Prospective randomized clinical trial comparing patient-controlled intravenous analgesia with patient-controlled epidural analgesia after lumbar spinal fusion. *Spine (Phila Pa 1976)*. 2003;28:739–743.

39. Jellish WS, Abodeely A, Fluder EM, Shea J. The effect of spinal bupivacaine in combination with either epidural clonidine and/or 0.5% bupivacaine administered at the incision site on postoperative outcome in patients undergoing lumbar laminectomy. *Anesth Analg.* 2003;96:874–880.

40. Ekatodramis G, Min K, Cathrein P, Borgeat A. Use of a double epidural catheter provides effective postoperative analgesia after spine deformity surgery. *Reg Anesth Pain Med.* 2002;49:173–177.

41. Farmery AD, Wilson-MacDonald J. The analgesic effect of epidural clonidine after spinal surgery: a randomized placebo-controlled trial. *Anesth Analg.* 2009;108:631–634.

42. Saravana Babu M, Verma AK, Agarwal A, Tyagi CM, Upadhyay M, Tripathi S. A comparative study in the post-operative spine surgeries: epidural ropivacaine with dexmedetomidine and ropivacaine with clonidine for post-operative analgesia. *Indian J Anaesth.* 2013;57:371–376.

43. Hwang W, Lee J, Park J, Joo J. Dexmedetomidine versus remifentanil in postoperative pain control after spinal surgery: a randomized controlled study. *BMC Anesthesiol.* 2015;15:21.

44. Tong YC, Kaye AD, Urman RD. Liposomal bupivacaine and clinical outcomes. *Best Pract Res Clin Anaesthesiol.* 2014;28:15–27.

45. Candiotti K. Liposomal bupivacaine: an innovative nonopioid local analgesic for the management of postsurgical pain. *Pharmacotherapy.* 2012;32:19S–26S.

46. Hartrick CT, Hartrick KA. Extended—Release epidural morphine (DepoDur): review and safety analysis. *Expert Rev Neurother.* 2008;8:1641–1648.

47. Vineyard JC, Toohey JS, Neidre A, Fogel G, Joyner R. Evaluation of a single-dose, extended-release epidural morphine formulation for pain control after lumbar spine surgery. *J Surg Orthop Adv.* 2014;23:9–12.

48. Gerbershagen HJ, Aduckathil S, van Wijck AJ, Peelen LM, Kalkman CJ, Meissner W. Pain intensity on the first day after surgery: a prospective cohort study comparing 179 surgical procedures. *Anesthesiology.* 2013;118:934–944.

49. Devin CJ, McGirt MJ. Best evidence in multimodal pain management in spine surgery and means of assessing postoperative pain and functional outcomes. *J Clin Neurosci.* 2015;22:930–938.

Postcraniotomy Pain

Zulfiqar Ali[1], Hemanshu Prabhakar[2]

[1]Division of Neuroanesthesiology, Department of Anesthesiology, SKIMS, Srinagar, Jammu and Kashmir, India; [2]Department of Neuroanaesthesiology and Critical Care, All India Institute of Medical Sciences, New Delhi, India

DEFINITION

Acute postoperative pain is defined as the pain occurring within first 24–48h after a craniotomy.

In a pilot study, De Benedittis et al. found that 60% of postcraniotomy patients suffered from moderate to severe postoperative pain.[1] In two-thirds of the patients, the intensity of pain was moderate to severe. Pain was mainly seen in the first 48 h after surgery, with subtemporal and suboccipital craniotomies associated with the highest incidence of postoperative pain.[2-5] Despite the advances in the treatment of acute pain, a gold standard for analgesic therapy in this subgroup of patients is still lacking.[6,7]

ANATOMICAL AND PHYSIOLOGICAL BASIS OF PAIN FOLLOWING CRANIOTOMY

The calvarium encloses and protects the brain. The facial skeleton forms the lower part of the skull and articulates with the mandible. The scalp consists of five layers: skin, subcutaneous tissue, epicranium, subaponeurotic areolar tissue, and the pericranium.

The interior of the cranium is lined with a fibrous membrane, the endocranium, which is the outer zone of the dura mater. It becomes continuous with the periosteum on the outer surface of the skull, the pericranium. The brain is enveloped by three layers of meninges: the dura mater, the arachnoid, and the pia mater.

Innervation of the scalp and the dura is mainly arising from:

1. The trigeminal nerve, and its three principal divisions (mandibular, maxillary, and ophthalmic) and their branches;
2. The upper three cervical nerves and the cervical sympathetic trunk;
3. Minor branches from the vagus, hypoglossus, facial, and glossopharyngeal nerves.

The anterior scalp region is innervated by the supraorbital and supratrochlear nerves (branches of the frontal nerve). The temporal scalp region is supplied by the zygomaticotemporal, temporomandibular, and auriculotemporal nerves (branches of the trigeminal nerve; Figure 1). The occiput and scalp regions receive their sensory innervations from the greater auricular and the greater and lesser occipital nerves (originating from the cervical plexus). The dura mater is innervated by nerves that accompany the meningeal arteries.

Surgical approaches to the skull are mainly supratentorial and infratentorial. Supratentorial craniotomies are mainly frontal, frontotemporal, temporal, and pterional.

PATHOGENESIS OF POSTCRANIOTOMY PAIN

Postcraniotomy pain is superficial in character,[1] suggesting a somatic rather than a visceral origin. The pain mainly originates from the pericranial muscles and soft tissues. The suboccipital and subtemporal

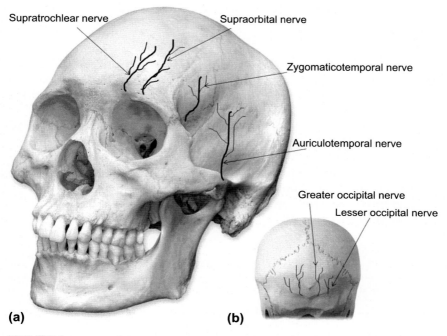

Supratrochlear nerve

Supraorbital nerve

Zygomaticotemporal nerve

Auriculotemporal nerve

Greater occipital nerve

Lesser occipital nerve

(a)   **(b)**

FIGURE 1   Nerves of the scalp that are blocked to produce the "scalp block": (a) nerves in the frontotemporal region; (b) nerves in the occipital region.

craniotomies have the highest incidence of pain due to nociceptive pain from surgical incision and reflection of major muscles as temporal, splenium capitis, and cervicis. The skull can be drilled and opened without discomfort to the patient (no sensory innervation). Pain is not thought to arise from the dissection of the brain tissue itself.[1,8]

Compared to the traditional theory of pain perception, where it was believed that pain is directly transmitted from somatic receptors to the brain, clinical and experimental evidence shows that noxious stimuli may sensitize the central neural structures involved in pain perception. Experimental evidence shows the development of sensitization, wind-up, or expansion of receptive fields of central nervous system neurons.

PREEMPTION OF PAIN

The concept of preemptive analgesia was suggested by Walls,[9] who found that the effects of preemptive analgesia may even outlast the presence of drugs.[10] Severe or prolonged acute pain in the postoperative period along with postsurgical complications may lead to increased nociception. This may lead to the development of the chronic pain.

TREATMENT OF ACUTE PAIN

Infiltration with Local Anesthetic

Preincisional local anesthetic scalp infiltration blunts the hemodynamic responses to craniotomy and minimizes bleeding from the skin incision by vasoconstrictive properties of the adrenaline added to the local anesthetic.

The infiltration of the scalp for skeletal fixation, skin incision, and wound closure has been found to reduce the postoperative pain scores, though there has been little effect on hemodynamics.[11] The postoperative scalp block with ropivacaine (Table 1) has been found to decrease the severity of postcraniotomy pain, even up to 48 h, possibly through a preemptive mechanism.[12] A reduced stress response has been associated with scalp block using 0.5% bupivacaine. Lower plasma

TABLE 1   Commonly Used Drugs and Their Doses Used for Postcraniotomy Pain

Local anesthetics and their doses that can be used for scalp blocks			
Agent	Concentration available	Maximum dose (mg/kg)	Typical duration of the nerve block
Bupivacaine	0.25%,0.5%,0.75%	3	Long
Lidocaine (Lignocaine)	0.2%,1%,1.5%,2%,4%	4.5, 7 (with epinephrine)	Medium
Mepivacaine	1%,1.5%,2%,3%	4.5, 7 (with epinephrine)	Medium
Ropivacaine	0.2%,0.5%,0.75%	3	Long

Opioids			
Agent	Dose and duration	Route of administration	Lock out interval (minutes)
Codeine phosphate	30–60 mg 4 h	Oral/rectal intramuscular[17,18]	
Morphine	Intravenously through PCA pump	1–1.5 mgs	8–10 min with a 4 h limit of 40 mg[20]
Fentanyl	Intravenously through PCA pump	(0.2 μg/kg/h)	6–8 min with a 4 h limit of 300 μg[28]
Tramadol PCA set to deliver 10 mg boluses with a 5 min lockout and a 4 h limit of 200 mg.		10 mg	5 min lockout and a 4 h limit of 200 mg[29]

PCA, patient-controlled analgesia; μg, micrograms.

cortisol and adrenocorticotropic hormone levels were seen with the scalp block when compared with local infiltration at pin sites using 0.5% bupivacaine.[13]

Use of Opioids

Parenteral opioids are mainly used for intraoperative pain during craniotomy surgeries.

During the postoperative period in spontaneously-breathing patients, there are fears of excessive sedation and respiratory depression with the use of parenteral opioids. Opioids may lead to respiratory depression, CO_2 retention, increased blood flow, and increased intracranial pressure.[14,15]

Intermittent systemic administration of opioids for postoperative pain relief may result in alternate periods of oversedation and inadequate analgesia. Patient-controlled analgesia (PCA) with morphine or oxycodone may be effective for postcraniotomy pain.[16] However, the occurrence of postoperative sedation may be troublesome because of the need of frequent postoperative neurological examinations.

Morphine, when used for postcraniotomy pain, may produce miosis, sedation, nausea, and respiratory depression. However, in the published clinical studies, none of these effects have been seen to be of clinical significance. Also, there are no clinical studies to date that have evaluated the safety of intravenous morphine in clinical doses that provide adequate postcraniotomy pain control.

Codeine phosphate, 30–60 mg 4-hourly is used in the immediate postoperative period by oral, rectal, or intramuscular routes because of its ceiling to its respiratory depressant effects.[17,18] It has an added advantage that it does not mask the pupillary signs. Following absorption, codeine undergoes demethylation with a cytochrome P450 enzyme to form morphine. Those patients with a cytochrome P450 gene with inactivating mutations are poor metabolizers. They have a severely compromised ability to metabolize codeine. The traditional use of codeine has shown to have inadequate analgesia.[19] Stoneham and Walters[19,20] recommend the use of PCA with morphine as a better alternative to codeine.

Jellish et al. published their experience of morphine use over 2 years by PCA. The authors found that a dosing regimen of 1.5 mg morphine with a lockout period of 8 min was associated with no incidence of respiratory depression or reintubation. The authors recommended that the total dose of morphine in 4 h should not exceed 40 mg.[21] Goldsack et al.[22] compared the use of intramuscular morphine with that of intramuscular codeine in a double-blind trial. The authors found that 10 mgs of intramuscular morphine was more efficacious than 60 mgs of intramuscular codeine in terms of pain relief. None of their patients exhibited any form of respiratory depression, sedation, pupillary constriction, or unwanted cardiovascular effects.

Nonsteroidal Antiinflammatory Drugs

The three major concerns about the use of NSAIDs for postoperative pain relief mainly after a craniotomy include: (1) effects on myocardial ischemia; (2) effects on platelet function and consequent increase in the incidence of postoperative hematoma; and (3) effects on renal function. These concerns are mainly from data collected from studies conducted in patients receiving NSAIDs from a few days to several weeks or months preoperatively.[23]

The effect of perioperative NSAIDs on blood coagulation is a major concern after a craniotomy. Palmer et al. in their study conducted over a period of 5 years found that the incidence of postoperative hematoma was 1.1% in a retrospective series of 6668 neurosurgical procedures. NSAID use in the 2 weeks preceding surgery was reported as a possible cause of postoperative hematoma. All but one patient with postoperative wound hematoma received either aspirin or NSAIDs within 2 weeks before surgery.[15]

There is a significant difference between nonselective NSAIDs and COX-2 inhibitors with regards to their potential to cause hemostatic complications. The likelihood of developing various complications was higher by 5.8 times for patients using NSAIDs 24 h before surgery.[24] In contrast to nonselective NSAIDs, celecoxib in doses of 1200 mg per day administered for 10 consecutive days in healthy adults demonstrated no effect on platelet aggregation or bleeding time.[25]

More clarity is required with regards to the safety and efficacy of NSAIDs for postcraniotomy pain relief. It seems to be clear that preoperative NSAIDs should be stopped prior to intracranial surgery. Also, COX-2 inhibitors in the postoperative period should be avoided in patients with cardiac disease.

Repeated use of paracetamol may not be sufficient for adequate pain relief in adult postcraniotomy patients unlike that in the pediatric population.[6]

POSTCRANIOTOMY PAIN MANAGEMENT IN THE PEDIATRIC POPULATION

There is scanty information about analgesia use or pain experienced in children after neurosurgical procedures. The children undergoing neurosurgical procedures may be inadequately treated due to a presumed lack of need, and a concern that opioids will adversely affect postoperative outcome and interfere with the neurologic examination.[26] Maxwell et al. conducted a study at three university hospitals to see the incidence of pain, the prescribed analgesics, methods of analgesic delivery, and patient/parent satisfaction in pediatric patients undergoing cranial surgery. In 284 pediatric patients studied, they found that the commonly-used analgesics in the postoperative period were oral oxycodone and/or acetaminophen. Patients were evaluated daily by a study investigator and by chart review for pain scores using age appropriate, validated tools. Pain scores in the studied children were low, side effects were minimal, and parental satisfaction was high.[26]

Another study conducted by Teo et al.[27] also tried to assess the degree of pain experienced by children after neurosurgery and the analgesic regimens used. The authors also tried to identify factors associated with significant pain in children undergoing neurosurgical procedures. Data for 52 children who underwent craniotomy were collected over 72h. The authors observed that for most of the time the children had little or no pain. Over the 72h, the median pain score recorded by nursing staff was 0.7 and 1.3 by the auditor. However, in spite of the low median scores, 42% of children had at least one episode of a pain score > or =3. Postoperatively, 71% of children received parenteral morphine, 92% of children received paracetamol, 35% oxycodone, 19% oral codeine, 4% tramadol, and 2% ibuprofen. Using multivariate regression, duration of procedure was the only factor associated with parenteral morphine use for >24h, and older age was the only factor associated with having an episode of pain scoring >3.

Commonly used drugs and their doses in the pediatric neurosurgical population are summarized in Table 2. Paracetamol is used in neurosurgical patients but may cause increased bleeding time due to dysfunction of the platelet. Therefore, paracetamol should be used carefully in the early postcraniotomy period to avoid devastating bleeding after neurosurgery.

CONCLUSION

Perioperative pain management in neurosurgical patients has been inadequately recognized and under treated. An increased awareness and a better understanding of pain modulation has led to improved practices and a better perioperative care of patients following craniotomy. The greatest challenge in managing postcraniotomy pain is the need to assess the neurological function while providing adequate analgesia with minimal respiratory depression. To achieve this goal, a multimodal approach to analgesia using various drugs and techniques may be practiced. Randomized controlled trials are needed so as to determine the best combination of drugs or techniques for treating perioperative pain in this patient population.

TABLE 2   Drugs and Their Doses in Pediatric Neurosurgical Population

Drug	Route	Dose
Paracetamol	Suspension Tablets Suppositories	20 mg/kg 6-hourly PO/PR for 48 h, then reduce to 15/mg/kg 6-hourly Maximum daily dose 75 mg/kg, not exceeding 4 g/day
Intravenous paracetamol	Only to be prescribed if oral route not available	≤10 kg–7.5 mg/kg 6-hourly
	50 mLs–500 mg	>10 kg–15 mg/kg 6-hourly
	100 mLs–1 g	>50 kg–1 g max 6-hourly
Morphine	Oramorph: 10 mg/5 mL	Orally
	Tablets: 10, 20 mg	≤12 months: 50 µg/kg 4-hourly
	Injection: 15 mg/mL	>12 months: 100–300 µg/kg 4-hourly
		Intravenous
		≤6 months 100 µg/kg 6-hourly
		>6 months 100 µg/kg 6-hourly
		Oramorph
		>12 months–100 µg/kg 6-hourly
		If OSA/altered respiratory drive: 50 µg/kg 6-hourly

INTRAVENOUS MORPHINE INFUSION

Any patient requiring a morphine infusion with needs admission in a high dependency unit.	Ensure adequate loading dose of 100 µg/kg	0–1 months: Maximum of 5 µg/kg/h 1–3 months: Maximum of 10 µg/kg/h Over 3 months: Maximum of 40 µg/kg/h Maximum infusion rate should be 2 mL/h, which is equal to 40 µg/kg/h.

MORPHINE PCA

For use in 4 years and above; usually have the ability to understand and push the button.	Loading dose: 100 µg/kg Bolus: 20 µg/kg Lockout 5 min.	

References

1. De Benedittis G, Lorenzetti A, Migliore M, et al. Postoperative pain in neurosurgery: a pilot study in brain surgery. *Neurosurgery*. 1996;38:466–469.
2. Klimek M, Ubben JF, Ammann J, et al. Pain in neurosurgically treated patients: a prospective observational study. *J Neurosurg*. 2006;104:350–359.
3. Gottschalk A, Berkow LC, Stevens RD, et al. Prospective evaluation of pain and analgesic use following major elective intracranial surgery. *J Neurosurg*. 2007;106:210–216.
4. Quiney N, Cooper R, Stoneham M, et al. Pain after craniotomy. A time for reappraisal? *Br J Neurosurg*. 1996;10:295–299.
5. Mordhorst C, Latz B, Kerz T, et al. Prospective assessment of postoperative pain after craniotomy. *J Neurosurg Anesthesiol*. 2010;22:202–206.
6. Nemergut EC, Durieux ME, Missaghi NB, et al. Pain management after craniotomy. *Best Pract Res Clin Anaesthesiol*. 2007;21:557–573.
7. Hansen MS, Brennum J, Moltke FB, et al. Pain treatment after craniotomy: where is the (procedure-specific) evidence? A qualitative systematic review. *Eur J Anaesthesiol*. 2011;28:821–829.
8. Bonica JJ. In: Wilkins WA, ed. *The Management of Pain*. 3rd ed. Philadelphia: Lippincott; 2001:1805–1831, 1842–1847.
9. Wall PD. The prevention of postoperative pain. *Pain*. 1988;33:289–290.
10. Wilder-Smith OHG, Tassonyi EC, Ben JP, Arendt-Nielsen L. Quantitative sensory testing and human surgery: effects of analgesic management on postoperative neuroplasticity. *Anesthesiology*. 2003;98:1214–1222.
11. Bloomfield EL, Schubert A, Secic M, Barnett G, Shutway F, Ebrahim ZY. The influence of scalp infiltration with bupivacaine on haemodynamics and postoperative pain in adult patients undergoing craniotomy. *Anesth Analg*. 1998;87:579–582.
12. Nguyen A, Girard F, Boudreault D, et al. Scalp nerve blocks decrease the severity of pain after craniotomy. *Anesth Analg*. 2001;93:1272–1276.
13. Geze S, Yilmaz AA, Tuzuner F. The effect of scalp block and local infiltration on the haemodynamic and stress response to skull-pin placement for craniotomy. *Eur J Anaesthesiol*. 2009;26:298–303.
14. Cold GE, Felding M. Even small doses of morphine might provoke "luxury perfusion" in the postoperative period after craniotomy (letter). *Neurosurgery*. 1993;32:327.
15. Palmer JD, Sparrow OC, Iannotti F. Postoperative hematoma: a 5-year survey and identification of avoidable risk factors. *Neurosurgery*. 1994;35:1061–1064.
16. Jellish WS, Leonetti JP, Sawicki K, Anderson D, Origitano TC. Morphine/ondansetron PCA for postoperative pain. Nausea and vomiting after skull base surgery. *Otolaryngol Head Neck Surg*. 2006;135:175–181.
17. MacEwan A, Sigston PE, Andrews KA. A comparison of rectal and intramuscular codeine phosphate in children following neurosurgery. *Paediatr Anaesth*. 2000;10:189–193.
18. Cunliffe M. Codeine phosphate in children: time for re-evaluation? *Br J Anaesth*. 2001;86:329–331.
19. Williams DG, Hatch DJ, Howard RF. Codeine phosphate in paediatric medicine. *Br J Anaesth*. 2001;86:413–421.
20. Stoneham MD, Cooper R, Quiney NF, Walters FJ. Pain following craniotomy: a preliminary study comparing PCA morphine with intramuscular codeine phosphate. *Anaesthesia*. 1996;51:1176–1178.
21. Scott Jellish W, Murdoch J, Leonetti JP. Peri-operative management of complex skull base surgery. *Neurosurg Focus*. 2002;12.
22. Goldsack C, Scuplak SM, Smith M. A double blind comparison of codeine and morphine for postoperative analgesia following intracranial surgery. *Anaesthesia*. 1996;51:1029–1032.

32. POSTCRANIOTOMY PAIN

23. Umamaheswara Rao GS, Gelb AW. To use or not to use: the dilemma of NSAIDs and craniotomy. *Eur J Anaesthesiol*. August 2009;26(8):625–626.
24. Robinson CM, Christie J, Malcom-Smith N. Nonsteroidal antiinflamatory drugs, perioperative blood loss, and transfusion requirements in elective hip arthroplasty. *J Arthroplasty*. 1993;8:607–610.
25. Leese PT, Hubbard RC, Karim A, et al. Effects of celecoxib, a novel cyclooxygenase-2 inhibitor, on platelet function in healthy adults: a randomized, controlled trial. *J Clin Pharmacol*. 2000;40:124–132.
26. Maxwell LG, Buckley GM, Kudchadkar SR, et al. Pain management following major intracranial surgery in pediatric patients: a prospective cohort study in three academic children's hospitals. *Paediatr Anaesth*. 2014;24:1132–1140.
27. Teo JH, Palmer GM, Davidson AJ. Post-craniotomy pain in a paediatric population. *Anaesth Intensive Care*. 2011;39:89–94.
28. Na HS, An SB, Park HP, et al. Intravenous patient-controlled analgesia to manage the postoperative pain in patients undergoing craniotomy. *Korean J Anesthesiol*. 2011;60:30–35.
29. Sudheer PS, Logan SW, Terblanche C, Ateleanu B, Hall JE. Comparison of the analgesic efficacy and respiratory effects of morphine, tramadol and codeine after craniotomy. *Anaesthesia*. 2007;62:555–560.

MISCELLANEOUS

33

Anaphylaxis

Ranadhir Mitra, Hemanshu Prabhakar

Department of Neuroanaesthesiology and Critical Care, All India Institute
of Medical Sciences, New Delhi, India

OUTLINE

DEFINITION

The term "anaphylaxis" infuses a sense of dread irrespective of place or person but with proper information in place, it can be treated in time.

The European Academy of Allergology and Clinical Immunology defines anaphylaxis as "a severe, life-threatening, generalized, or systemic hypersensitivity reaction" primarily mediated by type E immunoglobulin (IgE), while the National Institute of Allergy and Infectious Disease/Food Allergy and Anaphylaxis Network symposium defines it as "a serious allergic reaction that is rapid in onset and may cause death." Symptoms may start within 5–30 min of coming into contact with a sensitive allergen, while in some cases it manifests more than an hour.

Anaphylaxis was recognized and named at the beginning of the twentieth century by Charles Richet and Paul Portier[1] while attempting to immunize dogs with extracts of *Physalia* species in order to develop antitoxin to venom of Portuguese man of war.

VARIANT

Another term used quite frequently is the "anaphylactoid" reaction. The difference lies in the underlying mechanism. Anaphylaxis is an **antibody-mediated** systemic immediate type I hypersensitivity reaction where there is release of inflammatory mediators from basophils and mast cells causing severe manifestations in one or more organ systems. Anaphylactoid is a nonimmune-mediated mechanism where there are similar signs and symptoms due to **direct allergen-induced mast cell degranulation** (e.g., vancomycin, opioids, contrast media). According to Laxenaire's group, the French experts on anaphylaxis during anesthesia, all reactions should be described as anaphylactoid until an immune mechanism has been discovered, stressing the need for proper clinical investigation and reporting.[2]

The overall incidence of anaphylaxis during anesthesia has been reported to vary between 1 in 3500 and 1 in 13,000 procedures in a French series and between 1 in 10,000 and 1 in 20,000 in an Australian study.[3] The mortality from these reactions is in the range of 3–6%, and an additional 2% of patients experience significant residual brain damage. These figures can be higher in India given the connotation of drugs used in private anesthesia practice and the underreporting that follows.

CAUSE

In susceptible individuals, initial exposure to an allergen results in the production of IgE antibodies that bind to high-affinity $Fc\epsilon RI$ receptors located in the plasma membrane of tissue mast cells and blood basophils, which may be clinically silent in the initial phase of sensitization. Upon reexposure, the multimeric allergen cross-links two specific IgE receptors and produces a signal transduction cascade releasing systemically preformed biochemical mediators, including histamine, neutral proteases (tryptase, chymase), and proteoglycans (heparin) from intracellular granules leading to systemic manifestations. The target organs commonly include the skin, mucous membranes, cardiovascular and respiratory systems, and the gastrointestinal tract.[4]

To describe the clinical grade and severity of perioperative anaphylactic reactions the Ring and Messmmer scale is used.

Grade	Clinical signs
I	Cutaneous–mucous signs: Erythema, urticaria with or without angioedema
II	Moderate multivisceral signs: Cutaneous–mucous signs ± hypotension ± tachycardia ± dyspnea ± gastrointestinal disturbances
III	Life-threatening mono- or multivisceral signs: Cardiovascular collapse, tachycardia, or bradycardia ± cardiac dysrhythmia ± bronchospasm ± cutaneous–mucous signs ± gastrointestinal disturbances
IV	Cardiac arrest

Most of the immediate hypersensitivity reactions occurring during anesthesia (60%) are IgE-mediated in which neuromuscular blocking agents (NMBAs) is the most common causative agent involved, followed by latex and antibiotics.[5] Colloid solutions may be implicated in 3–4% of cases. Other drugs implicated are opioids and amide local anesthetics, while the only anesthetic agents that have not been found to cause anaphylaxis are potent inhalation agents.

Induction agents	Neuromuscular relaxants	Opioid	Local anesthetics
Barbiturates (e.g., thiopentone sodium)	Succinylcholine	Intravenous (IV) morphine or codeine (rare)	Ester local anesthetics (more commonly)
Benzodiazepines	Nondepolarizing neuromuscular blockers		Amide local anesthetics (rare)
Etomidate			Methylparaben or propylparaben preservatives
Ketamine			Sulfite, metabisulfite antioxidants
Propofol			

SIGNS AND SYMPTOMS

Anaphylaxis can involve multiple organ systems the manifestations such as:

1. Cutaneous: Pruritus, burning, tingling, erythema, urticaria, periorbital edema.
2. Respiratory: Nasal stuffiness, breathing difficulty, chest tightness, discomfort, coughing, sneezing, intercoastal recession, stridor, tachypnea, respiratory distress.
3. Cardiovascular: Dizziness, malaise, confusion, retrosternal oppression, diaphoresis, hypotension, tachycardia, arrhythmia, decreased vascular resistance, pulmonary hypertension, allergic angina, and myocardial infarction (Kounis syndrome).[10]
4. Other organ systems: Aura, nausea, abdominal pain, vomiting, diarrhea, acute intravascular coagulation, etc.

DIFFERENTIAL DIAGNOSIS

Skin and mucosa: Direct histamine release, venous obstruction, head low position, C1-esterase inhibitor deficiency, mastocytosis.

Airway: Direct histamine release (e.g., propofol), acid aspiration, acute exacerbation of asthma, intubation stress response, esophageal or bronchial intubation.

Fall in blood pressure: Direct histamine release, visceral traction (e.g., peritoneal stretch, fallopian tube ligation), vasodilatation by drugs (e.g., oxytocin), cardiac drug effects, concealed hypovolemia, drug overdose and interactions, gas embolism (laparoscopy), hypoxemia, neurocardiogenic syncope, vasovagal reaction, electrolyte disorders.

ANAPHYLAXIS IN NEUROSURGERY

A review of the literature regarding anaphylaxis during neurosurgical procedures shows isolated events pertaining to topical vancomycin powder,[13] bacitracin,[14] intravenous administration of fluorescein sodium,[15] etc. A special mention needs to be made regarding predisposition to latex allergy in patients with myelomeningoceles where number of surgeries and a history of atopy[16] have been shown to be the most important risk factors.

DIAGNOSIS

The pathway to diagnosis is based on clinical signs and symptoms and, according to consensus statements by the Australian and New Zealand Anesthetic Allergy Group,[6] anaphylaxis should be considered if skin signs are there along with bronchospasm or hypotension. Symptoms start within seconds to 10 min after intravenous injection of the allergen. Even hypotension or tachycardia alone, unresponsive to vasopressors or unexpected for the stage of operation, is an indicator for anaphylaxis. NMBA (58.2%), latex (16.7%), and antibiotics (15.1%) are the most frequent culprits.[3,7,8] Bronchospasm or difficulty with ventilation may be the only presenting feature in certain cases. Importantly, the absence of skin signs does not rule out the diagnosis of anaphylaxis, as skin signs may not appear until circulation is restored.

Diagnosis of anaphylaxis is based on a chain of events and the clinical picture. The follow-up investigations (biochemical and skin tests) are used to identify both the mechanism of reaction and, more importantly, the culprit allergen to prevent a future fatal reexposure.

Biochemical Tests (In Vivo and In Vitro)[5,9]

In Vivo Tests

Serum Tryptase Levels

Mast cell tryptase levels are important in cases where the diagnosis is unclear and are used to differentiate from other causes of perioperative adverse reaction. Tryptase is a mast cell tetrameric neutral serine protease consisting of two major forms: α and β-tryptase. Pro-β-tryptase is secreted constitutively and is a measure for mast cell number, whereas mature β-tryptase reflects mast cell activation. An elevated total serum tryptase level ($>25 \mu g/L = \text{pro-}\beta + \text{pro-}\alpha + \text{mature } \beta\text{-tryptase}$) is therefore highly indicative of mast cell degranulation, as seen in systemic anaphylaxis where sampling is recommended within 15–60 min for grades I and II, and 30 min to 2 h for grades III and IV. The results remain positive for more than 6 h in severe cases. To enable comparison with baseline levels, a new sample should be collected >2 days after the reaction. Tryptase levels can remain elevated in cases of late-onset, biphasic, or protracted cell activation and also in underlying mastocytosis. Discrimination between mature β-tryptase and total serum tryptase leads to greater specificity in the diagnosis of anaphylaxis.

Serum Histamine Test

An increase in serum histamine without an accompanying rise of tryptase indicates hypersensitivity reaction (allergenic/nonallergenic) caused exclusively by basophils. A combination of serum histamine and tryptase test is more sensitive than when used alone.

In Vitro Test: Radioallergosorbent Test (RAST)

RASTs detect the presence of IgE antibodies. The indications for specific IgE assays are currently restricted to the diagnosis of anaphylaxis to NMBAs, thiopental, and latex.

Skin Tests

Skin test is the gold standard for the detection of IgE-mediated reactions by exposing the mast cells of the skin to the suspected allergen. Skin tests should be preferentially performed after a delay of 4–6 weeks after the reaction because of mast cell depletion giving rise to false negative tests. Skin test reactivity should be first verified by negative (saline solution) control test (prick test or intradermal test (IDT), using an equal volume of the solvent) and a positive control test (prick test or IDT using an extract of 9% codeine phosphate solution and a 10 mg/mL solution of histamine) that produces a wheal with a diameter of at least 3 mm at 20 min. The IDT is performed on the patient's back or on the forearm by injecting 0.02–0.03 mL of the drug at a diluted concentration ranging from 10^{-4} to the pure solution, raising a wheal of about 3 mm. The IDT is considered positive if within 20 min after injection, an erythematous and pruriginous wheal appears surrounded by a flare, at least doubling the size of the injection wheal. The prick test is considered positive if within 20 min of injecting the allergen on forearm there is a wheal of at least half the positive control or 3 mm greater than the negative control. Investigation of anesthetic agents is performed by prick tests and/or IDTs. The most sensitive techniques must be used; currently these are the specific antiquaternary test or p-aminophenyl phosphoryl choline radioimmunoassay.

PREDISPOSING FACTORS

1. For latex allergy: Atopy, occupational contact or repeated exposure to latex, multiple surgical interventions, urinary abnormalities (e.g., spina bifida and neurogenic bladder).
2. For anesthetics:
   a. Unexplained reaction to an unidentified allergen during previous anesthesia.
   b. Allergy to classes of drugs that may be used during the anesthetic period.
   c. Patients at risk of latex allergy.

TREATMENT

Treatment for anaphylaxis during anesthesia should be flexible based on clinical severity, the patient's history, availability, and response to emergency treatment with obligatory monitoring throughout.

Anaphylaxis in Adults

1. General measures of resuscitation applicable to all cases:
   a. Withdrawal of suspect drug.
   b. Communicate with the surgical team and propose an appropriate course of action.
   c. Administration of 100% oxygen.
2. Grade I reactions:
   Same as in group A along with administration of H_1 antihistamines (diphenhydramine at doses of 25–50 mg or 0.5–1 mg/kg IV) and H_2 antihistamines (ranitidine 50 mg diluted and injected over 5 min) or as a substitute dexchlorpheniramine 5 mg IV can be administered and repeated once.
3. More severe cases (grade II or III):
   a. Oxygenation and rapid airway control.
   b. Injection of adrenaline in intravenous boluses the initial dose of which depends on the severity of hypotension (10–20 μg for grade II, 100–200 μg for grade III). This must be repeated every 1–2 min to maintain adequate blood pressure. Alternatively intravenous infusion at a dose of 0.05–0.1 μg/kg/min can also be used. If there is no effective intravenous access, the intramuscular route may be used (0.3–0.5 mg) and repeated after 5–10 min, depending on the hemodynamic effects. Similarly, the intratracheal route may be used in the intubated patient (it must be remembered that only one-third of the dose administered by this route reaches the bloodstream).
   c. Lower limbs are elevated.
   d. Rapid transfusion of intravenous crystalloids followed by colloids if volume infused exceeds 30 mL/kg.
   e. For bronchospasm without arterial hypotension salbutamol (using a metered dose inhaler) or nebulized adrenaline are used.
   f. In cases of extreme refractoriness to high-dose adrenaline: noradrenaline at a starting dose of 0.1 μg/kg/min or drugs such as terlipressin (a synthetic analog of vasopressin) in a 2 mg bolus may be used.
4. Cardiac arrest (grade IV):
   Cardiopulmonary resuscitation is initiated followed by 1 mg bolus of adrenaline every 1–2 min.[11]
5. Second-line treatment in severe reactions: Corticosteroids may decrease the late manifestations of shock: 200 mg of hydrocortisone hemisuccinate IV every 6 h (in spite of recommendations for steroids in anaphylaxis a Cochrane review did not find any eligible study assessing the benefits and harms of glucocorticoid treatment during episodes of anaphylaxis.
6. Due to risk of labile blood pressures, intensive monitoring should be maintained for at least 24 h.

Anaphylaxis in Children

The principles are identical to those described in adults with particular emphasis on dosage.

1. In the case of circulatory arrest (grade IV): A bolus of adrenaline (10 μg/kg) is usually recommended. Repeated boluses may be replaced by a continuous infusion, as with adults. The initial dosage is 0.1 μg/kg/min.
2. For grade II and III anaphylactic reactions: Titration of doses of adrenaline against the hemodynamic response.
3. Hypotension can be regarded as a systolic blood pressure with the following values: <70 mmHg in children up to age of 12 months; 70 mmHg + 2 times the age (in years) in children aged between 1 and 10 years; and <90 mmHg in children aged over 10 years.
4. Vascular volume is maintained with crystalloids (20 mL/kg) and colloids (10 mL/kg). A net cumulative dose of 60 mL/kg can be used.
5. Corticosteroids can be used as a second-line treatment same as in adults. The recommended doses are similar to those used in acute exacerbation of asthma, i.e., 1–2 mg/kg of methylprednisolone or hydrocortisone; 200 mg in children aged >12 years, 100 mg in children aged between 6 and 12 years, 50 mg in children aged between 6 months and 6 years, and 25 mg in children aged <6 months.
6. In cases of anaphylaxis with a predominance of respiratory symptoms, the recommended dose of salbutamol is 50 μg/kg to a maximum of 1000–1500 μg, which is almost equal to 4–15 puffs of salbutamol which should be repeated every 10–15 min.

PREVENTION

As they say "prevention is better than cure" and this is apt for anaphylaxis. A proper history regarding any previous incidence of hypersensitivity reaction and the offending agent should be keenly elicited with stress on physical manifestations which are more noticeable. When these incidences occur in emergency situations, it is unlikely the patient's anesthesia records will be available, therefore, it is advisable to use regional anesthesia for the patient and if general anesthesia is unavoidable then one should avoid agents known to cause histamine release and ensure the working environment is latex free. For incidences reported in elective cases with proper documentation, then it is compared with the patient's history and if found true then a referral to the allergy department (or skin and venereal disease) is sent for intradermal tests with the IgE of the offending agent. For common offenders like muscle relaxants intradermal tests are carried out and for local anesthetics a skin test followed by a

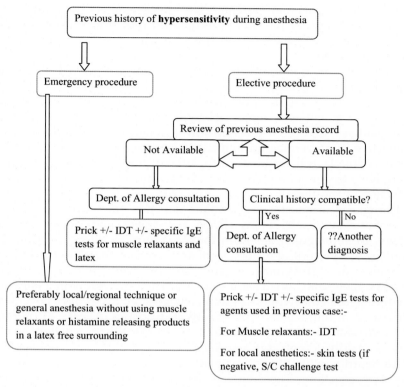

FIGURE 1   Algorithm for management of patients with history of hypersensitivity during anesthesia.

subcutaneous challenge test is done. In case of unavailability of anesthesia records the referral followed by testing should be done (Figure 1).

At the same time, some of the currently held beliefs must be reviewed.[12] There are no data to support the avoidance of propofol in patients with egg allergy, soy allergy, or peanut allergy. There is no cross-reactivity between povidone iodine, iodinated contrast media, and shellfish. The main risk factor for perioperative anaphylaxis is a previous immediate perioperative reaction.

1. Primary prevention: This is achieved by ensuring there is no exposure to the drug or material. It is not possible for anesthetic agents, but can be used for materials such as latex. The choice of drugs for anesthesia should be determined rationally.
2. Secondary prevention: The optimum mode of secondary prevention is to withhold the medication to which a patient is sensitized along with identification of the offending allergen. Patients sensitized to latex must be scheduled at the beginning of the operating list and in a latex-free environment.

It is not necessary to systematically investigate sensitization before anesthesia, except for patients in recognized risk groups (as mentioned above). Prior to anesthesia, a consultation with the allergy department needs to be taken.

Premedication is not effective in preventing an immediate allergic hypersensitivity reaction.

Though the use of H_1 antihistamines has reduced the incidence and intensity of nonallergic immediate hypersensitivity reactions but there is no evidence that premedication with a single dose of a corticosteroid is effective in preventing an immediate hypersensitivity. For patients at risk of anaphylaxis the antibiotic prophylaxis should be administered preoperatively to a monitored awake patient in the operating room prior to induction of anesthesia.

The choice of anesthetic technique depends on the patient (clinical history and the results of any allergy assessment) and the surgical procedure. In an emergency, and in the absence of an allergy workup but with suggestive clinical history, local and regional anesthesia techniques are preferred. NMBAs and histamine-releasing drugs are to be avoided as far as possible, and surgery must be conducted preferably in a latex-free environment. In the hypnotics group, halogenated drugs have never been implicated in immediate hypersensitivity reactions. Allergy to propofol and benzodiazepines can occur rarely. Hypersensitivity reactions to opiates are mainly described in association with morphine and codeine.

All neuromuscular blocking agents can induce immediate type hypersensitivity reactions. The choices of neuromuscular agent will depend on the indications for neuromuscular blockade and skin tests. Any patient with an allergy to one NMBA should be tested for cross-reactivity with others in the group.

CONCLUSION

Anaphylaxis under anesthesia is a diagnosis either self-declaratory due to rapidity of signs and symptoms or deceptive if mild. It is the latter that needs investigation. The cornerstone to avoiding anaphylaxis is proper history pertaining to drug allergy, review of the same prior to anesthesia with special focus on cross-reactivity, and alternate planning for drugs.

References

1. Ring J, Behrendt H, de Weck A. History and classification of anaphylaxis. *Chem Immunol Allergy*. 2010;95:1–11.
2. Mertes PM, Laxenaire MC, Alla F. Anaphylactic and anaphylactoid reactions occurring during anesthesia in France in 1999–2000. *Anesthesiology*. 2003;99:536–545.

3. Ebo DG, Fisher MM, Hagendorens MM, Bridts CH, Stevens WJ. Anaphylaxis during anaesthesia: diagnostic approach. *Allergy*. 2007;62:471–487.
4. Dewachter P, Mouton-Faivre C, Emala CW. Anaphylaxis and anesthesia controversies and new insights. *Anesthesiology*. 2009;111:1141–1150.
5. Dewachtera P, Mouton-Faivre C. What investigation after an anaphylactic reaction during anaesthesia? *Curr Opin Anaesthesiol*. 2008;21:363–368.
6. *ANZAAG-anzca Anaphylaxis Management Guidelines: Introduction Version 1.1*. June 2013.
7. Harboe T, Guttormsen AB, Irgens A, Dybendal T, Florvaag E. Anaphylaxis during anesthesia in Norway a 6-year single-center follow-up study. *Anesthesiology*. 2005;102: 897–903.
8. Karila C, Brunet-Langot D, Labbez F, et al. Anaphylaxis during anesthesia: results of a 12-year survey at a French pediatric center. *Allergy*. 2005;60:828–834.
9. Mertes PM, Malinovsky JM, Jouffroy L, et al. Reducing the risk of anaphylaxis during anesthesia: 2011 updated guidelines for clinical practice. *J Investig Allergol Clin Immunol*. 2011;21(6):442–453.
10. Kounis NG. Kounis syndrome (allergic angina and allergic myocardial infarction): a natural paradigm? *Int J Cardiol*. 2006;110:7–14.
11. Choo KJL, Simons FER, Sheikh A. Glucocorticoids for the treatment of anaphylaxis (review). *Cochrane Libr*. 2012;(8).
12. Dewachtera P, Mouton-Faivreb C, Castellsc MC, Hepner DL. Anesthesia in the patient with multiple drug allergies: are all allergies the same? *Curr Opin Anesthesiol*. 2011;24: 320–325.
13. Mariappan R, Manninen P, Massicotte EM, Bhatia A. Circulatory collapse after topical application of vancomycin powder during spine surgery. *J Neurosurg Spine*. 2013;19: 381–383.
14. Carver ED, Braude BM, Atkinson AR, Gold M. Anaphylaxis during insertion of a ventriculoperitoneal shunt. *Anesthesiology*. 2000;93:578–579.
15. Dilek O, Ihsan A, Tulay H. Anaphylactic reaction after fluorescein sodium administration during intracranial surgery. *Case Rep/J Clin Neurosci*. 2011;18:431–434.
16. Majed M, Nejat F, Khashab ME, et al. Risk factors for latex sensitization in young children with myelomeningocele. Clinical article. *J Neurosurg Pediatr*. 2009;4:285–288.

34

Hazards of Advanced Neuromonitoring

M. Srilata, Kavitha Jayaram

Department of Anesthesia and Intensive Care, Nizam's Institute of Medical Sciences, Hyderabad, India

Physiologic monitors are tools that enable the "vigilance" described in the motto of the American Society of Anesthesiologists (ASA) and guide the patient "safety" (*securitas*) in the motto of the Association of the Anesthetists of Great Britain and Ireland. The term is derived from *monere*, which in Latin means to warn, remind, or admonish. In perioperative care, monitoring implies the following four essential features: observation and vigilance, instrumentation, interpretation of data, and initiation of corrective therapy when indicated.[1] The principal objectives of intraoperative monitoring are to improve perioperative outcome, facilitate surgery, and reduce adverse events using continuously corrected data of cardiopulmonary, neurological, and metabolic functions to guide pharmacologic and physiologic therapy. Although sophisticated and reliable apparatuses may be used to collect these data, they are useless or even harmful without proper interpretation.

Advanced neuromonitoring has been broadly used in most operating rooms. This multimodal monitoring has evolved good outcomes with the advent of new and updated monitoring techniques in neurocritical intensive care. Advanced neuromonitoring allows sophisticated and individually focused treatment, thus contributing to patient safety. They not only provide real time information regarding the affected site but also guide us toward goal-directed, proactive preventive strategy with the interpretation of the available physiologic end points. But these are not without any disadvantages, as it always is with any advanced method.

The hazards of neuromonitoring include complications associated with the particular system, apart from its disadvantages. The distinguished limitation of these monitors is that it gives either an overall global measure or a regional measure of the cerebral function monitored.

Standard monitors used commonly are invasive lines for arterial and central venous pressure (CVP) monitoring. The complications associated with these monitors include:

1. Invasive arterial lines: Complications include thrombosis, infection, and disconnection. Inappropriate administration of medications into the arterial line may exacerbate thrombosis, sometimes leading to amputation of the limb. Mismanagement of arterial lines during positioning may lead to disconnection and unexpected blood loss. Sometimes, over- and underdamping of arterial lines may lead to false readings and inappropriate management. The incidence of serious complications with radial, femoral, and axillary artery cannulations like permanent ischemic damage, sepsis, and pseudoaneurysm formation is very low, i.e., <1%.[2]
2. Central venous and pulmonary artery catheters (PACs): The complications include arterial puncture, infection, thrombosis, kinking and knotting of the catheter, retained guidewire, entrapment with sutures or by cannulas, irritation of the right heart leading to arrhythmias, heart block, ventricular tachycardia, and ventricular fibrillation.[3] Fatal and rare complications include perforation of the sinus coronarius with resultant cardiac tamponade, and laceration of the subclavian artery. PACs are rarely indicated in neurosurgical cases with significant cardiac dysfunction. Apart from the complications seen with CVP catheters, this also includes some serious complications like pulmonary artery (PA) rupture, air embolism, torsion of the catheter, endocarditis, and pulmonary infarction.

TABLE 1   Comparison of Intracranial Pressure Monitors

Intracranial pressure monitoring	Intraventricular catheter (IVC)	Subarachnoid bolt	Fiber optic sensor
Accuracy of readings	Good	Less accurate	Better
Drainage of CSF	Possible	May or may not	Not possible
Risk of infection	Increased risk	Less risk compared to IVC	No risk
Recalibration	Possible	Possible	Not possible
Disruption of brain tissue	Yes	No	Yes; comparatively less than IVC

INTRACRANIAL PRESSURE MONITORS

These are most valuable in managing critically ill neurosurgical patients in the intensive care unit. The various intracranial pressure (ICP) monitors are seldom used intraoperatively. Potential complications of **intraventricular ICP catheters** include bleeding and infection leading to intracerebral hematomas and meningitis, respectively (Table 1).[4] On the other hand, **intraparenchymal fiber optic catheters** are costlier with the disadvantages of inability to zero and not able to drain cerebrospinal fluid (CSF) at times of emergency. Technical complications include dislocation of the transducer, breakage of the fiber optic cable, dislocation of the fixation screw, and defective probe for unknown reasons. Rare but disastrous complications include injury to vital structures like brain, important nerves, and vessels. The main disadvantage of these devices is that they cannot be recalibrated in situ. Another limitation is that they cannot be used for CSF drainage or compliance testing unless inserted in conjunction with a ventriculostomy. **Subdural devices** are easily inserted but can malfunction if they are not coplanar to the brain surface or if they become loose. The major complication of this procedure is infection, commonly meningitis, osteomyelitis, or a localized infection. Epidural bleeding and focal seizures, if the bolt is inserted too deeply, can also occur. With an **epidural transducer**, technical problems in positioning and calibrating the transducer in situ can also occur. Another shortcoming of the epidural transducer is that intracranial compliance testing and therapeutic CSF drainage cannot be performed.

CEREBRAL PERFUSION MONITORING

Either the functionality of parts of the brain are monitored (and the assumption is made that continued function implies an adequate oxygen supply) or the blood flow or pressure at one or more points in the brain are measured (and the assumption is made that the flow or pressure is equivalent elsewhere). Neither assumption is always correct, and despite monitoring, ischemia may sometimes occur without detection and may result in stroke.[5]

Noninvasive methods of monitoring cerebral blood flow (CBF): This involves injection of intravascular radioactive isotope followed by measurement of radioactivity using gamma detectors. Drawbacks of the methods are the patient's exposure to radioactive compounds and a need for externally placed, potentially cumbersome detector equipment, which may interfere with the surgery itself in case of intracranial surgery.

Transcranial Doppler (TCD): An important limitation of TCD results from the feeling that most of the examination is done through the temporal bone, which may be thick enough to preclude an adequate examination in 10–20% of patients.[6,7] Blood flow velocity is directly related to blood flow only if the diameter of the artery where it is measured and the measurement angle of Doppler probe remains constant. The difficulty is to find a means to affix the probe in a way that prevents dislodgement or movement during monitoring. Limitations of this technique include between-subject variation of TCD velocities, within-subject variation if vessel diameter changes in response to vasoactive agents or conditions, and error from changing the angle of insonation.

Near infrared spectroscopy: The main disadvantage is increase of the temperature because of the heating of the semiconductor junction.[8] The increase in temperature is seen around 1–10 °C. This may sometimes lead to intracranial heat injuries. Its major limitations include intersubject variability, variable optical path length, potential contamination from extracranial blood, and lack of a definable threshold. At present, it is considered a trend monitor, with each patient acting as his or her own control. In situations of potential regional ischemia—for example, carotid endarterectomy and temporary clip application during intracranial aneurysm surgery—bilateral monitoring should be used.

INVASIVE METHODS FOR CEREBRAL PERFUSION

Tissue-level monitoring of brain: By definition, this involves an invasive technique. All monitors in clinical or research use are implanted through a burr hole, extend into the white matter or into the ventricular system, and typically use a bolt for stabilization. They all share a 1–2% risk of bleeding, ischemia, or infection owing to the implantation procedure.[9] Also, they have a limited spatial resolution, i.e., each probe monitors only a limited area of brain surrounding the probe.

Cerebral oximetry: Contamination of oximetry signals by extracranial blood sources is a serious concern, although two sensing diodes with different distances from the light source within one sensor patch and adjustment of the algorithms of the oximeter may minimize the problems.[10]

Jugular venous bulb oxygen saturation: This is done by placing a fiber optic catheter in retrograde fashion into the jugular bulb. Correct tip placement is crucial to minimize admixture of extracranial venous blood to reduce the risk of complication. Usually, only one side is monitored. There are several theoretical limitations that should be borne in mind during interpretation of the values and trends. This is particularly because of improper admixture of extracranial venous blood in the jugular bulb, and there can be difference in saturations between the right side and the left. The dominant jugular vein drains cortical blood, whereas the nondominant one drains more subcortical blood.[11]

Thermal diffusion-based CBF monitoring: This works by placing double thermistor probes in the white matter. The distal thermistor is heated 2 °C above the proximal passive thermistor. In order to avoid thermal injury, the heating is stopped automatically when the temperature is more than 39.1 °C. Since fever is the most common complication, particularly in severe brain disease, the monitor may not work during febrile episodes.[12]

Laser Doppler flowmetry-based measurement of CBF: This is also an invasive technique. It does not give a quantal measure; rather, it provides a qualitative parameter.

Microdialysis catheter: This is an invasive technique of providing a regional measure of metabolic status of the brain following an insult. Potential complications include alteration of tissue morphology due to its invasiveness, delayed dialysate recovery, and low temporal and spatial resolution.[13]

ELECTROPHYSIOLOGICAL MONITORING

Invasive electrophysiological monitoring: This is commonly used perioperatively for an accurate definition of the epileptic focus in the intraoperative period. Complications include an additional risk of damage to the cortex, reaction to the implant electrodes, wound infection, CSF leak, intracranial bleeding, and pneumocephalus.

Intraoperative motor-evoked potentials (MEPs): There is increased risk of activation of the seizure focus in patients with epilepsy, tongue lacerations, bite block, and sometimes dysfunctioning of the pacemakers and implantable cardioverter defibrillators (ICDs).

Electroencephalogram (EEG) and evoked potentials: The increasing usage of the different types of monitoring, particularly evoked potentials, has raised the essentiality of increasing the point of care in anesthetic management. To minimize the effects of a multitude of potential artifacts and sources of noise in the operating room, the EEG signal of each channel must be preconditioned prior to digital sampling. The length of unshielded leads from the electrodes to the first amplifier should be minimized, and other electrical wires and electromagnetic sources should be kept away from the wires leading to the amplifier. The first-stage amplifiers must be completely isolated from the patient to provide electrical safety and prevent potential burns from intraoperative electrocautery, and the amplifiers should be capable of handling extensive saturation, which may be caused by high-amplitude signals from sources such as electrocautery. Relatively narrow frequency filtering is often necessary to produce satisfactory EEG recordings in the operating room.[14] When employing any form of processed EEG monitoring, care must be taken that the EEG signal is of high quality prior to further levels of processing and abstraction, otherwise the risk is that a noisy signal contaminated with significant artifacts may produce a display subject to significant misinterpretation. Alternating current (AC) power noise is a common contaminant, which can be minimized by good isolation, the use of well-shielded power supplies, keeping power cords removed from the unamplified EEG signal, the use of differential inputs to the amplifier, and the use of an AC notch filter when necessary. The somatosensory-evoked potentials (SSEPs) are very sensitive to electromagnetic interference, although it remains useful during mild hypothermia (32°C). Although the occurrence of false negatives and positives is well documented, SSEPs remain an integral component of the cord protection regimen in some centers.[15,16] Like SSEPs, MEPs are susceptible to mechanical and electromagnetic interference in the operating room, and the extracranial magnetic coil is unwieldy. A pilot study by Lin A has reported a decrease in the EEG burst suppression ratio with intraoperative SSEP monitoring during general anesthesia.[17]

SURGERY-ASSOCIATED HAZARDS

Cerebral angiography: There are several risks and problems associated with angiography itself, including an incidence of neurologic problems from inadvertent occlusion of normal vessels.[18] In addition, arterial spasm, hematoma, and local infection can occur at the site of needle puncture. Subintimal dissection or occlusion of the vessel may result from injection into the vessel wall. Iodine-containing contrast media produces vasodilation and a burning sensation in the distribution of the injected vessel. Septicemia, cerebral embolism, vessel perforation, subarachnoid hemorrhage, transient ischemic attacks, pulmonary embolism from systemic shunting of particulate material, anaphylactic reactions to the iodinated contrast material, and, rarely, seizures or death are all potential complications of cerebral angiography.

Interventional neuroradiology: Endovascular procedures performed by interventional neuroradiologists include placement of procoagulant coils in the intracranial aneurysms. In wide-necked aneurysms, wherein detachable coils are placed after the placement of coil and angiographic confirmation of position, a short electrical impulse is sent through the coil so that it attaches to a new position. We should be aware of the potential hazards of such new techniques and the electrical issues of macro/micro-shock in these procedures.[19]

INTRAOPERATIVE MAGNETIC RESONANCE IMAGING

The development of hybrid operating rooms have specific hazards both on patients as well as on operating room professionals. Incorporating magnetic resonance imaging (MRI) technology into the operating room presents new challenges in the transdisciplinary environment.

Advances in technologies like magnetic resonance (MR) image-guided surgery is now possible, providing the surgeon with dynamic high-resolution images during intricate stereotactic neurosurgery. Various MR systems have been configured for this application, including "doughnut"-shaped magnets permitting surgery with real-time concurrent imaging and portable systems set up to allow easy and rapid interchange between scanning and surgery. All the hazards associated with diagnostic MR also apply to interventional procedures. There are additional risks from patient repositioning, contamination of the sterile field, and the proximity of ferromagnetic surgical instruments, including scalpels, to the magnetic field. Incorporating MR technology into the operating room provides new challenges.[20] Anesthetists who are involved with 3-T systems, open scanners, or interventional and intraoperative procedure should remain acquainted with the constantly changing recommendations relating to occupational exposure. They should take all practical steps to minimize the risk from exposure.

Intraoperative MRI: Intraoperative MRI guides the neurosurgeon for the exact location of the tumor, helps in navigating the neurosurgeon to the tumor site, and allows for adequate resection of tumors. The incorporation of this technology requires MRI-compatible consoles in the operating room. In 2007, safety guidelines were updated by the Medicines and Healthcare Products Regulatory Agency (MHRA) regarding MRI. The old MRI-compatible system is replaced by three terms as follows: MR conditional, MR safe, and MR unsafe.

MR conditional: objects that are deemed to pose no known hazards in a specified MR environment with specified conditions of use.

MR safe: equipment presenting no safety hazard to patients or personnel when this is inside the MRI room, provided instructions are correctly followed regarding its use, e.g., infusion pumps, warming mattresses, and temperature probes.

The hazards include noise pollution, strong impact of the magnet leading to failure of pacemakers, ICDs, long tubings, which are prone for damage, and dark rooms during scanning leading to disconnection problems and loud acoustic noise. Adequate hearing protection should be provided to all patients. The threshold exposure to impulsive noise in adults for permanent acoustic trauma is 140 dB, and for children, 120 dB. It is advisable to provide ear protection to others in the scan room if the levels reach 80 dB.

Static magnetic field gradients liberate electric potentials. This, along with the related effects during physical movements, may result in sensations of vertigo, nausea, phosphenes, and a metallic taste in the mouth. Patients and attending staff should be slowly and gradually shifted inside the scanner to decrease the incidence of such biological effects. Sometimes time-varying magnetic field strengths with frequencies >30 MHz interfere with normal function of nerve cells and muscle fibers. The response varies from less serious responses, such as the sensation of flashes of light due to stimulation of the retina, to more serious responses such as ventricular fibrillation.

A wide variety of neurostimulators are now in use. Concerns about MR safety relate to the radio frequency (RF) and gradient fields that may interfere with the operation of these devices or cause thermal injury. The risk of overheating the patient is increased in the presence of high ambient temperatures and high relative humidity. Precautions should be taken to minimize the RF deposition, to ensure good air flow, and to maintain moderate environmental conditions of relative humidity and ambient temperature. Quench hazards due to cryogens are explained by the dysfunction of external vent pipes. In such an event, low liquefied gases normally present around the magnet expand and boil off to the outside.

It is recommended that patients implanted with neurostimulators should not undergo MR. However, some manufacturers are suggesting that MR examinations of specific devices may be safe if strict guidelines relating to scanning parameters, in particular to RF exposure, are followed. All patients and personnel should be screened for any ferromagnetic devices such as pacemakers, ICDs, and aneurysm clips, or avoid wearing/carrying them to prohibit movement or malfunction of these devices.[21]

Radiosurgery: Modern neurosurgery develops toward minimally invasive procedures; therefore, radiosurgery has gained space. The multidisciplinary nature of the procedure involving the neurosurgeon, radiation oncologist, and medical physicist aims to minimize the risks and to improve the treatment success rate. Understanding all of the steps of the radiosurgery procedure is essential to optimize results and reduce risks. Regardless of the approach, the fundamental concepts of radiosurgery include high doses of radiation, minimal doses in surrounding structures, stereotactic localization, use of computerized dosimetry planning and a highly accurate radiation delivery system.[22,23] These precision techniques pose more hazards apart from the radiation hazards to the healthcare professionals. Regardless of the method of delivery, it is important to follow all the safety steps of the procedure, because there is no equipment that is error proof. Moreover, radiosurgery is prone to repetitive errors. Because the effects of the treatment are not immediately seen, a large number of patients can be treated based on a single human error.[24,25] The first step is a daily quality assurance routine to check basic aspects of the delivery system and software, and the precision of the delivery device. This should be followed by correct application of the stereotactic guiding device, either frameless or with a frame. A routine protocol of treatment delivery followed harmonically by all team members is essential to avoid any mishaps.

Endoscopies: Modern stereotactic systems and small endoscopes have added a significant margin of safety to the procedure when it is performed in a narrow ventricular system. Knowledge of the relevant anatomy is crucial because it allows the trajectory of the endoscope to be visualized before surgery and the procedure to be mentally "rehearsed" before making the incision.[26,27] Once the patient is draped, the surgeon loses access to most of the external landmarks that define the trajectory of the endoscope, and reorientation may be difficult. Although the technique has been greatly refined since its advent in the twentieth century, today's neurosurgeons must never forget that this seemingly simple procedure holds the potential for a number of devastating complications. Careful and thorough sterilization of the endoscopic equipment and the use of perioperative antibiotics can minimize the occurrence of infection. Prompt diagnosis and treatment of ventriculitis are essential.[28]

TRANSPORTATION

This is the most hazardous region in the hospital care and more important value it has and the least taken care. Maximizing the medical management of the patient can minimize secondary injury.[29] Prehospital spinal immobilization should be a standard of care in the tertiary care centers, but not so in the primary centers wherein the patients are attended to first. The various measures include placement of a rigid cervical collar, logrolling of the patient, and transportation on a rigid spine board. These patients are often multitrauma victims, and being insensate, they may lack physical signs of intraabdominal or thoracic trauma. A high index of suspicion must be maintained, and the diagnosis must often be made radiographically. Potential hazards do occur due to improper transport.[30] Also, none of the monitors available are transportable because of size and cost.

Although there is a wealth of clinical experience with many of the monitoring modalities, there is little in the way of randomized prospective studies evaluating the efficacy of neurological monitoring. Based on clinical experience with neurological monitoring and nonrandomized clinical studies in which neurological monitoring is used and generally compared with historical controls, practice patterns for use of neurological monitoring are developed. Of these, some may be practiced in few areas, as it is mostly based on availability of the equipment as well as technical expertise. Vigilance is now used more appropriately to describe the virtues of sophisticated electronic monitors and alarms in the operating room.

References

1. The Association of Australian and New Zealand College of Anaesthetists. *Recommendations on Monitoring During Anaesthesia*; 2013. Available at: http://www.anzca.edu.au/resources/professional-documents/pdfs/ps18-2013-recommendations-on-monitoring-during-anaesthesia.pdf. Accessed 10.07.14.
2. Scheer B, Perel A, Pfeiffer UJ. Clinical review: complications and risk factors of peripheral arterial catheters used for haemodynamic monitoring in anaesthesia and intensive care medicine. *Crit Care*. 2002;6:199–204.
3. Csanky-Treels JC. Hazards of central venous pressure monitoring. *Anaesthesia*. 1978;33:172–177.
4. Blei AT, Olafsson S, Webster S, Levy R. Complications of intracranial pressure monitoring in fulminant hepatic failure. *Lancet*. 1993;341:157–158.
5. Papworth D. Intraoperative monitoring during vascular surgery. *Anesthesiol Clin N Am*. 2004;22:223–250. vi.
6. Bass A, Krupski WC, Schneider PA, Otis SM, Dilley RB, Bernstein EF. Intraoperative transcranial Doppler: limitations of the method. *J Vasc Surg*. 1989;10:549–553.
7. Manno EM. Transcranial Doppler ultrasonography in the neurocritical care unit. *Crit Care Clin*. 1997;13:79–104.
8. Murkin JM, Arango M. Near-infrared spectroscopy as an index of brain and tissue oxygenation. *Br J Anaesth*. 2009;103(suppl 1):i3–i13.
9. Haitsma IK, Maas AI. Advanced monitoring in the intensive care unit: brain tissue oxygen tension. *Curr Opin Crit Care*. 2002;8:115–120.
10. Samra SK, Stanley JC, Zelenock GB, Dorje P. An assessment of contributions made by extracranial tissues during cerebral oximetry. *J Neurosurg Anesthesiol*. 1999;11:1–5.
11. White H, Baker A. Continuous jugular venous oximetry in the neurointensive care unit–a brief review. *Can J Anaesth*. 2002;49:623–629.
12. Verdu-Lopez F, Gonzalez-Darder JM, Gonzalez-Lopez P, Botella Macia L. Using thermal diffusion flowmetry in the assessment of regional cerebral blood flow in cerebral aneurysm microsurgery. *Neurocir Astur*. 2010;21:373–380.
13. Baldini F. Microdialysis-based sensing in clinical applications. *Anal Bioanal Chem*. 2010;397:909–916.
14. Schneider G, Jordan D, Schwarz G, et al. Monitoring depth of anesthesia utilizing a combination of electroencephalographic and standard measures. *Anesthesiology*. 2014;120:819–828.
15. Guerit JM, Dion RA. State-of-the-art of neuromonitoring for prevention of immediate and delayed paraplegia in thoracic and thoracoabdominal aorta surgery. *Ann Thorac Surg*. 2002;74:S1867–S1869. discussion S1892–S1898.

16. Sharan A, Groff MW, Dailey AT, et al. Guideline update for the performance of fusion procedures for degenerative disease of the lumbar spine. Part 15: Electrophysiological monitoring and lumbar fusion. *J Neurosurg Spine*. 2014;21:102–105.

17. Călin A, Kumaraswamy VM, Braver D, Nair DG, Moldovan M, Simon MV. Intraoperative somatosensory evoked potential monitoring decreases EEG burst suppression ratio during deep general anesthesia. *J Clin Neurophysiol*. 2014;31:133–137.

18. Kaufmann TJ, Huston 3rd J, Mandrekar JN, Schleck CD, Thielen KR, Kallmes DF. Complications of diagnostic cerebral angiography: evaluation of 19,826 consecutive patients. *Radiology*. 2007;243:812–819.

19. Young WL. Anesthesia for endovascular neurosurgery and interventional neuroradiology. *Anesthesiol Clin*. 2007;25:391–412. vii.

20. Bergese SD, Puente EG. Anesthesia in the intraoperative MRI environment. *Neurosurg Clin N Am*. 2009;20:155–162.

21. Safety in magnetic resonance imaging. *Responsible Person: Alexandra Lipton* Published.; Thursday, March 14, 2013. ISBN: 1-871101-95-6.

22. Vesper J, Bolke B, Wille C, et al. Current concepts in stereotactic radiosurgery - a neurosurgical and radiooncological point of view. *Eur J Med Res*. 2009;14:93–101.

23. Levivier M, Gevaert T, Negretti L. Gamma Knife, CyberKnife, TomoTherapy: gadgets or useful tools? *Curr Opin Neurol*. 2011;24:616–625.

24. Berkowitz O, Jones K, Lunsford LD, Kondziolka D. Determining the elements of procedural quality. *J Neurosurg*. 2013;119:373–380.

25. Guckenberger M, Roesch J, Baier K, Sweeney RA, Flentje M. Dosimetric consequences of translational and rotational errors in frame-less image-guided radiosurgery. *Radiat Oncol*. 2012;7:63.

26. Kulkarni AV, Riva-Cambrin J, Browd SR, et al. Endoscopic third ventriculostomy and choroid plexus cauterization in infants with hydrocephalus: a retrospective Hydrocephalus Clinical Research Network study. *J Neurosurg Pediatr*. 2014:1–6.

27. Walker ML. Complications of third ventriculostomy. *Neurosurg Clin N Am*. 2004;15:61–66.

28. Fukuhara T, Vorster SJ, Luciano MG. Risk factors for failure of endoscopic third ventriculostomy for obstructive hydrocephalus. *Neurosurgery*. 2000;46:1100–1109. discussion 1109–1111.

29. Esposito TJ, Reed 2nd RL, Gamelli RL, Luchette FA. Neurosurgical coverage: essential, desired, or irrelevant for good patient care and trauma center status. *Ann Surg*. 2005;242:364–370. discussion 370–374.

30. Sollid S, Sundstrom T, Kock-Jensen C, et al. Scandinavian guidelines for prehospital management of severe traumatic brain injury. *Tidsskr Nor Laegeforen*. 2008;128:1524–1527.

Hypothermia

M. Srilata, Kavitha Jayaram

Department of Anesthesia and Intensive Care, Nizam's Institute of Medical Sciences, Hyderabad, India

OUTLINE

Hypothermia is characterized by fall of at least 1 °C below normal core temperature. This becomes clinically relevant when the core temperature starts to fall below 36 °C. This usually occurs either with a decrease in heat production, an increase in heat loss, or with dysfunctional thermoregulation. The maximum fall of temperature ranges from 2 to even 6 °C. This is a common but preventable complication of neurosurgical anesthesia. However, if not treated in time may lead to increased morbidity and poor outcome. This is clinically categorized as:[1]

Normothermia: 36–38 °C

Mild hypothermia: 32.2–35 °C
Moderate hypothermia: 28–32.2 °C
Profound hypothermia: <28 °C
Electrical silence: 12–18 °C

HISTORY

The use of therapeutic hypothermia started from old and ancient mythology. This was first introduced in neurosurgical practice by Temple Fay in 1940s for treating tumors in neurosurgical patients and in patients with head injuries.[2] Later, Bigelow pioneered the same for heart operations in animals and Drew et al. used the same principle for cardiac surgery in humans where circulatory arrest is planned under profound hypothermia to ensure low cerebral metabolic rate and to optimize oxygen delivery accordingly.[3,4] This was then advocated by Drake et al. in 1964 in surgical clipping of giant intracranial aneurysms where the benefits outweigh the disadvantages of hypothermia and is still in use.[5] Currently, mild therapeutic hypothermia is gaining recognition in the field of cerebral resuscitation.

NORMAL COMPENSATORY RESPONSE MECHANISMS

Whenever a patient experiences changes in temperature, this is sensed by the thermoreceptors at specific temperature thresholds. The sensory input from these thermoreceptors is then relayed to the hypothalamus[6] (Figure 1). The effect is either via autonomic (anterior hypothalamus) or behavioral changes (posterior hypothalamus). The autonomic response is predominant in anesthetized patients whereas the latter response is seen in normal individuals.

PATHOPHYSIOLOGY

1. Alterations in the nervous system.[7,8]
   Changes in the nervous system include:
   a. Cerebral metabolic rate ($CMRO_2$) for oxygen is reduced by approximately 8% per °C fall in temperature; normal $CMRO_2$ is almost halved at 28 °C.
   b. Oxygen demand is reduced; oxygen consumption, especially by the brain is also reduced, thus indirectly improving brain oxygenation without compromising aerobic metabolism.
   c. This reduces the production of oxygen-free radicals and lactate, proinflammatory cytokines, excitatory neurotransmitters, and finally decreases apoptosis.

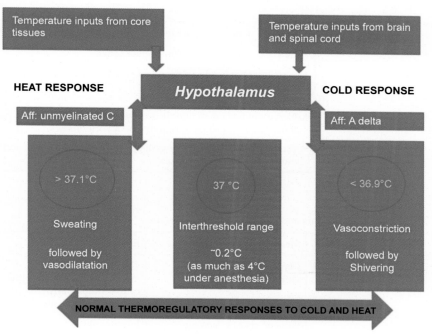

FIGURE 1   Normal thermoregulatory responses to cold and heat.

d. These two factors are responsible for sustaining aerobic metabolism even during periods of compromised oxygen supply.

e. Decreased metabolic rate also contributes to important effects like membrane stabilization and decreased release of toxic metabolites and excitatory amino acids.

f. Decreased cerebral metabolic rate leads to a compensatory increase in cerebrovascular resistance due to autoregulation, this in turn further decreases the cerebral blood flow. Hence, there is no change in the arteriovenous partial pressure of oxygen difference and no increase in the venous lactate concentrations.

g. Altered mental status may result with hypothermia.

h. Functional changes with fall of temperature are depicted in Table 1.

2. Changes in other systems: Hypothermia produces a swarm of harmful and lethal effects on other systems of the body, which are concisely tabulated[9,10] in Table 2.

GENESIS OF PERIOPERATIVE INADVERTENT HYPOTHERMIA

1. Type, duration of surgery, and fluids: All neurosurgical operations usually last more than 60 min and hence are prone to perioperative

TABLE 1   Functional Changes in the Nervous System during Hypothermia

• Hypothermia	• Changes in neurological function
• >33 °C	• Cerebral activity is maintained and normal
• <33 °C	• Somatosensory and audio-evoked potentials are reduced
• <28 °C	• Consciousness is lost
• 26 °C	• Nerve conduction amplitude decreases; peripheral muscle tone increases leading to rigidity and myoclonus
• <25 °C	• Primitive reflexes are lost, e.g., gag, pupillary constriction, and monosynaptic spinal reflexes

TABLE 2   Hypothermia and Its Effect on Other Systems

	Mechanism	Effects
Cardiovascular system[11]	Depression of the cardiac output and heart rate	Threefold increase in morbid cardiac events—low cardiac output, arrhythmias, ventricular fibrillation
	Vasoconstriction leading to increased peripheral resistance—increased contractility and maintenance of stroke volume	Increased blood pressure and afterload leading to ischemia
	Increases coronary vascular resistance and reduces coronary perfusion pressure	Angina, ischemia
	<28 °C disrupts sinoatrial pacing	Ventricular irritability, fibrillation
	Enhanced levels of circulating catecholamines like norepinephrine	Increased blood pressure and heart rate followed by compensatory bradycardia
Immunity	Impairs both antibody- and cell-mediated immunity	Poor wound healing
	Thermoregulatory vasoconstriction leading to impaired oxygen delivery to damaged tissues	Several fold increase in surgical wound infection rate
	Impaired leukocyte mobilization	
	Increase in cortisol levels due to cold stress	

TABLE 2   Hypothermia and Its Effect on Other Systems—cont'd

	Mechanism	Effects
Coagulation system[12]	• Qualitative platelet dysfunction • Impaired activity of the enzymes driving the coagulation cascade • Increased viscosity and increased peripheral vascular resistance • Reduced blood flow to the extremities leading to blood stasis	• Blood clotting is disturbed • Increases blood loss by 20% • Necessitating intra and postoperative allogeneic transfusions by 20% Enhances blood clots Prone for postoperative deep vein thrombosis and pulmonary embolus
Pharmacokinetics and pharmacodynamics	Decreased hepatic blood flow leads to decreased drug metabolism	Prolonged effects of inhalational, intravenous anesthetics, and neuromuscular blocking drugs[13]
Protein metabolism	Postoperative protein catabolism and stress response	Shivering, increase in heart rate and blood pressure
Renal system	Increased renovascular resistance leads to decreased renal blood flow—impairs the glomerular filtration rate	Increased blood urea nitrogen and creatinine
	Sodium and potassium reabsorption is inhibited	Antidiuretic hormone-mediated cold diuresis
Respiratory system	Stimulation of the respiratory center following cold stress	Hyperventilation followed by hypoventilation/abnormal respiratory pattern
	Left ward shift of the hemoglobin oxygen dissociation curve—decreased oxygen delivery	Hypoxia, anaerobic metabolism, and lactic acidosis; further worsened in patients with shivering.
	Bronchial arterial blood flow is also diminished and may further cause delay in oxygen uptake and delivery to tissues	Aggravates hypoxia
	<33°C diminishes respiratory strength	Delayed muscle recovery
Physiological comfort		Impaired thermal comfort in the postoperative period is quite stressful; may sometimes lead to increased heart rate, blood pressure, and elevated levels of catecholamines.

hypothermia. The complexity of the surgery with its evident increased requirement of intravenous fluids and blood is another important predictor for perioperative hypothermia in neuroanesthesia. The severity is more evident in pediatric patients undergoing craniotomies where the comparatively large head is completely exposed to the atmosphere. Neuroendoscopic procedures require continuous irrigation either with ringers lactate or normal saline for optimal visualization of the surgical field. Though the time is limited, these patients are comparatively more prone to hypothermia than the usual craniotomies. Other neurosurgical conditions like subarachnoid hemorrhage, hypothalamic injury, and infection are associated with temperature dysregulation.[8] Hypothermia occurs in several settings outside the operating room, such as magnetic resonance imaging, stereotactic procedures, deep brain stimulations (elderly), radiotherapy, and imaging neuroradiology, the particularly vulnerable group being extremes of age.[14] Prolonged duration of these procedures especially under anesthesia causes a drastic fall in temperature in these situations.

2. Anesthetic agents and hypothermia: General anesthesia impairs thermoregulation and reduces cold response thresholds.[15] The use of intravenous induction agents like propofol has shown to cause vasodilation thus promotes drifting of temperature from core to periphery. This is responsible for the initial fall of core temperature by 0.5–1.5 °C in the first 30 min following induction of anesthesia.[16] On the other hand, barbiturates decrease both cerebral metabolic rate and flow and therefore decrease the brain temperature specifically, independent of core temperature.[17] Inhalational agents like isoflurane, sevoflurane, and desflurane have been shown to reduce shivering and vasoconstriction thresholds.[18–20] Current neuroanesthesia practice involves more of propofol for induction and maintenance rather than inhalational agents thus redistribution of temperature contributing to hypothermia to a larger extent.

3. Exposure to cold operating room: Operating room standards prescribe a room temperature of 20–23 °C.[21] This set temperature invariably leads to hypothermia because of the temperature gradient between the operating room and patient.

4. Others include failure to actively warm the patient and inadequate insulation.[15]

TEMPERATURE MONITORING AND INDICATIONS

Temperature monitoring becomes mandatory for all neurosurgical cases as duration mostly lasts longer than 1 h and anesthesia time invariably exceeds 30 min.[22] Core temperature is more reliable to be monitored and documented to quantify change of temperature. Skin surface temperature monitoring is preferred wherever core temperature monitoring is not feasible or available, especially in pediatric patients.

The most commonly used probes for temperature monitoring are thermocouples and thermistors. These probes should be capable of discriminating a minimum difference of 0.5 °C, because this difference of temperature has shown to affect blood loss.[23] Temperature probes used for monitoring should be in the unadjusted mode and the same site of monitor should be used as far as possible.[24] The core temperature is best monitored with esophageal probes, nasopharyngeal probe, rectal probes, pulmonary artery catheter (PAC), tympanic membrane, bladder, and jugular bulb probe. The American Heart Association (ASA) recommends PAC as reliable and the gold standard for monitoring of core temperature during therapeutic hypothermia, e.g., deep hypothermic circulatory arrest (DHCA). Neither core sites other than PAC nor skin sites are recommended during therapeutic hypothermia. Skin probes are also used frequently in neurosurgical practice. The tympanic membrane is the recommended site for measurement as it is close to the hypothalamus and responds to changes in the set temperature.[25] Axillary and forehead sites are no longer recommended but easy to use.[24] The advantages and disadvantages of commonly used sites, physics related are described in Table 3.[23]

PREVENTION OF HYPOTHERMIA

This should start from the preoperative phase (1 h before induction) where the patient is kept covered and warm with temperature >36 °C. All the fluids, blood, and blood products are warmed to 37 °C before administration. The patient is covered with blankets and their temperature is not allowed to drift below 36 °C.[31]

Redistribution is thought to be the primary cause for initial drift in the core temperature. Active prewarming in the preoperative period 30 min before induction is shown to be effective in minimizing redistribution hypothermia. The ambient room temperature of the operating theater should be set at >21 °C. This is the threshold below which patients are prone to hypothermia.

The ASA guidelines advocate monitoring of temperature for all cases exceeding duration of surgery >30 min and to be documented every 15 min.[22] Firstly, vasodilation following the use of anesthetic agents, and secondly, due to the initial thermoregulatory vasodilatation contribute to better control of hypothermia in the intraoperative period rather than in the postoperative period when vasoconstriction predominates. This explains the effectiveness of intraoperative warming in treating the hypothermia compared with in the postoperative period and thus reducing the

TABLE 3   Sites of Temperature Monitoring: Physics, Advantages, and Disadvantages

Temperature Probe sites	Physical principles	Advantages	Disadvantages
Nasopharyngeal probe	Thermistor	Correlates well with the temperature of the hypothalamus	Slowly adjusts to rapid changes in brain temperature; bleeding from the nose
Pulmonary artery catheter	Thermistor	Correlates well with the brain temperature	Invasive; affected by cardiopulmonary bypass and profound hypothermia
Jugular bulb	Thermistor	Correlates well with the brain temperature in nonhead injury patients; reliable in deep hypothermic circulatory arrest	Invasive; affected by rapid changes in local temperature like fever and the severity of head injury
Tympanic membrane	Thermocouple	Correlates well with the nasopharyngeal temperature[25]	Affected by air currents, presence of wax, changes in local skin temperature; correct placement difficult; perforation of the tympanic membrane is a possibility
	Infrared	Used for monitoring in the pre and postoperative time; useful in pediatric patients[26]	Difficult to place Not recommended for monitoring during therapeutic hypothermia
Rectal[10]	Thermistor	Normally correlates closely with core temperature	Not reliable as it responds too slowly compared with other methods, especially in warm patients; sometimes gets lodged in the fecal matter
Deep tissue thermometry[27]	Thermistor	Shown to reflect the temperature at a depth of 18 mm or greater below the skin surface, i.e., the core temperature. Sites include upper sternum and forehead	Long equilibration time; unpredictable response to change in temperature

TABLE 3 Sites of Temperature Monitoring: Physics, Advantages, and Disadvantages—cont'd

Temperature Probe sites	Physical principles	Advantages	Disadvantages
Skin[28]	Thermistor or thermocouple (liquid crystal device)	Easily accessible	Less reliable; slowly adjusts to changes in temperature
Airway devices, e.g., cuff of endotracheal tube, perilaryngeal airway[29]	Thermocouple	Correlates well with the tympanic temperatures	Affected by gas flows
Brain tissue (intraparenchymal)	Thermocouple; Invasive, e.g., paratrend[30]	Reliable	Invasiveness of paratrend
	Noninvasive, e.g., Near infrared spectroscopy, ultrasound, microwave radiometry		Detects only focal changes in cerebral metabolism including temperature

incidence of complications following hypothermia.[9] Techniques used in the intraoperative period to prevent hypothermia include:

1. Regulating temperature of operation theaters: Raising the operation theater temperature to 24 °C is helpful in minimizing the heat loss due to radiation, convection, and redistribution. This is done especially from the time of patient transferring to the theater, during induction, and until the patient is positioned and draped.[32]
2. Forced air warming: This is the most efficient technique to maintain normothermia and avoid redistribution hypothermia, especially for lengthy neurosurgical cases.[33] This is also found to be effective in pediatric patients thus reducing the incidence of intraoperative complications.[34] Other alternatives include resistive polymer warming devices and underbody resistive heating which have found to be equally effective in preventing hypothermia.[35,36]
3. Fluid warming devices: These are indicated especially when large amounts of intravenous fluids or blood and blood products are administered.[37]
4. Use of warm fluids for intravenous infusion and for continuous irrigation: Fluid sets are placed in warm cabinets to achieve the required temperature and used accordingly.[38]

5. Breathing circuits and heat and moisture exchange filters: Closed and semiclosed circuits with low flows are ideal for conservation of both heat and moisture. Active inspired gas humidification has also shown to be effective in decreasing the magnitude of hypothermia in long duration surgeries.[39]
6. Warmed cotton blankets: If most of the surgery is in the head and neck area, the rest of the body can be covered with blankets to preserve body heat.
7. Gel-coated circulating mattress are especially useful in pediatric patients.[40]
8. Electric heating pads and convective warm blankets.
9. Amino acid infusions have shown to be effective in reducing the incidence of hypothermia and shivering, decreasing infection rate, and in turn decreasing the hospital stay and cost.[41] This may be beneficial especially in patients undergoing lengthy surgical procedures.
10. Avoiding or minimizing unnecessary exposure of the surgical field to the atmosphere.
11. New devices include circulating water garments and negative pressure devices. These have the benefit of covering large surface areas and for improving subcutaneous perfusion for effective warming, respectively.[33]

POSTANESTHETIC SHIVERING

The shivering response is part of the centrally mediated thermoregulatory defense mechanism that can have a significant detrimental impact on systemic oxygen consumption, brain tissue oxygenation, and intracranial pressure.[42] The overall metabolic consequences of shivering may eliminate many of the clinical benefits of temperature control. This is a common phenomenon following any surgery. This consists of two patterns: (1) tonic pattern, at a frequency of 4–8 cycles/min with both waxing and waning phenomena, this resembles normal shivering, and (2) clonic or phasic pattern-burst pattern of 5–7 Hz frequency. This occurs as a thermoregulatory response to intraoperative hypothermia. Appropriate initiation of pre- and intraoperative preventive and treatment measures for hypothermia has decreased the incidence of postoperative shivering. Once this occurs it has its own adverse effects like increased oxygen consumption and increased sympathetic tone. In neurosurgery, this may occasionally cause increased intracranial pressure which may further aggravate the primary condition especially in head injury victims.

Treatment:

1. Cutaneous warming, e.g., blankets, forced air warming.
2. Treatment of shivering includes drugs like meperidine (25–50 mg), clonidine (30–150 μg), ketanserin (10 mg), tramadol (0.5–1 mg/kg),

physostigmine (0.04 mg/kg), dexmedetomidine, magnesium sulfate (30 mg/kg), doxapram (25–100 mg), nalbhupine (0.05–0.1 m/kg), and nefopam.[43] Drugs like clonidine and dexmedetomidine act on the central thermoregulatory center and reset the shivering and vasoconstriction thresholds to a lower level.[44,45]

3. Oxygen supplementation to counteract the increased oxygen consumption.

4. Propofol is frequently used in the intensive care unit (ICU) for sedation. In addition to sedative and amnestic actions it mildly reduces the vasoconstriction and shivering thresholds.[46] Hypotension, negative cardiac ionotropy, sedation, and propofol infusion syndrome are limiting factors in the use of propofol for shivering.

5. We consider the use of paralytics as the last step because of the considerable side effects including loss of the neurologic examination and increased incidence of prolonged weakness associated with critical illness.[47]

THERAPEUTIC HYPOTHERMIA

1. Mild hypothermia is found to be beneficial in patients with head injury who sustained cardiac arrest with evidence of global ischemia.[48]

2. Patients following sudden cardiac arrest including those with nonshockable rhythm would benefit from therapeutic mild hypothermia.[49] This is seen especially in patients with prehospital evidence of return of spontaneous circulation.

3. The clipping and excision of giant intracranial aneurysms requires extensive dissection of the feeding artery and other surrounding vessels. DHCA is advocated for surgical treatment of such cases.[50] In contrast, intraoperative hypothermia for aneurysm surgery trial has not shown any beneficial effect of hypothermia in patients following surgical clipping of approachable intracranial aneurysms.[51,52]

4. Hypothermia has been proven to be beneficial in neonates postcardiac arrest who had experienced hypoxic–ischemic encephalopathy.[53]

HYPOTHERMIA IN CRITICAL CARE

Most of the indications for maintaining hypothermia warrant its continuation in the ICU as well. There has been an increasing use of advanced temperature modulating devices to achieve both therapeutic hypothermia and normothermia as a treatment.[54] Each device works by promoting conductive heat loss either by surface or intravascular cooling and maintains a tightly regulated temperature (±0.1 °C) through a feedback mechanism linked to a continuous core body temperature measurement. Therapeutic temperature modulation can be performed with intravascular cooling methods or external cooling.[55] Each device is regulated to a core temperature measured either by a bladder thermistor or esophageal probe.

During the cooling period, shivering has to be scored intermittently as shivering negates the advantages of hypothermia.[56] Also antishivering therapies are associated with prolonged sedation which may result in prolonged observation of the neurological examination and increase in the length of stay in the ICU. Hence, it would be appropriate if stepwise protocol is being followed which emphasizes the utilization of the least sedating regimen to achieve adequate shivering control.[57]

References

1. Hanania NA, Zimmerman JL. Hypothermia. In: Hall JB, Schmidt GA, Wood LDN, eds. *Principles of Critical Care*. 3rd ed. New York: McGraw-Hill; 2005.
2. Fay T. Observations on prolonged human refrigeration. *NY State J Med*. 1940;40:1351–1354.
3. Bigelow WG, Lindsay WK, et al. Oxygen transport and utilization in dogs at low body temperatures. *Am J Physiol*. 1950;160:125–137.
4. Drew CE, Keen G, Benazon DB. Profound hypothermia. *Lancet*. 1959;1:745–747.
5. Drake CG, Barr HW, Coles JC, Gergely NF. The use of extracorporeal circulation and profound hypothermia in the treatment of ruptured intracranial aneurysm. *J Neurosurg*. 1964;21:575–581.
6. Kurz A. Thermoregulation in anesthesia and intensive care medicine. Preface. *Best Pract Res Clin Anaesthesiol*. 2008;22:vii–viii.
7. Sessler DI. Temperature regulation and monitoring. In: Miller RD, Eriksson LI, Fleisher LA, Weiner-Kronis PJ, Young WL, eds. *Miller's Anesthesia*. Philadelphia: Churchill Livingstone Elsevier; 2010:1534–1556.
8. Cottrell JE, Young WL. *Cottrell and Young's Neuroanesthesia*. 5th ed. PHiladelphia: Mosby Elsevier; 2010.
9. Journeaux M. Peri-operative hypothermia: implications for practice. *Nurs Stand*. 2013;27:33–38.
10. Sessler DI. Temperature monitoring and perioperative thermoregulation. *Anesthesiology*. 2008;109:318–338.
11. Frank SM, Fleisher LA, Breslow MJ, Higgins MS, Olson KF, Kelly S, et al. Perioperative maintenance of normothermia reduces the incidence of morbid cardiac events. A randomized clinical trial. *JAMA*. 1997;277:1127–1134.
12. Schmied H, Kurz A, Sessler DI, Kozek S, Reiter A. Mild hypothermia increases blood loss and transfusion requirements during total hip arthroplasty. *Lancet*. 1996;347:289–292.
13. Bjelland TW, Klepstad P, Haugen BO, Nilsen T, Dale O. Effects of hypothermia on the disposition of morphine, midazolam, fentanyl, and propofol in intensive care unit patients. *Drug Metab Dispos*. 2013;41:214–223.
14. Lo C, Ormond G, McDougall R, Sheppard S, Davidson A. Effect of magnetic resonance imaging on core body temperature in anaesthetised children. *Anaesth Intensive Care*. 2014;42:333–339.
15. Horosz B, Malec-Milewska M. Inadvertent intraoperative hypothermia. *Anaesthesiol Intensive Ther*. 2013;45:38–43.
16. Ikeda T, Sessler DI, Kikura M, Kazama T, Ikeda K, Sato S. Less core hypothermia when anesthesia is induced with inhaled sevoflurane than with intravenous propofol. *Anesth Analg*. 1999;88:921–924.

17. Erickson KM, Lanier WL. Anesthetic technique influences brain temperature, independently of core temperature, during craniotomy in cats. *Anesth Analg.* 2003;96:1460–1466. [Table of contents].

18. Annadata R, Sessler DI, Tayefeh F, Kurz A, Dechert M. Desflurane slightly increases the sweating threshold but produces marked, nonlinear decreases in the vasoconstriction and shivering thresholds. *Anesthesiology.* 1995;83:1205–1211.

19. Xiong J, Kurz A, Sessler DI, Plattner O, Christensen R, Dechert M, et al. Isoflurane produces marked and nonlinear decreases in the vasoconstriction and shivering thresholds. *Anesthesiology.* 1996;85:240–245.

20. Hanagata K, Matsukawa T, Sessler DI, Miyaji T, Funayama T, Koshimizu M, et al. Isoflurane and sevoflurane produce a dose-dependent reduction in the shivering threshold in rabbits. *Anesth Analg.* 1995;81:581–584.

21. Recommended practices for sterilization. In: *Perioperative Standards and Recommended Practices.* Denver, CO: AORN, Inc.; 2013:513–540.

22. American Society of Anesthesiologists. *Standards for Basic Anesthetic Monitoring;* 2010. http://www.asahq.org/for-members/~/media/For%20Members/documents/Standards%20Guidelines%20Stmts/Basic%20Anesthetic%20Monitoring%202011.ashx. Accessed 09.05.14.

23. Sappenfield, et al. Perioperative temperature measurement and management:moving beyond the surgical care improvement project. *J Anesthesiol Clin Sci.* 2013;2.

24. Sund-Levander M, Grodzinsky E. Assessment of body temperature measurement options. *Br J Nurs.* 2013;22(942):44–50.

25. Drake-Brockman T, Hegarty M, Chambers N, von Ungern-Sternberg B. Monitoring temperature in children undergoing anaesthesia: a comparison of methods. *Anaesth Intensive Care.* 2014;42:315–320.

26. El-Radhi AS, Barry W. Thermometry in paediatric practice. *Arch Dis Child.* 2006;91:351–356.

27. Akata T, Machida Y, Yoshino J, Hirai T, Sato M, Takamatsu J, et al. Usefulness of monitoring forehead deep-tissue temperature as an index of core temperature in adult patients undergoing laparotomies under general anesthesia–investigation in operating rooms with air-movement control system using vertical flow. *Masui.* 2003;52:1066–1073.

28. Insler SR, Sessler DI. Perioperative thermoregulation and temperature monitoring. *Anesthesiol Clin.* 2006;24:823–837.

29. Wadhwa A, Sessler DI, Sengupta P, Hanni K, Akca O. Core temperature measurements through a new airway device, perilaryngeal airway (CobraPLA). *J Clin Anesth.* 2005;17:358–362.

30. Feuerstein TH, Langemann H, Gratzl O, Mendelowitsch A. A four lumen screwing device for multiparametric brain monitoring. *Acta Neurochir (Wien).* 2000;142:909–912.

31. Bernard H. Patient warming in surgery and the enhanced recovery. *Br J Nurs.* 2013;22: 319–320, 322–325.

32. Hardcastle TC, Stander M, Kalafatis N, Hodgson RE, Gopalan D. External patient temperature control in emergency centres, trauma centres, intensive care units and operating theatres: a multi-society literature review. *S Afr Med J.* 2013;103:609–611.

33. John M, Ford J, Harper M. Peri-operative warming devices: performance and clinical application. *Anaesthesia.* 2014.

34. Sessler DI. Forced-air warming in infants and children. *Paediatr Anaesth.* 2013;23:467–468.

35. Brandt S, Oguz R, Huttner H, Waglechner G, Chiari A, Greif R, et al. Resistive-polymer versus forced-air warming: comparable efficacy in orthopedic patients. *Anesth Analg.* 2010;110:834–838.

36. Egan C, Bernstein E, Reddy D, Ali M, Paul J, Yang D, et al. A randomized comparison of intraoperative PerfecTemp and forced-air warming during open abdominal surgery. *Anesth Analg.* 2011;113:1076–1081.

37. Moola S, Lockwood C. Effectiveness of strategies for the management and/or prevention of hypothermia within the adult perioperative environment. *Int J Evid Based Health.* 2011;9:337–345.

IX. MISCELLANEOUS

38. Shao L, Zheng H, Jia FJ, Wang HQ, Liu L, Sun Q, et al. Methods of patient warming during abdominal surgery. *PLoS One*. 2012;7:e39622.
39. Han SB, Gwak MS, Choi SJ, Kim MH, Ko JS, Kim GS, et al. Effect of active airway warming on body core temperature during adult liver transplantation. *Transpl Proc*. 2013;45:251–254.
40. Mathew B, Lakshminrusimha S, Sengupta S, Carrion V. Randomized controlled trial of vinyl bags versus thermal mattress to prevent hypothermia in extremely low-gestational-age infants. *Am J Perinatol*. 2013;30:317–322.
41. Moriyama T, Tsuneyoshi I, Omae T, Takeyama M, Kanmura Y. The effect of amino-acid infusion during off-pump coronary arterial bypass surgery on thermogenic and hormonal regulation. *J Anesth*. 2008;22:354–360.
42. Miller CA. *Pharmacological Treatment of Post-Anesthetic Shivering: An Educational Outreach Project*; 2011.
43. Charuluxananan S, et al. *Pharmacological Treatment of Post-anesthetic shivering: A Systematic Review and Meta-analysis*; 2010.
44. Delaunay L, Bonnet F, Liu N, Beydon L, Catoire P, Sessler DI. Clonidine comparably decreases the thermoregulatory thresholds for vasoconstriction and shivering in humans. *Anesthesiology*. 1993;79:470–474.
45. Talke P, Tayefeh F, Sessler DI, Jeffrey R, Noursalehi M, Richardson C. Dexmedetomidine does not alter the sweating threshold, but comparably and linearly decreases the vasoconstriction and shivering thresholds. *Anesthesiology*. 1997;87:835–841.
46. Matsukawa T, Kurz A, Sessler DI, Bjorksten AR, Merrifield B, Cheng C. Propofol linearly reduces the vasoconstriction and shivering thresholds. *Anesthesiology*. 1995;82:1169–1180.
47. Oehmichen F, Pohl M, Schlosser R, Stogowski D, Toppel D, Mehrholz J. Critical illness polyneuropathy und polymyopathy. How certain is the clinical diagnosis in patients with weaning failure? *Nervenarzt*. 2012;83:220–225.
48. Kimberger O, Kurz A. Thermoregulatory management for mild therapeutic hypothermia. *Best Pract Res Clin Anaesthesiol*. 2008;22:729–744.
49. Shinada T, Hata N, Kobayashi N, Tomita K, Shirakabe A, Tsurumi M, et al. Efficacy of therapeutic hypothermia for neurological salvage in patients with cardiogenic sudden cardiac arrest: the importance of prehospital return of spontaneous circulation. *J Nippon Med Sch*. 2013;80:287–295.
50. Ponce FA, Spetzler RF, Han PP, Wait SD, Killory BD, Nakaji P, et al. Cardiac standstill for cerebral aneurysms in 103 patients: an update on the experience at the Barrow Neurological Institute. Clinical article. *J Neurosurg*. 2011;114:877–884.
51. Mahaney KB, Todd MM, Bayman EO, Torner JC. Acute postoperative neurological deterioration associated with surgery for ruptured intracranial aneurysm: incidence, predictors, and outcomes. *J Neurosurg*. 2012;116:1267–1278.
52. Todd MM, Hindman BJ, Clarke WR, Torner JC. Mild intraoperative hypothermia during surgery for intracranial aneurysm. *N Engl J Med*. 2005;352:135–145.
53. Wassink G, Gunn ER, Drury PP, Bennet L, Gunn AJ. The mechanisms and treatment of asphyxial encephalopathy. *Front Neurosci*. 2014;8:40.
54. Atkins CM, Truettner JS, Lotocki G, Sanchez-Molano J, Kang Y, Alonso OF, et al. Post-traumatic seizure susceptibility is attenuated by hypothermia therapy. *Eur J Neurosci*. 2010;32:1912–1920.
55. Taniguchi Y, Lenhardt R, Sessler DI, Kurz A. The effect of altering skin-surface cooling speeds on vasoconstriction and shivering thresholds. *Anesth Analg*. 2011;113:540–544.
56. Sessler DI. Defeating normal thermoregulatory defenses: induction of therapeutic hypothermia. *Stroke*. 2009;40:e614–e621.
57. Choi HA, Ko SB, Presciutti M, Fernandez L, Carpenter AM, Lesch C, et al. Prevention of shivering during therapeutic temperature modulation: the Columbia anti-shivering protocol. *Neurocrit Care*. 2011;14:389–394.

Nausea and Vomiting

M. Srilata, Kavitha Jayaram

**Department of Anesthesia and Intensive Care, Nizam's
Institute of Medical Sciences, Hyderabad, India**

DEFINITION

Nausea is defined as a subjective feeling of unpleasant sensation of urge to vomit. Vomiting is defined as dynamic expulsion of stomach contents from the mouth.[1]

VARIANTS

Retching is defined as strenuous, spasmodic, and periodic contractions of the respiratory muscles (diaphragm and muscles of the chest and abdominal wall) without expulsion of the stomach contents.

Postoperative nausea and vomiting (PONV) is a common complication following surgery and anesthesia.[1,2] Patients often rate PONV as equivalent to, or sometimes worse than, postoperative pain.[3–5] This is found to be an important factor predicting the delay in discharge from the hospital with increased costs following most surgeries including ambulatory surgery. At the same time, it is associated with psychological disturbance and dissatisfaction to the patient. Therefore, preventing PONV improves satisfaction in patients likely to experience it.[6] Nausea and vomiting pose significant medical risk particularly in neurosurgery patients as they increase both intracranial pressure and cerebrospinal fluid pressure.

AETIOLOGY

Various pathways are involved in the aetiology of nausea and vomiting.[7,8] The main sensory stimulus includes local gastrointestinal irritants, absorbed toxins and drugs, and vestibular movement. Pharyngeal stimulation and other factors like pain, emotions leading to direct cortical stimulation also contribute to nausea and vomiting. The integrative mechanism involves mechanoreceptors, chemoreceptors, and afferent pathways ending in higher centers for vomiting like the chemoreceptor trigger zone (CRTZ; area postrema) and vomiting center (medulla). The efferent output is generated via visceral and somatic nuclei in the form of nausea, dizziness, vomiting, and other sympathetic and vagal symptoms[9] (Figure 1).

INCIDENCE

The global incidence of PONV is around 20–30%[2] and specifically in neurosurgical practice is found to be around 40–50%.[10]

CONTRIBUTING FACTORS[4,11–16]

1. PONV is more prevalent in females compared with males (3:1). Sex is a strong predictor of PONV but there is no clear cut rationalization.[4,10,17]

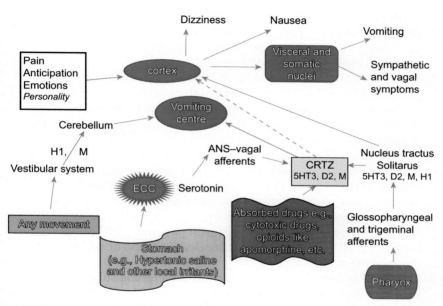

FIGURE 1 Pathophysiology and pathways for nausea and vomiting. Text in italics and dotted line indicates indirect evidence. Abbreviations: ECC, enterochromaffin cells; CRTZ, chemoreceptor trigger zone; ANS, autonomic nervous system; H, histaminic; M, muscarinic; 5-HT, 5-hydroxytrytamine; D, dopaminergic.

2. History of motion sickness or PONV plays an important role. Patients with a history of migraine also have increased susceptibility to PONV.[18]
3. Nonsmokers have depleted stores of dopamine compared with smokers whereas indirect γ-aminobutyric acid-mediated cerebral dopamine levels are increased due to nicotine. Reduced activation of dopaminergic circuits in the CRTZ is responsible for the increased incidence of PONV in nonsmokers and in patients with nicotine withdrawal in the perioperative period.[18]
4. Postoperative opioids increase the incidence of PONV in a dose-dependent manner[19] and this effect lasts as long as opioids are used for pain.[13]
5. The most likely causes of PONV are volatile anesthetics, nitrous oxide, and postoperative opioids.[14,20] The effect of volatile anesthetics on PONV is dose-dependent and particularly prominent in the first 2–6 h after surgery. Recent evidence has shown nonsignificant difference in PONV when inhalational anesthetics like sevoflurane, isoflurane, enflurane, and desflurane were compared.[14] Use of nitrous oxide enhanced the emetogenic effect of inhalational agents thus adding the incidence of PONV.[21]

6. As the duration of surgery is increased, the incidence of PONV is further increased.[21] This is due to obvious reasons like increased exposure to anesthetic agents, use of intraoperative opioids, and increased exposure to hemodynamic instability.

7. Type of surgery also influences likelihood of PONV. The most consistent surgeries found to have high predilection for PONV are laparoscopic cholecystectomy and hysterectomy in adults and strabismus surgery in children.[15,22–24] For other types of surgeries, the increased incidence is thought to be due to increased duration of surgery and hence increased exposure to anesthetic agents and opioids and patient-related factors like female gender, smoking history, and history of PONV. Infratentorial surgery, midline posterior fossa tumors, microvascular decompression, acoustic neuroma surgery, and epilepsy surgery are found to be surgical risk factors for PONV in neurosurgical patients.[17,25–27] Most neurosurgical operations with increased duration of surgery will be more prone to PONV.

8. Hypoxia[28] is especially seen in patients undergoing surgery under spinal or epidural anesthesia exhibiting severe hypotension. Severe fall in blood pressure decreases cerebral perfusion pressure which in turn is responsible for hypoxia-induced nausea and sometimes vomiting; this may be exacerbated where nitrous oxide is used to supplement analgesia.

The multifactorial origin of PONV explains validation of different risk models with the above described variables for prediction of PONV both in inpatients and outpatients following surgery under anesthesia (Table 1).

PREVENTION

1. Preanesthetic assessment should include proper identification of high-risk patients, like female patients with nonsmoking history.

2. Hydration in the perioperative period (level of evidence A1)[29–31] is especially controversial in neurosurgical practice. Restrictive fluid strategy has shown to have beneficial effects in overall outcome following craniotomies. Administration of intraoperative fluids should be guided by the urinary output and insensible losses.[32]

3. Avoid use of nitrous oxide (level of evidence A1).[33,34]

4. Avoid inhalational agents (level of evidence A2).[14,35]

5. Minimizing the duration of surgery and anesthesia.[21]

6. The incidence of PONV is reduced in opioid-free regional anesthesia[36] and with reduced opioid consumption by the use of nonopioid analgesics,[37] perioperative α2-agonists,[38] and β-blockers.[39]

TABLE 1   Risk Factors and Current Evidence

Evidence	Risk factors (level of evidence)
Positive overall	Female sex (B1)
	History of PONV or motion sickness (B1)
	Nonsmoking (B1)
	Younger age (B1)
	General versus regional anesthesia (A1)
	Use of volatile anesthetics and nitrous oxide (A1)
	Postoperative opioids (A1)
	Duration of anesthesia (B1)
Conflicting	ASA physical status (B1)
	Menstrual cycle (B1)
	Level of anesthetist's experience (B1)
	Muscle relaxant antagonists (A2)
Disproven or of limited relevance	BMI (B1)
	Anxiety (B1)
	Nasogastric tube (A1)
	Supplemental oxygen (A1)
	Perioperative fasting (A2)
	Migraine (B1)

Abbreviations: PONV, postoperative nausea and vomiting; ASA, American Society of Anesthesiologists; BMI, body mass index.

7. In neurosurgery, the use of regional nerve blocks[12,40] such as scalp nerve blocks, cervical plexus block, maxillary blocks, and infiltration analgesia may help in reducing the incidence of PONV following craniotomies, cervical surgeries, and transsphenoidal excision of tumors.[41] The incidence of PONV is comparatively less in patients undergoing central neuraxial block like spinal and epidural anesthesia.[42]
8. Prophylactic use of antiemetics.
9. Use of intravenous agents like propofol both for induction and maintenance. In children subhypnotic doses of propofol infusion in combination with an antiemetic significantly reduces the incidence of PONV[35,43,44] (level of evidence A1).
10. Minimization of neostigmine dosage has been removed from the list of strategies to reduce baseline risk as new evidence did not find this to be helpful, and the evidence is contradictory.[2]

11. Nonpharmacologic prophylaxis includes acupuncture guided P6 stimulation and neuromuscular titanic stimulation over the median nerve[45,46] (level of evidence A1).
12. Systematic reviews of randomized controlled trials show that supplemental oxygen had no effect on nausea or overall vomiting, although it may reduce the risk of early vomiting. As a result, supplemental oxygen is not recommended for the prevention of PONV.[2,47]

MEASUREMENT OF NAUSEA AND VOMITING

PONV should be assessed separately both for nausea and vomiting. Uses of antiemetics have adverse effects ranging from headache to corrected QT interval (QTc) prolongation and rarely cardiac arrest.[48] Therefore, patients risk has to be assessed using validated risk score based on independent risk predictors. Use of risk scores significantly reduce institutional rate of PONV.[35,49,50] Two scores are commonly used: the Koivuranta score[4] and the Apfel score.[11]

For nausea, the Visual Analog Scale is the most widely accepted scale for measurement of severity of nausea, 10 cm horizontal scale, with the lower end corresponding to no nausea and upper end corresponding to the worst imaginable nausea. Other approach is the 11 point numeric rating scale (0–10) with 0 corresponding to no symptoms and 10 to worst possible symptoms. The other approach is the categorical verbal rating scale which is easy to use and has moderate sensitivity. It is divided into four categories: none, mild, moderate, and severe.

For vomiting, this is better described as an emetic episode as this includes the lesser variety, i.e., retching, in its description. This measurement is simpler compared with the measurement of nausea and its severity is best evaluated by the number of episodes.

TREATMENT

The algorithm for management of PONV as per published guidelines is given in Figure 2.[2] Antiemetics used for PONV are described as below and tabulated (Table 2).

5-HT$_3$ Antagonists

Ondansetron is as effective as other 5-HT$_3$ receptor antagonists including ramosetron 0.3 mg.[51] However, it is less effective than aprepitant for reducing emesis and palonosetron for the incidence of PONV.[52] In December 2010, the United States Food and Drug Administration (US FDA) announced

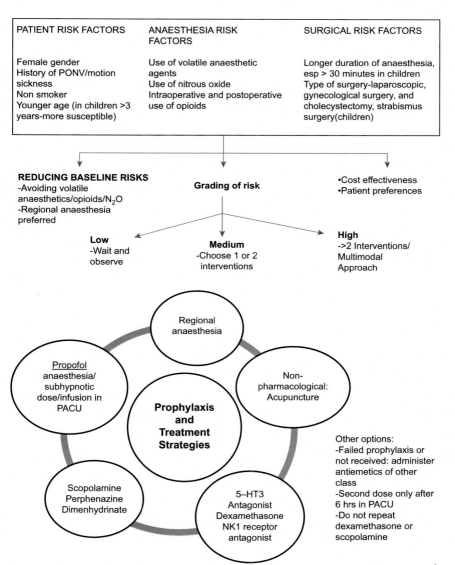

FIGURE 2   Algorithm for PONV. Abbreviations: PONV, postoperative nausea and vomiting; PACU, postanesthesia care unit.

that intravenous dolasetron should no longer be used for chemotherapy-induced nausea and vomiting in adults and children because of concerns of QT prolongation and torsade de pointes. Palonosetron 0.075 mg is more effective than granisetron 1 mg and ondansetron 4 mg in preventing PONV.[53] The 5-HT$_3$ receptor antagonists have a favorable side effect profile, and while generally considered equally safe, all except palonosetron

TABLE 2   Commonly Used Antiemetics: Class, Mechanism of Action, Dose, Side Effects, and Timing of Administration

Dopamine antagonists	Site and mechanism of action	Dosage	Side effects	Timing of administration
Metaclopromide	D_2, prokinetic, (5-HT$_3$)	25, 50 mg	Hypotension, tachycardia, extra-pyramidal side effects	
Droperidol	D_2 antagonist	0.625–1.25 mg	Sedation, anxiety, restlessness, torsades de pointes	End of surgery
Serotonin receptor antagonists Ondansetron Palonosetron Dolasetron Granisetron Tropisetron Ramosetron	5-HT$_3$ receptor antagonists	4 mg IV, 8 mg ODT 0.075 mg IV 12.5 mg IV 0.35–3 mg IV 2 mg IV 0.3 mg IV	Allergic reactions, bronchospasm, blurred vision, dysrrythmias, QT interval prolongation	End of surgery At induction End of surgery End of surgery End of surgery End of surgery
NK1 receptor antagonist, aprepitant Casopitant Rolapitant	NK 1 receptors	40–80 mg oral 50–150 mg oral 70–200 mg oral		At induction At induction At induction
Steroids Dexamethasone Methyprednisolone		4–5 mg IV 40 mg IV	Hyperglycaemia, increased infection	At induction At induction
Scopalamine		Transdermal patch	Visual disturbances, dry mouth and dizziness	Prior evening–12 h before surgery

Abbreviations: 5-HT, 5-hydroxytryptamine; D, dopaminergic; NK, neurokinin.

affect the QTc interval. In June 2012, the US FDA recommended the dose of ondansetron for chemotherapy-induced nausea and vomiting should not exceed 16 mg in a single dose because of risks of QT prolongation.

NK1 Receptor Antagonists

Aprepitant is an NK1 receptor antagonist with a 40-hour half-life. Aprepitant was significantly more effective than ondansetron for preventing vomiting at 24 and 48 h after surgery and in reducing nausea severity in the first 48 h after surgery.[54] Casopitant and rolapitant has not been approved for use though they have longer half-lives and are under phase III trial.

Corticosteroids

The corticosteroid dexamethasone effectively prevents nausea and vomiting in postoperative patients.[55,56] Studies are increasingly using the higher dose of 8 mg dexamethasone IV rather than the minimum effective dose of 4–5 mg.[57,58] A metaanalysis evaluating the dose-dependent analgesic effects of perioperative dexamethasone found that doses >0.1 mg/kg are an effective adjunct in multimodal strategies to reduce postoperative pain and opioid consumption.[59,60] Use of dexamethasone in labile diabetes patients is relatively contraindicated.[61]

Butyrophenones

Many physicians stopped using droperidol in 2001 due to the FDA "black box" restrictions on its use. However, the droperidol doses used for the management of PONV are extremely low, and it is believed that at these dosing levels, droperidol is unlikely to be associated with significant cardiovascular events. It is recommended to use droperidol as in hospital treatment and in children only if other therapy fails.[2] Haloperidol has antiemetic properties when used in low doses and has been investigated as an alternative to droperidol only in adults.[62] Its efficacy can be increased when combined with other antiemetics such as dexamethasone or ondansetron.

Antihistamines

Dimenhydrinate is an antihistamine with antiemetic effects. The recommended dose is 1 mg/kg IV. Meclizine has a longer duration of PONV effect than ondansetron.

Other Antiemetics

Metoclopramide is a weak antiemetic and at a dose of 10 mg is not effective in reducing the incidence of nausea and vomiting.[63] Numerous studies have demonstrated antiemetic properties of propofol. Propofol used as part of Total intravenous anesthesia (TIVA) is recommended to reduce baseline risk for PONV.[64] In a metaanalysis, perioperative systemic $\alpha 2$-adrenoceptor agonists (clonidine and dexmedetomidine) showed a significant albeit weak and short-lived antinausea effect.[65] Mirtazapine is a noradrenergic and specific serotonergic antidepressant. Prophylactic mirtazapine delays the onset of PONV.[66] Gabapentin doses of 600 mg per os given 2 h before surgery effectively decreases PONV.[67] Midazolam decreases nausea and vomiting compared with placebo.[68,69] Midazolam 2 mg when administered 30 min before the end of surgery was as effective against PONV as ondansetron 4 mg.

References

1. Kovac AL. Update on the management of postoperative nausea and vomiting. *Drugs.* 2013;73:1525–1547.
2. Gan TJ, Diemunsch P, Habib AS, et al. Consensus guidelines for the management of postoperative nausea and vomiting. *Anesth Analg.* 2014;118:85–113.
3. Andion O, Canellas M, Banos JE. Physical well-being in postoperative period: a survey in patients, nurses and physicians. *J Clin Nurs.* 2014;23:1421–1429.
4. Koivuranta M, Laara E, Snare L, Alahuhta S. A survey of postoperative nausea and vomiting. *Anaesthesia.* 1997;52:443–449.
5. Macario A, Weinger M, Truong P, Lee M. Which clinical anesthesia outcomes are both common and important to avoid? the perspective of a panel of expert anesthesiologists. *Anesth Analg.* 1999;88:1085–1091.
6. Darkow T, Gora-Harper ML, Goulson DT, Record KE. Impact of antiemetic selection on postoperative nausea and vomiting and patient satisfaction. *Pharmacotherapy.* 2001;21:540–548.
7. Andrews PL, Horn CC. Signals for nausea and emesis: Implications for models of upper gastrointestinal diseases. *Auton Neurosci.* 2006;125:100–115.
8. Sanger GJ, Broad J, Andrews PL. The relationship between gastric motility and nausea: gastric prokinetic agents as treatments. *Eur J Pharmacol.* 2013;715:10–14.
9. Sanger GJ, Andrews PL. Treatment of nausea and vomiting: gaps in our knowledge. *Auton Neurosci.* 2006;129:3–16.
10. Neufeld SM, Newburn-Cook CV. What are the risk factors for nausea and vomiting after neurosurgery? A systematic review. *Can J Neurosci Nurs.* 2008;30:23–34.
11. Apfel CC, Laara E, Koivuranta M, Greim CA, Roewer N. A simplified risk score for predicting postoperative nausea and vomiting: conclusions from cross-validations between two centers. *Anesthesiology.* 1999;91:693–700.
12. Sinclair DR, Chung F, Mezei G. Can postoperative nausea and vomiting be predicted? *Anesthesiology.* 1999;91:109–118.
13. Apfel CC, Philip BK, Cakmakkaya OS, et al. Who is at risk for postdischarge nausea and vomiting after ambulatory surgery? *Anesthesiology.* 2012;117:475–486.
14. Apfel CC, Kranke P, Katz MH, et al. Volatile anaesthetics may be the main cause of early but not delayed postoperative vomiting: a randomized controlled trial of factorial design. *Br J Anaesth.* 2002;88:659–668.
15. Apfel CC, Kranke P, Eberhart LH. Comparison of surgical site and patient's history with a simplified risk score for the prediction of postoperative nausea and vomiting. *Anaesthesia.* 2004;59:1078–1082.
16. Leslie K, Myles PS, Chan MT, et al. Risk factors for severe postoperative nausea and vomiting in a randomized trial of nitrous oxide-based vs nitrous oxide-free anaesthesia. *Br J Anaesth.* 2008;101:498–505.
17. Audibert G, Vial V. Postoperative nausea and vomiting after neurosurgery (infratentorial and supratentorial surgery). *Ann Fr Anesth Reanim.* 2004;23:422–427.
18. Rusch D, Eberhart LH, Wallenborn J, Kranke P. Nausea and vomiting after surgery under general anesthesia: an evidence-based review concerning risk assessment, prevention, and treatment. *Dtsch Arztebl Int.* 2010;107:733–741.
19. Roberts GW, Bekker TB, Carlsen HH, Moffatt CH, Slattery PJ, McClure AF. Postoperative nausea and vomiting are strongly influenced by postoperative opioid use in a dose-related manner. *Anesth Analg.* 2005;101:1343–1348.

20. Myles PS, Leslie K, Chan MT, et al. Avoidance of nitrous oxide for patients undergoing major surgery: a randomized controlled trial. *Anesthesiology.* 2007;107:221–231.
21. Apfel CC, Heidrich FM, Jukar-Rao S, et al. Evidence-based analysis of risk factors for postoperative nausea and vomiting. *Br J Anaesth.* 2012;109:742–753.
22. Stadler M, Bardiau F, Seidel L, Albert A, Boogaerts JG. Difference in risk factors for post-operative nausea and vomiting. *Anesthesiology.* 2003;98:46–52.
23. Cohen MM, Duncan PG, DeBoer DP, Tweed WA. The postoperative interview: assessing risk factors for nausea and vomiting. *Anesth Analg.* 1994;78:7–16.
24. Wallenborn J, Gelbrich G, Bulst D, et al. Prevention of postoperative nausea and vomiting by metoclopramide combined with dexamethasone: randomised double blind multicentre trial. *BMJ.* 2006;333:324.
25. Tan C, Ries CR, Mayson K, Gharapetian A, Griesdale DE. Indication for surgery and the risk of postoperative nausea and vomiting after craniotomy: a case-control study. *J Neurosurg Anesthesiol.* 2012;24:325–330.
26. Neufeld S, Dundon B, Yu H, Newburn-Cook C, Drummond J. Midline location of tumour is a risk factor for postoperative vomiting in children requiring posterior fossa tumour resection. *Can J Neurosci Nurs.* 2009;31:10–14.
27. Kurita N, Kawaguchi M, Nakahashi K, et al. Retrospective analysis of postoperative nausea and vomiting after craniotomy. *Masui.* 2004;53:150–155.
28. Purhonen S, Niskanen M, Wustefeld M, Mustonen P, Hynynen M. Supplemental oxygen for prevention of nausea and vomiting after breast surgery. *Br J Anaesth.* 2003;91:284–287.
29. Scuderi PE, James RL, Harris L, Mims 3rd GR. Multimodal antiemetic management prevents early postoperative vomiting after outpatient laparoscopy. *Anesth Analg.* 2000;91:1408–1414.
30. Apfel CC, Meyer A, Orhan-Sungur M, Jalota L, Whelan RP, Jukar-Rao S. Supplemental intravenous crystalloids for the prevention of postoperative nausea and vomiting: quantitative review. *Br J Anaesth.* 2012;108:893–902.
31. Goodarzi M, Matar MM, Shafa M, Townsend JE, Gonzalez I. A prospective randomized blinded study of the effect of intravenous fluid therapy on postoperative nausea and vomiting in children undergoing strabismus surgery. *Paediatr Anaesth.* 2006;16:49–53.
32. Tommasino C. Fluids and the neurosurgical patient. *Anesthesiol Clin N Am.* 2002;20: 329–346, vi.
33. Tramer M, Moore A, McQuay H. Meta-analytic comparison of prophylactic antiemetic efficacy for postoperative nausea and vomiting: propofol anaesthesia vs omitting nitrous oxide vs total i.v. anaesthesia with propofol. *Br J Anaesth.* 1997;78:256–259.
34. Tramer M, Moore A, McQuay H. Omitting nitrous oxide in general anaesthesia: meta-analysis of intraoperative awareness and postoperative emesis in randomized controlled trials. *Br J Anaesth.* 1996;76:186–193.
35. Apfel CC, Korttila K, Abdalla M, et al. A factorial trial of six interventions for the prevention of postoperative nausea and vomiting. *N Engl J Med.* 2004;350:2441–2451.
36. Liu SS, Strodtbeck WM, Richman JM, Wu CL. A comparison of regional versus general anesthesia for ambulatory anesthesia: a meta-analysis of randomized controlled trials. *Anesth Analg.* 2005;101:1634–1642.
37. Marret E, Kurdi O, Zufferey P, Bonnet F. Effects of nonsteroidal antiinflammatory drugs on patient-controlled analgesia morphine side effects: meta-analysis of randomized controlled trials. *Anesthesiology.* 2005;102:1249–1260.
38. Gurbet A, Basagan-Mogol E, Turker G, Ugun F, Kaya FN, Ozcan B. Intraoperative infusion of dexmedetomidine reduces perioperative analgesic requirements. *Can J Anaesth.* 2006;53:646–652.
39. Collard V, Mistraletti G, Taqi A, et al. Intraoperative esmolol infusion in the absence of opioids spares postoperative fentanyl in patients undergoing ambulatory laparoscopic cholecystectomy. *Anesth Analg.* 2007;105:1255–1262. [table of contents].
40. Rowley MP, Brown TC. Postoperative vomiting in children. *Anaesth Intensive Care.* 1982;10:309–313.

41. Sinha PK, Koshy T, Gayatri P, Smitha V, Abraham M, Rathod RC. Anesthesia for awake craniotomy: a retrospective study. *Neurol India*. 2007;55:376–381.

42. Moore JG, Ross SM, Williams BA. Regional anesthesia and ambulatory surgery. *Curr Opin Anaesthesiol*. 2013;26:652–660.

43. Erdem AF, Yoruk O, Alici HA, et al. Subhypnotic propofol infusion plus dexamethasone is more effective than dexamethasone alone for the prevention of vomiting in children after tonsillectomy. *Paediatr Anaesth*. 2008;18:878–883.

44. Erdem AF, Yoruk O, Silbir F, et al. Tropisetron plus subhypnotic propofol infusion is more effective than tropisetron alone for the prevention of vomiting in children after tonsillectomy. *Anaesth Intensive Care*. 2009;37:54–59.

45. Lee A, Fan LT. Stimulation of the wrist acupuncture point P6 for preventing postoperative nausea and vomiting. *Cochrane Database Syst Rev*. 2009:CD003281.

46. Kim YH, Kim KS, Lee HJ, Shim JC, Yoon SW. The efficacy of several neuromuscular monitoring modes at the P6 acupuncture point in preventing postoperative nausea and vomiting. *Anesth Analg*. 2011;112:819–823.

47. Orhan-Sungur M, Kranke P, Sessler D, Apfel CC. Does supplemental oxygen reduce postoperative nausea and vomiting? A meta-analysis of randomized controlled trials. *Anesth Analg*. 2008;106:1733–1738.

48. Charbit B, Albaladejo P, Funck-Brentano C, Legrand M, Samain E, Marty J. Prolongation of QTc interval after postoperative nausea and vomiting treatment by droperidol or ondansetron. *Anesthesiology*. 2005;102:1094–1100.

49. Pierre S, Benais H, Pouymayou J. Apfel's simplified score may favourably predict the risk of postoperative nausea and vomiting. *Can J Anaesth*. 2002;49:237–242.

50. Pierre S, Corno G, Benais H, Apfel CC. A risk score-dependent antiemetic approach effectively reduces postoperative nausea and vomiting–a continuous quality improvement initiative. *Can J Anaesth*. 2004;51:320–325.

51. Ryu J, So YM, Hwang J, Do SH. Ramosetron versus ondansetron for the prevention of postoperative nausea and vomiting after laparoscopic cholecystectomy. *Surg Endosc*. 2010;24:812–817.

52. Diemunsch P, Gan TJ, Philip BK, et al. Single-dose aprepitant vs ondansetron for the prevention of postoperative nausea and vomiting: a randomized, double-blind phase III trial in patients undergoing open abdominal surgery. *Br J Anaesth*. 2007;99:202–211.

53. Park SK, Cho EJ. A randomized, double-blind trial of palonosetron compared with ondansetron in preventing postoperative nausea and vomiting after gynaecological laparoscopic surgery. *J Int Med Res*. 2011;39:399–407.

54. Gan TJ, Apfel CC, Kovac A, et al. A randomized, double-blind comparison of the NK1 antagonist, aprepitant, versus ondansetron for the prevention of postoperative nausea and vomiting. *Anesth Analg*. 2007;104:1082–1089. [table of contents].

55. Henzi I, Walder B, Tramer MR. Dexamethasone for the prevention of postoperative nausea and vomiting: a quantitative systematic review. *Anesth Analg*. 2000;90:186–194.

56. Wang JJ, Ho ST, Lee SC, Liu YC, Ho CM. The use of dexamethasone for preventing postoperative nausea and vomiting in females undergoing thyroidectomy: a dose-ranging study. *Anesth Analg*. 2000;91:1404–1407.

57. Arslan M, Cicek R, Kalender HU, Yilmaz H. Preventing postoperative nausea and vomiting after laparoscopic cholecystectomy: a prospective, randomized, double-blind study. *Curr Ther Res Clin Exp*. 2011;72:1–12.

58. Arslan M, Demir ME. Prevention of postoperative nausea and vomiting with a small dose of propofol combined with dexamethasone 4 mg or dexamethasone 8 mg in patients undergoing middle ear surgery: a prospective, randomized, double-blind study. *Bratisl Lek Listy*. 2011;112:332–336.

59. De Oliveira Jr GS, Almeida MD, Benzon HT, McCarthy RJ. Perioperative single dose systemic dexamethasone for postoperative pain: a meta-analysis of randomized controlled trials. *Anesthesiology*. 2011;115:575–588.

60. Waldron NH, Jones CA, Gan TJ, Allen TK, Habib AS. Impact of perioperative dexamethasone on postoperative analgesia and side-effects: systematic review and meta-analysis. *Br J Anaesth.* 2013;110:191–200.
61. Miyagawa Y, Ejiri M, Kuzuya T, Osada T, Ishiguro N, Yamada K. Methylprednisolone reduces postoperative nausea in total knee and hip arthroplasty. *J Clin Pharm Ther.* 2010;35:679–684.
62. Smith 2nd JC, Wright EL. Haloperidol: an alternative butyrophenone for nausea and vomiting prophylaxis in anesthesia. *AANA J.* 2005;73:273–275.
63. Henzi I, Walder B, Tramer MR. Metoclopramide in the prevention of postoperative nausea and vomiting: a quantitative systematic review of randomized, placebo-controlled studies. *Br J Anaesth.* 1999;83:761–771.
64. Tramer M, Moore A, McQuay H. Propofol anaesthesia and postoperative nausea and vomiting: quantitative systematic review of randomized controlled studies. *Br J Anaesth.* 1997;78:247–255.
65. Blaudszun G, Lysakowski C, Elia N, Tramer MR. Effect of perioperative systemic alpha2 agonists on postoperative morphine consumption and pain intensity: systematic review and meta-analysis of randomized controlled trials. *Anesthesiology.* 2012;116:1312–1322.
66. Chen CC, Lin CS, Ko YP, Hung YC, Lao HC, Hsu YW. Premedication with mirtazapine reduces preoperative anxiety and postoperative nausea and vomiting. *Anesth Analg.* 2008;106:109–113. [table of contents].
67. Khademi S, Ghaffarpasand F, Heiran HR, Asefi A. Effects of preoperative gabapentin on postoperative nausea and vomiting after open cholecystectomy: a prospective randomized double-blind placebo-controlled study. *Med Princ Pract.* 2010;19:57–60.
68. Jung JS, Park JS, Kim SO, et al. Prophylactic antiemetic effect of midazolam after middle ear surgery. *Otolaryngol Head Neck Surg.* 2007;137:753–756.
69. Tarhan O, Canbay O, Celebi N, et al. Subhypnotic doses of midazolam prevent nausea and vomiting during spinal anesthesia for cesarean section. *Minerva Anestesiol.* 2007;73:629–633.

Peripheral Nerve Injuries

M.V.S. Satya Prakash, Prasanna Udupi Bidkar
Department of Anaesthesiology and Critical Care, JIPMER,
Puducherry, India

OUTLINE

Various positions are used in neurosurgery, including supine, lateral, prone, and sitting as well as many modifications of these positions. If positioning is not performed properly, position-related nerve injuries can occur more commonly in neurosurgery than in other surgeries as the majority of these surgeries are of longer duration. Dhuner et al. published a retrospective review of more than 30,000 patients in 1950 and found that the incidence of peripheral nerve injury was 1/1000. The majority (83%) of these cases were ulnar nerve injury.[1,2] The American Society of Anesthesiologists (ASA) closed claim studies showed that 15% of the total claims were related to nerve injuries; one-third were for ulnar nerve, 23% for brachial plexus, and 16% for lumbosacral roots.[3] The nerve injuries that can occur due to improper positioning are as described below (Table 1).

PREDISPOSING FACTORS

The factors predisposing to peripheral nerve injuries can be divided into:

1. Patient factors;
2. Surgical factors; and
3. Anesthetic factors.

PATIENT FACTORS

The predisposing factors that can increase the chance of perioperative peripheral neuropathies due to improper positioning are smoking,

TABLE 1 Peripheral Nerves at Risk in Different Positions

Position	Nerves at risk
Supine	Ulnar nerve at elbow, brachial plexus injuries.
Lateral	Radial nerve, common peroneal nerve.
Prone	Optic neuropathy, brachial plexus injuries.
Sitting	Sciatic nerve injury, common peroneal nerve.

diabetes mellitus, peripheral vascular disease, extremes of body weight, extremes of age, preexisting neurological symptoms, alcohol dependency, arthritis, and gender.[4,5] Males are more prone to peripheral nerve injuries than females as they have less subcutaneous fat. Some other factors like abnormal course of the nerve or congenital anomalies of that region can also influence perioperative peripheral nerve injuries. The superficial course of the nerve also increases the risk of nerve injury.

SURGICAL FACTORS

The majority of neurosurgeries last for a prolonged duration, i.e., more than 2–4 h. If positioning is not properly performed, this prolonged surgery itself may increase the risk of nerve injury. In 1979, Keykhah et al. studied foot drop after craniotomy. They concluded that the frequency was approximately 1% from a series of 488 patients.[2,6] Recurrent laryngeal nerve injury might happen due to prolonged use of transesophageal echocardiography. In patients undergoing anterior cervical discectomies, prolonged application of retractors may increase the risk of recurrent laryngeal nerve injury.

The perioperative factors that may have a role in causing peripheral nerve injuries are blood loss leading to prolonged hypovolemia and hypotension, dehydration, hypoxia, and electrolyte disturbance.[2,7–9] Induced hypothermia can also cause perioperative peripheral nerve injury.[10,11]

ANESTHETIC FACTORS

Lingual nerve damage has been associated with prolonged intubation and use of laryngeal mask airway.[12,13]

ETIOLOGY

There are many mechanisms that can cause perioperative peripheral nerve injuries. They can be classified as follows:

1. Direct nerve damage may occur due to surgery or regional anesthetic techniques. Blunt needles are less likely to cause nerve damage than other types of needles.
2. Stretch and compression: poor padding, poor positioning of limbs and body.
3. Ischemia is the final common pathway for perioperative peripheral nerve injuries. It may be caused by prolonged immobility and hematoma surrounding the nerves.

4. Injection of high concentrations of local anesthetic or intrafascicular injection of local anesthetics may predispose to perioperative peripheral nerve injury.
5. A nerve with predisposing neuropathy may have a high chance of damage when a second insult occurs during surgery.
6. Unknown factors and combination of above factors.

CLASSIFICATION OF NERVE INJURIES

There are two classifications which are commonly used for the degree of nerve damage: Seddon classification and Sunderland classification (Table 2).[2]

SPECIFIC NERVE INJURIES

Ulnar Nerve Injury

In general, incidence of ulnar nerve injury is 0.037%.[5] The ulnar nerve has a superficial course near the medial condyle at the elbow makes it most commonly affected nerve. Males are more commonly affected than females as males have larger tubercles than females and males have less fat. Prolonged forearm flexion causes direct pressure on the ulnar nerve in the ulnar groove makes it most common cause of etiology. Compression of the ulnar nerve can occur against the operating table if the forearm is extended and pronated. Injury can also occur when the nerve is stretched around the medial epicondyle during extreme flexion of the elbow across the chest. It commonly presents as tingling and numbness along the little finger and weakness of abduction, adduction of fingers, or both. Examination of the hand reveals hyperextension of metacarpophalangeal joints and flexion at the distal and the proximal inter phalangeal joints of the ring and the little finger leading to ulnar claw.

ASA PRACTICE ADVISORY[4] TO REDUCE ULNAR NERVE INJURIES

1. Supine position with arm on the arm board: forearm should be positioned to decrease pressure on the posterior condylar groove of the humerus (ulnar groove). Either supination or the neutral forearm position meets the goal.
2. Supine position with arms tucked at side: forearm should be in neutral position.

TABLE 2 Classification of Nerve Injuries

Seddon	Sunderland	Function	Pathological basis	Prognosis
Neurapraxia	Type 1	Focal conduction block.	Local myelin injury. Large fibers. Axonal continuity, no Wallerian degeneration.	Recovery occurs in weeks to months.
Axonotmesis	Type 2	Loss of nerve conduction at injury site and distally.	Disruption of axonal continuity with Wallerian degeneration.	Axonal regeneration is required for recovery. Good prognosis as original end organs are reached.
	Type 3	Loss of nerve conduction at injury site and distally.	Loss of axonal continuity and endoneural tubes. Perineurium and epineurium preserved.	Disruption of endo neural tubes, hemorrhage and edema produce scarring. Axonal misdirection. Poor prognosis. Surgery may be required.
	Type 4	Loss of nerve conduction at injury site and distally.	Loss of axonal continuity, endoneural tubes, and perineurium. Epineurium remains intact.	Total degeneration guiding elements. Intraneural scarring and axonal misdirection. Poor prognosis and surgery necessary.
Neurotmesis	Type 5	Loss of nerve conduction at injury site and distally.	Severance of entire nerve.	Surgical modification of nerve ends required. Prognosis guarded and dependent upon nature of injury and local factors.

3. Flexion of the elbow can increase the chances of ulnar nerve injury. However, there is no consensus on an acceptable degree of flexion of the forearm.

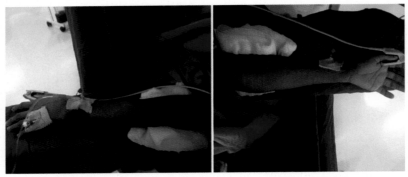

Improper position   **Right position**

BRACHIAL PLEXUS INJURY

The general incidence of brachial plexus injury is 0.2–0.6%. The brachial plexus has a superficial course running between two fixed points intervertebral foramen and axillary sheath. It has a course through limited space between the clavicle and the first rib. It has a course which is proximity to a number of mobile structures. All these points make it susceptible to injury. Injury can occur in the lateral decubitus position with compression against the thorax and humeral head. Stretch in the upper brachial plexus roots is caused by arm abduction, external rotation with posterior displacement. Extreme abduction of the arm more than 90° can also cause stretch of the brachial plexus roots. Extension and lateral flexion of the head to one side with the patient supine, and then abduction, external rotation, and extension of the arm by allowing it to drop away from the side of the body can also cause stretch of the brachial plexus roots. C5–C6 nerve root involvement leads to "waiter's tip position." C8–T1 lesions affect small muscle of the hand leading to claw hand and numbness in the ulnar distribution.

ASA PRACTICE ADVISORY TO REDUCE BRACHIAL PLEXUS INJURIES

1. Arm abduction in supine patient should be limited to 90°.
2. Arm abduction in prone patient: the prone position affects shoulder and brachial plexus mobility differently than the supine position.

These differences may allow patients to comfortably tolerate abduction of their arms greater than 90°.

3. There is no practice advisory issued for the prevention of brachial plexus injury in the lateral position. However, it is always safer not to hang the hand by the side of the patient to prevent brachial plexus injury.

RADIAL NERVE INJURY

Radial nerve injury commonly occurs at the spiral groove of the humerus. Injury occurs due to compression of the nerve between the edge of the operating table and the humerus, arterial pressure cuffs, compression against patient screen, or arm board positioned at an incorrect height creating step. It can also occur when the patient is in the lateral position and the upper arm is abducted beyond 90° and suspended from a vertical screen support. Wrist drop and numbness along the posterior surface of the lower part of the arm, posterior surface of the forearm, and a small area on the dorsum of the hand and lateral three and half fingers are the manifestations of the radial nerve injury. It is also a classical "Saturday night palsy."

The ASA practice advisory to prevent radial nerve injury recommends that prolonged pressure on the radial nerve in the spiral groove of the humerus should be avoided.

MEDIAN NERVE INJURY

The median nerve can be damaged due to invasive procedures around the elbow and compression in the carpal tunnel. It manifests as paraesthesia along the palmar aspect of the lateral three and half fingers, weakness of abduction and opposition of the thumb, weak wrist flexion, and wasting of the thenar eminence. ASA practice advisory says that extension of the elbow beyond the range that is comfortable during the preoperative assessment should be avoided to prevent stretch of the median nerve and its injury.

SCIATIC NERVE INJURY

Sciatic nerve injury commonly occurs in lower-weight patients on hard tables. Stretch, compression, and ischemia are the primary mechanisms. It can occur in frog leg position in vertebral surgeries, and in prolonged surgeries in the sitting position. Hyperflexion of the hip, and abduction and extension of the leg causes the stretching of sciatic nerve. Hyperflexion of the lower limbs is commonly done in patients with sitting position craniotomy. The common peroneal component is more frequently affected than the tibial component as it is the superficial part. Paralysis of the hamstring muscles and all the muscles below the knee leading to a weak knee flexion and foot drop are the common manifestations of sciatic nerve injury. All the sensations below the knee except the medial aspect of the leg and foot are impaired.

ASA PRACTICE ADVISORY TO REDUCE SCIATIC NERVE INJURY

1. Stretching of the hamstrings muscles group: positions that stretch hamstring muscle group beyond the range that is comfortable during preoperative assessment may stretch the sciatic nerve. Therefore, this should be avoided.
2. Limiting hip flexion: while determining the amount of hip flexion, flexion and extension of the knee joint should also be considered. This advisory is given as the sciatic nerve and its branches cross both the hip and knee joints.

FEMORAL NERVE INJURY

Femoral nerve injury can occur during invasive procedures on the femoral vessels. Loss of sensation at the front of the thigh and the medial aspect of the leg are the clinical presentations. It can also present as weak hip flexion and loss of extension of the knee causing difficulty in climbing the stairs. Diagnosis can be confirmed by decreased or absent knee jerk reflex. The ASA practice advisory says that neither extension nor flexion of the hip changes the risk of femoral nerve injury.

PERONEAL NERVE INJURY

Peroneal nerve is the most frequently damaged nerve in the lower limb. It can injure due to compression of the nerve between the hard surface of the operating table and fibular head at fibular groove. It can present as loss of dorsiflexion and eversion of the foot (equinovarus deformity), loss of sensations along the arterolateral border of the leg and dorsum of the digits except those supplied by saphenous nerve. Prolonged pressure at the fibular head should be avoided to prevent peroneal nerve injury.

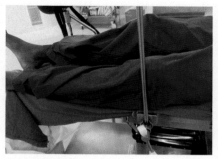

Improper position

COMMON MEASURES TO PREVENT PERIOPERATIVE PERIPHERAL NERVE INJURIES

1. During the preoperative visit, the anesthesiologist should check for any predisposing factors for perioperative peripheral nerve injury.
2. Whenever there are predisposing factors, as described above, the anesthesiologist should be careful during positioning to prevent prolonged compression on any nerve.
3. It is advisable to assess the desired position of the patient regularly and frequently during the intraoperative period.
4. Padded arm boards may decrease the risk of upper extremity neuropathy.
5. Whenever the patient is positioned in lateral position, it is better to use the chest rolls.
6. Proper padding is required at all at-risk areas during positioning and after positioning the patient during the intraoperative period. Improper padding may increase the chance of perioperative neuropathy.
7. Proper functioning automated blood pressure cuffs on the arm should be used.
8. Use of shoulder braces in steep head down position may increase the chance of perioperative neuropathy.
9. Simple postoperative assessment of the extremity nerve function can help in early recognition of the neuropathy.

INVESTIGATIONS

Clinical assessment of the patient is the first investigation to be done. It gives a good idea about the preoperative disposing factors of the patient. Electromyography can provide information about nerve supply to the muscle. Nerve conduction studies can identify the number of nerve fibers participating in the conduction of impulse. Electrophysiology can distinguish between nerve dysfunction due to axonal degeneration such as perioperative peripheral nerve injury and the nerve dysfunction due to demyelination. Timing of electrophysiological studies is more important to diagnose perioperative peripheral nerve injury. Fourteen days or more is required for nerve degeneration to complete. Therefore, it is recommended that electrophysiological studies should be done several weeks after the onset of symptoms to avoid false reassuring assessment.

If localization of nerve injury is undetermined by the electrophysiological studies 3T magnetic resonance imaging may be used to confirm the site of lesion.[5]

References

1. Dhuner KG. Nerve injuries following operations: survey of cases occurring during a 6 year period. *Anesthesiology*. 1950;11:289–293.
2. Sawyer RJ, Richmond MN, Hickey JD, Jarrratt JA. Peripheral nerve injuries associated with anaesthesia. *Anaesthesia*. 2000;55:980–991.
3. Kroll DA, Caplan RA, Posner K, Ward RJ, Cheney FW. Nerve injury associated with anaesthesia. *Anesthesiology*. 1990;73:202–207.
4. Practice advisory for the prevention of perioperative peripheral neuropathies. A report by the American Society of Anesthesiologists Task Force on prevention of perioperative peripheral neuropathies. *Anaesthesiology*. 2000;92:1168–1182.
5. Abdul GL, Kailash B. Perioperative peripheral nerve injuries. *Crit Care & Pain J*. 2012;12(1):38–42.
6. Keykhah HM, Rosenberg H. Bilateral foot drop after craniotomy in the sitting position. *Anesthesiology*. 1979;51:163–164.
7. Stoelting RK. Post operative ulnar nerve palsy—is it a preventable complication? *Anaesth Analg*. 1993;76:7–9.
8. Garriques HJ. Anaesthesia paralysis. *Am J Med Sci*. 1897;113:81–89.
9. Bartholomew LG, Scholz DA. Reversible post operative neurological symptoms; report of 5 cases secondary to water intoxication and sodium depletion. *J Am Med Assoc*. 1956;162:22–26.
10. Delorme EJ. Hypothermia. *Anaesthesia*. 1956;11:221–231.
11. Swan H, Virtue RW, Blount SG, Kircher LT. Hypothermia in surgery: analysis of 100 clinical cases. *Ann Surg*. 1953;142:382–400.
12. Ahmad NS, Yentis SM. Laryngeal mask airway and lingual nerve injury. *Anaesthesia*. 1996;51:707–708.
13. Laxton CH, Kipling R. Lingual nerve paralysis following the use of the laryngeal mask airway. *Anaesthesia*. 1996;51:869–870.

Pharmacological Complications

M. Srilata, Kavitha Jayaram

Department of Anesthesia and Intensive Care, Nizam's Institute
of Medical Sciences, Hyderabad, India

Oxygenation to the cerebrum carries the utmost priority above other organs of the body. Neuroanesthesia is mostly about maintaining the rheology and cerebral or spinal perfusion in order to maintain the milieu. Pharmacological complications due to the perioperative use of drugs or fluids may result in serious consequences. A thorough knowledge of the drug-related complications and fluid rheology is a requirement for the prevention of perioperative morbidity and mortality. The major goals in neurosurgical anesthesia are to provide adequate tissue perfusion to the brain (and spinal cord) so that the regional metabolic demand is

Complications in Neuroanesthesia
http://dx.doi.org/10.1016/B978-0-12-804075-1.00038-9

met and an adequate surgical condition (a "relaxed brain") is provided. If anesthetic drugs or anesthetic techniques are improperly used, they can worsen the existing intracranial pathologic condition and may produce new damage. Some anesthetics or anesthetic techniques may help protect the brain subjected to metabolic stress or even ameliorate damage from such an insult.[1,2] The various pharmacological issues discussed in this chapter include use of anesthetic drugs, surgical drugs, and intravenous (IV) fluids.

NEUROSURGICAL DRUGS AND COMPLICATIONS

These include:

1. Intracisternal instillation of papaverine is most commonly used to alleviate cerebral vasospasm following aneurysm surgery.[3] Complications include mild hypotension. Sometimes, it may precipitate severe hypotension and bradycardia, especially in patients undergoing a third ventriculostomy.[4]
2. Intrathecal baclofen treatment: This has shown a steep rise in the management of patients with spasticity.[5] Complications include sexual dysfunction, which is reversible,[6] and meningitis. Rarely, technical complications like a leaking tubule attachment may present with baclofen withdrawal syndrome resulting in near cardiac arrest.[7]
3. Increased risk of intracranial bleeding is seen with use of anticoagulants like low molecular weight heparin (LMWH).[8,9] National Institute for Health and Clinical Excellence (United Kingdom), Societé Française d'anesthesie et de Reanimation (France), and the American College of Physicians guidelines recommend the use of only mechanical prophylaxis in the form of compression stockings and pneumatic compression devices for thromboprophylaxis in patients undergoing neurosurgery.[10] Patients with one or more risk factors for venous thromboembolism and neurosurgery should have a combination of mechanical prophylaxis and LMWH.
4. Adenosine. Adenosine administration has emerged as a form of temporary flow arrest in various open surgical and interventional procedures, including cardiac surgery, embolization of cerebral arteriovenous malformations. Adenosine has negative cardiac dromotropic and chronotropic effects. Adenosine in large doses of 0.3–0.4 mg/kg is used as a loading dose to produce asystole for intracranial aneurysm surgeries where temporary clipping is difficult.[11] This may produce transient arrhythmias and increased cardiac morbidity.
5. Antiepileptic drugs (AEDs): These agents like phenytoin, carbamazepine, and valproic acid are commonly used in the perioperative period. Patients on long-term phenytoin and carbamazepine develop resistance to neuromuscular blocking drugs. This is mainly due to increased clearance of these blocking agents.

Patients on chronic treatment with AEDs may present with complications like thrombocytopenia or neutropenia to anemia, or red cell aplasia, until reaching bone marrow failure.[12] They seem to be related to an immunological mechanism. Other long-term effects include osteoporosis, gingival hyperplasia, or alterations in reproductive endocrine function.[13] The incidence of such effects is significantly curtailed with the advent of AEDs such as gabapentin, tiagabine, lamotrigine, oxcarbazepine, and levetiracetam, with a more favorable pharmacokinetic profile.

AEDs such as oxcarbazepine, felbamate, and topiramate are associated with some side effects.[13] Hyponatremia is common with oxcarbazepine when compared with carbamazepine use. The association of felbamate with aplastic anemia and liver failure and topiramate with acute angle closure glaucoma was observed. Prompt recognition and early intervention, such as discontinuation of topiramate, reverses the pathology. Awareness of such conditions by both the physician and the patient is very important.

Phenytoin: This is thought to be related to toxicity from its diluent propylene glycol. In these cases, patients developed hypotension, bradyarrhythmias, and even asystole. The therapeutic range of phenytoin is quite narrow. With increasing levels of phenytoin, symptoms range from nystagmus, ataxia, and altered mental status with mild impairment of neurophysiologic testing. This drug is also implicated in the causation of toxic epidermo necrolysis and Stevens–Johnson syndrome.[14] Fosphenytoin is devoid of propylene glycol toxicity. The side effects seen are minimal discomfort at the injection site, pruritus, and reactions typical of phenytoin (e.g., dizziness, somnolence, and ataxia).[15]

6. Current evidence has shown use of steroids only for peritumoral edema in neurosurgery. Preoperative corticosteroid use is associated with an increased risk of infectious complications after neurosurgery.[16] Use of steroids are also implicated for thick filament myopathies and delayed weaning in neurocritically ill patients.[17] Steroids should be used in the lowest dose possible for supportive therapy.

INTRAVENOUS ANESTHETIC DRUGS

Hypnotic/Sedative Agents

These are used both in the perioperative and critical care settings.[18] In patients with reduced cerebral compliance, a small increase in cerebral blood volume can cause a life-threatening increase in intracranial pressure (ICP). Most sedative–hypnotic drugs cause a proportional reduction in cerebral metabolism ($CMRO_2$) and cerebral blood flow (CBF), resulting in a decrease in ICP.[2] The effect of intravenous anesthetic drugs on cerebral dynamics is depicted in Table 1. Although a decrease in $CMRO_2$

TABLE 1 Anaesthetic Drugs and Pharmacological Complications

Pharmacy	Effect on cerebral hemodynamics	Autoregulation	CO_2 responsiveness	Untoward effects
IV INDUCTION AGENTS				
Thiopentone	↓CBF, ↓ICP, ↓$CMRO_2$ CBF/$CMRO_2$ ratio unchanged	Intact	Intact	Hypotension
Propofol	↓CBF, ↓ICP, ↓$CMRO_2$ CBF/$CMRO_2$ ratio unchanged	Intact	Intact	Hypotension; Propofol infusion syndrome in children; Pain on injection
Etomidate	↓CBF, ↓ICP, ↓$CMRO_2$ CBF/$CMRO_2$ ratio unchanged	-	Intact	Adrenocortical suppression; Myoclonic movements; Pain on injection
Benzodiazepines	Modest reduction in CBF (intermediate between narcotics and barbiturates)	Intact	Intact	Respiratory depression
Ketamine	↑CMR, ↑CBF, ↑ICP	Intact	Intact	Increased sympathetic activity; hallucinations
INHALATIONAL AGENTS				
Volatile anaesthetic agents 0.5 MAC < 1 -1.5MAC > 1 MAC	Dose related ↓$CMRO_2$ >> ↑CBF ↓$CMRO_2$ = ↑CBF ↑CBF >> ↓$CMRO_2$	Intact with < 1 MAC; Altered with > 1 MAC	Intact	Vasodilatory effect: halothane > enflurane > desflurane > sevoflurane > isoflurane; Halothane – hepato-toxicity; Enflurane – epileptogenic; Sevoflurane – Compound A formation, seizures
Nitrous oxide	Potent cerebral vasodilator - ↑ICP; variable effect as usually administered with other agents	Intact	Intact	Pneumocephalus
OPIOIDS				
Morphine	Modest ↓ of CMR and CBF	Intact; -	Intact; -	Respiratory depression, constipation; Histamine release

Fentanyl	Modest ↓ of CMR and CBF in quiescent brain; Larger reduction during arousal	-	-	Chest wall rigidity
Alfentanil	No significant changes	-	-	Augments temporal lobe spike activity
Sufentanil	↓ or = CMR and CBF	-	-	Sudden decrease in MAP may result in increase in ICP
Remifentanil	Low doses – minor ↑CBF	-	-	Hyperalgesia immediately after discontinuation of the drug
MUSCLE RELAXANTS				
Succinyl choline	↑ICP, ↑CBF	Intact	Intact	Hyperkalemia, fasciculations, myalgia
Pancuronium, vecuronium and rocuronium	Minimal effects	-	-	Interaction with AEDs and magnesium
Atracurium	Minimal effects	-	-	Histamine release
ALPHA 2 ADRENERGIC AGONISTS				
	Vasoconstrictor leading to ↓CBF	Intact	Intact	Bradycardia, hypertension, hypotension
LOCAL ANAESTHETICS				
	Dose related ↓$CMRO_2$	Intact	Intact	Seizures with large doses of lignocaine

*All intravenous agents do not alter the autoregulation or CO_2 responsiveness unless there is severe hypotension associated.

*Autoregulation is impaired more with use of vasodilators and in patients with hypercapnia.

Abbreviations: ICP, Intracranial pressure; CBF, Cerebral blood flow; CMR, Cerebral metabolic rate; $CMRO_2$, Cerebral metabolic oxygen demand; MAC, Minimum alveolar concentration; AED, Antiepileptogenic drugs; MAP, Mean arterial pressure.

IX. MISCELLANEOUS

probably provides only a modest degree of protection against cerebral ischemia or hypoxia, some hypnotics appear to possess cerebroprotective potential. Most IV hypnotics have similar electroencephalographic (EEG) effects. At high concentrations, a burst-suppressive pattern develops with an increase in the isoelectric periods.

Barbiturates produce a proportional decrease in $CMRO_2$ and CBF, thereby lowering ICP. The maximal decrease in $CMRO_2$ (55%) occurs when the EEG becomes isoelectric (burst-suppressive pattern). An isoelectric EEG can be maintained with a thiopental infusion rate of 4–6 mg/kg/h (resulting in plasma concentrations of 30–50mg/mL).[2] Because the decrease in systemic arterial pressure is usually less than the reduction in ICP, thiopental should improve cerebral perfusion and compliance. Therefore, thiopental is widely used to improve brain relaxation during neurosurgery and to improve cerebral perfusion pressure (CPP) after acute brain injury. Although barbiturate therapy is widely used to control ICP after brain injury, the results of outcome studies are no better than with other aggressive forms of cerebral antihypertensive therapy. Based on evidence from experimental studies, it has been concluded that barbiturates have no place in the therapy following resuscitation of a cardiac arrest patient. In contrast, barbiturates are frequently used for cerebroprotection during incomplete brain ischemia (e.g., carotid endarterectomy, temporary occlusion of cerebral arteries, profound hypotension, and cardiopulmonary bypass).

Continuous infusions of thiopental have been used to treat refractory status epilepticus. However, low doses of thiopental may induce spike wave activity in epileptic patients. Common complications seen with thiopental are hypotension and infections. A rare but serious complication of paralytic ileus leading to bowel ischemia was reported following continuous infusion of thiopental.[19] Methohexital has well-established epileptogenic effects in patients with psychomotor epilepsy. Low-dose methohexital infusions are frequently used to activate cortical EEG seizure discharges in patients with temporal lobe epilepsy. It is also the IV anesthetic of choice for electroconvulsive therapy.[20]

The true epileptogenic activity of methohexital needs to be differentiated from the myoclonic-like phenomena seen with etomidate.[21] Myoclonic activity is generally considered to be the result of an imbalance between excitatory and inhibitory subcortical centers, produced by an unequal degree of suppression of these brain centers by low concentrations of hypnotic drugs.

Evidence for a possible neuroprotective effect has been reported in in vitro preparations, and the use of propofol to produce EEG burst suppression has been proposed as a method for providing neuroprotection during aneurysm surgery. However, when larger doses are administered, the marked depressant effect on systemic arterial pressure can significantly decrease CPP. Propofol appears to possess profound anticonvulsant properties. Propofol has been reported to decrease spike activity in patients with cortical electrodes implanted for resection of epileptogenic foci and has been used successfully to terminate status epilepticus. Propofol produces a decrease in the early components of somatosensory (SSEPs) and motor evoked potentials (MEPs) but does not influence the early components of the auditory evoked potentials. On the other hand, propofol is not devoid of complications. They include pain on injection, hemodynamic instability especially in dehydrated patients, hypertriglyceridemia and propofol infusion syndrome. Use of propofol along with opioids like fentanyl results in hypotension with bradycardia. This may be detrimental in cases with increased ICP.

The other dreaded complication is propofol infusion syndrome, rarely seen with continuous infusion of propofol at a dose of 4mg/kg/h over 24–48h, especially in children and neurocritical care settings.[22] Continuous infusion of propofol is indicated in special situations like patients with severe traumatic brain injury (TBI), increasing ICP, and status epilepticus.[23] Other predisposing factors include young age, severe critical illness of other central nervous system or respiratory origin, exogenous catecholamine or glucocorticoid administration, inadequate carbohydrate intake, and subclinical mitochondrial disease. These patients may present with findings of cardiac decompensation such as acute bradycardia refractory, ultimately leading to asystole. This is associated with metabolic acidosis, rhabdomyolysis, hyperlipidemia, renal failure, hyperkalemia, and an enlarged or fatty liver. The proposed mechanism involves either a direct mitochondrial respiratory chain inhibition or impaired mitochondrial fatty acid metabolism. Management includes prompt recognition, early intervention in the form of discontinuation of propofol infusion, and supportive therapy in the form of hemodialysis or hemoperfusion with cardiorespiratory support.

Other rare complications include acute pancreatitis.[24] Cautious use of these agents in neurosurgical practice in both perioperative and critical care settings is warranted.

Analogous to the barbiturates, etomidate decreases $CMRO_2$, CBF, and ICP. However, the hemodynamic stability associated with etomidate will maintain adequate CPP.[2] Etomidate has been used successfully for both induction and maintenance of anesthesia for neurosurgery. Although clear evidence for a neuroprotective effect in humans is lacking, etomidate is frequently used during temporary arterial occlusion and intraoperative angiography (for the treatment of cerebral aneurysms). Etomidate's well-known inhibitory effect on adrenocortical synthetic function limits its clinical usefulness for long-term treatment of elevated ICP. Other complications include pain on injection and myoclonic movements. Etomidate can induce convulsion-like EEG potentials in epileptic patients without the appearance of myoclonic or convulsant-like motor activity, a property that has been proven useful for intraoperative mapping of seizure foci. Etomidate also possesses anticonvulsant properties and it has been used to terminate status epilepticus. Etomidate produces a significant increase of the amplitude of SSEPs while only minimally increasing their latency.

Consequently, etomidate can be used to facilitate the interpretation of SSEPs when the signal quality is poor.

Ketamine has been traditionally contraindicated for patients with increased ICP or reduced cerebral compliance because it increases $CMRO_2$, CBF, and ICP. Prior administration of thiopental or benzodiazepines can blunt ketamine-induced increases in CBF. Ketamine has been reported to have little effect on MEPs.

Benzodiazepines decrease both $CMRO_2$ and CBF analogous to the barbiturates and propofol. However, in contrast to these compounds, midazolam is unable to produce a burst-suppressive (isoelectric) pattern on the EEG. Accordingly, there is a "ceiling" effect with respect to the decrease in CMRO2 produced by increasing doses of midazolam. Midazolam induces dose-dependent changes in regional cerebral perfusion in the parts of the brain that subserve arousal, attention, and memory. In patients with severe head injury, a bolus dose of midazolam may decrease CPP with little effect on ICP. Although flumazenil does not appear to change CBF or $CMRO_2$ following midazolam anesthesia for a craniotomy, acute increases in ICP have been reported in head-injured patients receiving flumazenil.

Dexmedetomidine

It is a pure α_2 agonist, which is being increasingly used in neurosurgery cases and also in intensive care units in order to produce conscious sedation associated with minimal respiratory depression and mild analgesia. It decreases CBF without proportional reduction in $CMRO_2$.[25] The neuroprotective effect is primarily related to lower peripheral catecholamine levels. But its safety in patients with neurologic diseases or patients with severe sepsis is still not validated.

Dexmedetomidine causes a unique kind of sedation, acting on the subcortical areas, which resembles natural sleep without respiratory depression and thus creates an environment favoring weaning from mechanical ventilation. It also facilitates intermittent neurological monitoring as it does not interfere with electrophysiological monitoring. Hence, it can be used safely in neurocritical care settings. It creates an ideal sedation state for awake craniotomy, carotid endarterectomy under regional anesthesia, carotid angioplasty and stenting, microelectrode recording during implantation of deep-brain stimulators, and most of the neurological interventional procedures.[26] Complications include bradycardia with loading dose and hypotension. Other than this, no significant side effects have been reported.[18]

Opioids

Use of large doses may depress ventilation, and especially patients with low Glasgow coma scale (GCS) score are susceptible for aspiration and respiratory complications. A cautious use of opioids is advocated in patients with quadriparesis and with decreased consciousness.

Neuromuscular Blocking Drugs

These drugs are used in special situations in neurocritical care settings apart from the surgical relaxation provided in the perioperative period. Critical care indications include treatment of Acute lung injury/acute respiratory distress syndrome and status asthmaticus, management of elevated ICP, and provision of therapeutic hypothermia after cardiac arrest.[27] Continuous infusion of neuromuscular blocking drugs in neurocritical care has shown to increase the incidence of myopathies and delayed weaning.[17] Interaction of neuromuscular blocking drugs with AEDs has already been described.

Local Anesthetics

Local anesthetic toxicity is rarely seen in neurosurgical practice. Scalp nerve block, especially in pediatrics, requires a large volume. Lignocaine is found to be equally effective compared to thiopentone in attenuating increase in ICP without any significant effect on MAP. Higher doses are found to be seizure prone. Lidocaine dose should be restricted to amounts that target serum levels less than the seizure threshold (>5 to 10 μg/mL) in human volunteers. Bupivacaine in doses >5 mg/kg reduced the latency to N-methyl-D-asparate seizures compared to levobupivacaine.[28] Proper calculation of the toxic dose, preparation, and dilution is important to avoid such mishaps in children.

Magnesium

The multimodal role of Magnesium in anesthesia practice has been clearly elucidated. The neuroprotection properties of magnesium in patients with focal cerebral ischemia have been reported.[29] Serum concentrations of magnesium between 2 and 3 mmol/L offered the best brain tissue protection during procedures that are prone to the risk of temporary vessel occlusion. Magnesium is also an anticonvulsant, enhances the efficacy of analgesic agents and anesthesia, attenuates hemodynamic response to perioperative stimulation, and also attenuates arrhythmias with hemodynamic stability.[30] It possesses an excellent safety profile. The complications associated with magnesium are very rare and occur mainly due to overdosage. It potentiates the effects of neuromuscular blocking drugs. Neuromuscular junction monitoring is useful in titrating the dose of muscle relaxants in patients on magnesium therapy.

INHALATIONAL ANESTHETICS

All of the potent agents depress cerebral metabolic rate (CMR) to varying degrees in a nonlinear fashion (Table 1). For most of the potent agents, CMR is decreased only to the extent that spontaneous cortical neuronal activity (as reflected in the EEG) is decreased.[31] Once spontaneous cortical electrical activity is absent, there is no further decrease in the CMR by these agents except for halothane, which further reduces after the concentrations of 4.5% due to toxic metabolites of oxidative phosphorylation.[32] Isoflurane causes a larger minimum alveolar concentration (MAC)–dependent depression of CMR than halothane, and does not depress $CMRO_2$ once an isoelectric EEG is produced.[33] Because of this greater depression in neuronal activity, isoflurane abolishes EEG activity at doses used clinically and can usually be tolerated from a hemodynamic standpoint. Desflurane and sevoflurane both cause decreases in CMR similar to isoflurane.

The increase in ICP is far less for isoflurane than for halothane. Like isoflurane, both sevoflurane and desflurane above 1 MAC produces a mild increase in ICP, paralleling their mild increases in CBF.[34,35] Several studies in both children and adults suggest that increases in ICP from desflurane are slightly greater than from either isoflurane or sevoflurane.[36,37] Significant hypercapnia is associated with dramatic increases in CBF whether volatile anesthetics are administered or not. On the other hand, hypocapnia can blunt or abolish volatile anesthetic-induced increases in CBF depending on when the hypocapnia is produced.

The most compelling evidence for an advantage of isoflurane over halothane for neuroprotection was shown in patients undergoing carotid endarterectomy surgery.[38] In these patients, not only were the incidences of ischemic EEG changes less using isoflurane than halothane, but ischemic EEG changes occurred at a lower CBF with isoflurane than with halothane.[39,40] Human neuroprotection outcome studies for sevoflurane and desflurane have not been published.

Nitrous oxide causes cerebral vasodilatation. Nitrous oxide has variable effects on the cerebral metabolism as it is not used alone and its effects are usually blunted with the coadministration of other agents like premedicants, induction agents, voltatile agents, and benzodiazepines. The literature has reported its antineuroprotective effect, as addition of N_2O to isoflurane during temporary ischemia is associated with greater tissue damage and worsened neurologic outcome. It also expands the air-filled cavities in closed spaces, hence has a large propensity to aggravate pneumocephalus and venous air embolism. Air is a safe alternative to nitrous oxide, especially in patients undertaking surgeries in the sitting and prone position.[41]

A number of authors have demonstrated that inhalational anesthetics, including isoflurane, sevoflurane, halothane, enflurane, and desflurane, suppress myogenic MEPs in a dose-dependent manner.[42,43]

FLUID MANAGEMENT AND COMPLICATIONS

Patients presenting for neuroanesthesia pose special challenges with respect to the administration of fluids.[44] They may be on diuretics like mannitol with restricted fluids to decrease cerebral edema, or they may be on hypervolemic therapy due to SAH or hypotensive with absent blood–brain barrier (BBB) at many areas due to severe TBI or polytrauma. Their management involves specific problems in order to maintain hemostasis. Knowledge of fluid movement across the brain is essential for decision making with respect to what and how much fluids to use. As such, even improper usage leads to several complications. Little substantial human data exists concerning the impact of fluids on the brain or which can guide rational fluid management in neurosurgical patients.

With intravenous fluids, three properties of blood can be manipulated; osmolality, oncotic pressure and hematocrit. In the periphery, the pore size of the capillary endothelium is 65A° and it is permeable to small molecules and ions like sodium but are impermeable to proteins which are larger molecules. Hence, the movement of water in the periphery is governed by the concentration of larger molecules or the colloid oncotic pressure gradient. Whereas the BBB has a pore size of 7–9A°, which prevents not only the movement of proteins but also that of ions like sodium, potassium, and chloride ions.[45] Hence, fluid movement across the BBB depends mainly on the total osmotic gradient generated by the larger as well as the smaller molecules. As there are less protein molecules compared to that of inorganic ions, their effect is negligible. The influence of changes in osmolality on cerebral water distribution dwarfs the effect of alteration in colloid osmotic pressure (COP). This explains why large volumes of isotonic crystalloids do not cause cerebral edema whereas produces peripheral edema due to the dilutional reduction of COP.

This scenario may not be the same with patients having an alteration in their BBB due to various disease processes. The alteration may not be uniform globally, and hence we try to conserve that portion of the brain that is not affected. Presence of an intact BBB to some extent is essential for osmotherapy.

IV fluid administration can also cause hemodilution, which enhances CBF. But caution is necessary as the normal responses of CBF to hypoxia and hemodilution is attenuated with head injury, and these together may contribute to secondary injury. A hematocrit level of 30–33% gives optimal viscosity and oxygen-carrying capacity and may improve neurological outcome.[46] Aggressive hemodilution with hypervolemia may result again in hyponatremia and volume overload.[47]

Hypoosmolar crystalloids cause concomitant reduction in plasma osmolality and can result in cerebral edema. Fluid therapy with excess free water should be avoided to prevent cerebral as well as spinal cord ischemia. Isoosmolar solutions with an osmolality of approximately 300 mosm/L, such as plasmalyte, 0.9% saline, do not change the plasma osmolality and do not increase brain water content. The same does not apply for solutions that are not truly isoosmolar with respect to plasma, such as lactated Ringer's solution. Hyperosmolar crystalloids such as hypertonic saline exert beneficial effects by increasing the plasma osmolality, thereby enhancing movement of fluid from interstitial tissue to the vascular compartment. These solutions are used for volume resuscitations in hemorrhagic shock states. The concerns for using hypertonic saline solutions will be the development of hypernatremia, which is mostly tolerable, and intracranial tension rebounds when the saline solutions are stopped. The increased serum osmolality also decreases the secretion of the cerebrospinal fluid (CSF) and hence provides an improvement in the intracranial compliance.[48,49] choice of management fairly depends on the sodium levels and cerebral hemodynamics.

Colloids have an oncotic pressure similar to that of plasma. Colloidal solutions share the presence of larger molecules that are impermeable to capillary endothelium. These fluids in small volumes restore normovolemia in states of circulatory shock without increasing ICP and also avoiding secondary injury due to ischemia. They have been used successfully to treat intracranial hypertension in patients with head injury and stroke.[50,51] Colloids have shown to impair clot strength, and hence the effect of fluid therapy on coagulation should be considered to decrease the incidence of bleeding complications.[44]

Patients with head injuries will have three different types of areas: some where the osmotic and oncotic gradient are totally effective (normal BBB), some where only colloid oncotic gradient is effective (mild opening of the BBB, with pore sizes similar to periphery), and some areas where there is no effective osmotic or oncotic gradient effective (BBB breakdown). Hence, we must avoid and correct the decrease in both osmotic and oncotic pressures. This also ensures perfusion and hemostasis in other organs, which may indirectly influence cerebral perfusion.

Diuretics are commonly used in the management of ICP in neurosurgery. Mannitol is the preferred diuretic. Reported complications of mannitol therapy include fluid and electrolyte imbalance in the form of hypo/hyperkalemia or hyponatremia, acidosis, and hypotension.[52] This may be aggravated with added administration of furosemide in a high dose.[53] Chronic use of mannitol administration may result in a severe hyperosmolar state, leading to kidney failure.[54] Accumulation of mannitol in the interstitium reverses normal blood–brain gradient and may worsen the cerebral edema.[55] Mannitol in combination with colloids has shown to impair coagulation.[44]

Several studies have demonstrated that furosemide causes reduction in CSF production and hence improves intracranial compliance, but the action is delayed when compared to mannitol, and so its role is doubtful.

In neurosurgical patients, blood sugar levels should be controlled frequently, and the goal should be to avoid either hyper- or hypoglycemia, as both are detrimental. Blood sugar has to be maintained between 100 and 150 mg/dL in order to avoid secondary injury, postoperative morbidity, and mortality.

Apart from these, neurosurgical patients may also present with electrolyte and water disturbances due to conditions like diabetes insipidus, syndrome of inappropriate antidiuretic hormone secretion and cerebral salt wasting syndrome. All these conditions are to be identified and treated appropriately.

The available data indicate that volume replacement or expansion will have no effect on edema as long as normal serum osmolality and oncotic pressure are maintained, and as long as cerebral hydrostatic pressures are not markedly increased (due to volume overload). Whether this is achieved by crystalloids or colloids seems irrelevant.[56] Hence the goal of neuroanesthesiologist should be to maintain the patient's isovolemic, isoosmotic, isooncotic, and normoglycemic in order to have a better outcome.

ANESTHETIC NEUROTOXICITY AND NEUROAPOPTOSIS

The concept of neuroapoptosis has emerged, and the literature has shown the direct correlation of loss of neuronal network in the young and an increased use of general anesthesia in animal studies.[57] Activated cleaved caspase 3 is a marker of apoptotic cell death. This has been found to be significantly increased in certain areas of the smart tot brains leading to early cognitive dysfunction. Studies have found that the degree of these disastrous complications is increased when inhaled anesthetics were used in combination with ketamine, nitrous oxide, or midazolam. The usual presentations include problems with spatial learning and memory, decreased social interactions, and increased contextual fear of conditioning. Some recovery was seen by adulthood. Though it is quite dangerous, the studies need also to be substantiated in humans. At the same time, protective and preventive strategies were studied to attenuate this effect, thus limiting the potential brain injury.[58] Drugs that were found to be effective in ameliorating this neuroapoptosis are lithium, xenon, hypothermia, methazolamide, melatonin, N-arachidonoylethanolamine, and dexmedetomidine.

References

1. Schifilliti D, Grasso G, Conti A, Fodale V. Anaesthetic-related neuroprotection: intravenous or inhalational agents? *CNS Drugs.* 2010;24:893–907.
2. Turner BK, Wakim JH, Secrest J, Zachary R. Neuroprotective effects of thiopental, propofol, and etomidate. *AANA J.* 2005;73:297–302.
3. Chowdhury FH, Haque MR. Severe hypotension, cardiac arrest, and death after intracisternal instillation of papaverine during anterior communicating artery aneurysm clipping. A case report. *Acta Neurochir (Wien).* 2013;155:281–282.
4. Rath GP, Mukta, Prabhakar H, Dash HH, Suri A. Haemodynamic changes after intracisternal papaverine instillation during intracranial aneurysmal surgery. *Br J Anaesth.* 2006;97:848–850.
5. Morota N, Kubota M, Nemoto A, Katayama Y. Intrathecal baclofen treatment for spasticity in childhood. Initial report of long-term follow up in Japan. *No To Hattatsu.* 2014;46:179–186.
6. Calabro RS, D'Aleo G, Sessa E, Leo A, De Cola MC, Bramanti P. Sexual dysfunction induced by intrathecal baclofen Administration: Is this the price to pay for severe spasticity management? *J Sex Med.* 2014;11.
7. Cardoso AL, Quintaneiro C, Seabra H, Teixeira C. Cardiac arrest due to baclofen withdrawal syndrome. *BMJ Case Rep.* 2014.
8. Salmaggi A, Simonetti G, Trevisan E, et al. Perioperative thromboprophylaxis in patients with craniotomy for brain tumours: a systematic review. *J Neurooncol.* 2013;113:293–303.
9. Niemi T, Armstrong E. Thromboprophylactic management in the neurosurgical patient with high risk for both thrombosis and intracranial bleeding. *Curr Opin Anaesthesiol.* 2010;23:558–563.
10. Pollak AW, McBane 2nd RD. Succinct review of the new VTE prevention and management guidelines. *Mayo Clin Proc.* 2014;89:394–408.
11. Khan SA, McDonagh DL, Adogwa O, et al. Perioperative cardiac complications and 30-day mortality in patients undergoing intracranial aneurysmal surgery with adenosine-induced flow arrest: a retrospective comparative study. *Neurosurgery.* 2014;74:267–271. discussion 271–272.
12. Verrotti A, Scaparrotta A, Grosso S, Chiarelli F, Coppola G. Anticonvulsant drugs and hematological disease. *Neurol Sci.* 2014;35.
13. Asconape JJ. Some common issues in the use of antiepileptic drugs. *Semin Neurol.* 2002;22:27–39.
14. East-Innis AD, Thompson DS. Stevens-johnson syndrome and toxic epidermal necrolysis at the university hospital of the west indies, Jamaica. *West Indian Med J.* 2013;62:589–592.
15. Ramsay RE, DeToledo J. Intravenous administration of fosphenytoin: options for the management of seizures. *Neurology.* 1996;46:S17–S19.
16. Merkler AE, Saini V, Kamel H, Stieg PE. Preoperative steroid use and the risk of infectious complications after neurosurgery. *Neurohospitalist.* 2014;4:80–85.
17. Hund E. Neurological complications of sepsis: critical illness polyneuropathy and myopathy. *J Neurol.* 2001;248:929–934.
18. Roberts DJ, Haroon B, Hall RI. Sedation for critically ill or injured adults in the intensive care unit: a shifting paradigm. *Drugs.* 2012;72:1881–1916.
19. Cereda C, Berger MM, Rossetti AO. Bowel ischemia: a rare complication of thiopental treatment for status epilepticus. *Neurocrit Care.* 2009;10:355–358.
20. Kirchberger K, Schmitt H, Hummel C, et al. Clonidine- and methohexital-induced epileptiform discharges detected by magnetoencephalography (MEG) in patients with localization-related epilepsies. *Epilepsia.* 1998;39:1104–1112.
21. Valadao PA, Naves LA, Gomez RS, Guatimosim C. Etomidate evokes synaptic vesicle exocytosis without increasing miniature endplate potentials frequency at the mice neuromuscular junction. *Neurochem Int.* 2013;63:576–582.
22. Barbosa FT. Propofol infusion syndrome. *Rev Bras Anestesiol.* 2007;57:539–542.

23. Hwang WS, Gwak HM, Seo DW. Propofol infusion syndrome in refractory status epilepticus. *J Epilepsy Res*. 2013;3:21–27.
24. Scholten JG, Buijs E. Acute pancreatitis after propofol administration. *Ned Tijdschr Geneeskd*. 2014;158:A7115.
25. Karlsson BR, Forsman M, Roald OK, Heier MS, Steen PA. Effect of dexmedetomidine, a selective and potent alpha 2-agonist, on cerebral blood flow and oxygen consumption during halothane anaesthesia in dogs. *Anesth Analg*. 1990;71:125–129.
26. Farag E, Argalious M, Sessler DI, Kurz A, Ebrahim ZY, Schubert A. Use of alpha(2)-agonists in neuroanesthesia: an overview. *Ochsner J*. 2011;11:57–69.
27. Warr J, Thiboutot Z, Rose L, Mehta S, Burry LD. Current therapeutic uses, pharmacology, and clinical considerations of neuromuscular blocking agents for critically ill adults. *Ann Pharmacother*. 2011;45:1116–1126.
28. Marganella C, Bruno V, Matrisciano F, Reale C, Nicoletti F, Melchiorri D. Comparative effects of levobupivacaine and racemic bupivacaine on excitotoxic neuronal death in culture and N-methyl-D-aspartate-induced seizures in mice. *Eur J Pharmacol*. 2005;518:111–115.
29. Chang JJ, Mack WJ, Saver JL, Sanossian N. Magnesium: potential roles in neurovascular disease. *Front Neurol*. 2014;5:52.
30. James MF. Magnesium: an emerging drug in anaesthesia. *Br J Anaesth*. 2009;103:465–467.
31. Sanders RD, Ma D, Maze M. Anaesthesia induced neuroprotection. *Best Pract Res Clin Anaesthesiol*. 2005;19:461–474.
32. Michenfelder JD, Theye RA. In vivo toxic effects of halothane on canine cerebral metabolic pathways. *Am J Physiol*. 1975;229:1050–1055.
33. Miura Y, Amagasa S. Perioperative cerebral ischemia and the possibility of neuroprotection by inhalational anesthetics. *Masui*. 2003;52:116–127.
34. Talke P, Caldwell J, Dodsont B, Richardson CA. Desflurane and isoflurane increase lumbar cerebrospinal fluid pressure in normocapnic patients undergoing transsphenoidal hypophysectomy. *Anesthesiology*. 1996;85:999–1004.
35. Talke P, Caldwell JE, Richardson CA. Sevoflurane increases lumbar cerebrospinal fluid pressure in normocapnic patients undergoing transsphenoidal hypophysectomy. *Anesthesiology*. 1999;91:127–130.
36. De Deyne C, Joly LM, Ravussin P. Newer inhalation anaesthetics and neuro-anaesthesia: what is the place for sevoflurane or desflurane? *Ann Fr Anesth Reanim*. 2004;23:367–374.
37. Sponheim S, Skraastad O, Helseth E, Due-Tonnesen B, Aamodt G, Breivik H. Effects of 0.5 and 1.0 MAC isoflurane, sevoflurane and desflurane on intracranial and cerebral perfusion pressures in children. *Acta Anaesthesiol Scand*. 2003;47:932–938.
38. Rijsdijk M, Ferrier C, Laman M, Kesecioglu J, Stam K, Slooter A. Detection of ischemic electroencephalography changes during carotid endarterectomy using synchronization likelihood analysis. *J Neurosurg Anesthesiol*. 2009;21:302–306.
39. Michenfelder JD, Sundt TM, Fode N, Sharbrough FW. Isoflurane when compared to enflurane and halothane decreases the frequency of cerebral ischemia during carotid endarterectomy. *Anesthesiology*. 1987;67:336–340.
40. Messick Jr JM, Casement B, Sharbrough FW, Milde LN, Michenfelder JD, Sundt Jr TM. Correlation of regional cerebral blood flow (rCBF) with EEG changes during isoflurane anesthesia for carotid endarterectomy: critical rCBF. *Anesthesiology*. 1987;66: 344–349.
41. Hoffman WE, Miletich DJ, Albrecht RF. The effects of midazolam on cerebral blood flow and oxygen consumption and its interaction with nitrous oxide. *Anesth Analg*. 1986;65:729–733.
42. Chong CT, Manninen P, Sivanaser V, Subramanyam R, Lu N, Venkatraghavan L. Direct comparison of the effect of desflurane and sevoflurane on intraoperative motor-evoked potentials monitoring. *J Neurosurg Anesthesiol*. 2014;26.
43. Tamkus AA, Rice KS, Kim HL. Differential rates of false-positive findings in transcranial electric motor evoked potential monitoring when using inhalational anesthesia versus total intravenous anesthesia during spine surgeries. *Spine J*. 2013;14.

44. Lindroos A-C. *Perioperative Fluid Therapy in Neurosurgery: effects on Circulatory and Haemostatic Variables*; 2013.
45. Fenstermacher JD, Johnson JA. Filtration and reflection coefficients of the rabbit blood–brain barrier. *Am J Physiol*. 1966;211:341–346.
46. Xiong L, Lei C, Wang Q, Li W. Acute normovolaemic haemodilution with a novel hydroxyethyl starch (130/0.4) reduces focal cerebral ischaemic injury in rats. *Eur J Anaesthesiol*. 2008;25:581–588.
47. Gura M, Elmaci I, Cerci A, Sagiroglu E, Coskun KK. Haemodynamic augmentation in the treatment of vasospasm in aneurysmal subarachnoid hemorrhage. *Turk Neurosurg*. 2012;22:435–440.
48. Cottenceau V, Masson F, Mahamid E, et al. Comparison of effects of equiosmolar doses of mannitol and hypertonic saline on cerebral blood flow and metabolism in traumatic brain injury. *J Neurotrauma*. 2011;28:2003–2012.
49. Tseng MY, Al-Rawi PG, Pickard JD, Rasulo FA, Kirkpatrick PJ. Effect of hypertonic saline on cerebral blood flow in poor-grade patients with subarachnoid hemorrhage. *Stroke*. 2003;34:1389–1396.
50. Sekhon MS, Dhingra VK, Sekhon IS, Henderson WR, McLean N, Griesdale DE. The safety of synthetic colloid in critically ill patients with severe traumatic brain injuries. *J Crit Care*. 2011;26:357–362.
51. Schwarz S, Schwab S, Bertram M, Aschoff A, Hacke W. Effects of hypertonic saline hydroxyethyl starch solution and mannitol in patients with increased intracranial pressure after stroke. *Stroke*. 1998;29:1550–1555.
52. Ryu JH, Walcott BP, Kahle KT, et al. Induced and sustained hypernatremia for the prevention and treatment of cerebral edema following brain injury. *Neurocrit Care*. 2013;19:222–231.
53. Bebawy JF, Ramaiah VK, Zeeni C, Hemmer LB, Koht A, Gupta DK. The effect of furosemide on intravascular volume status and electrolytes in patients receiving mannitol: an intraoperative safety analysis. *J Neurosurg Anesthesiol*. 2013;25:51–54.
54. Karajala V, Mansour W, Kellum JA. Diuretics in acute kidney injury. *Minerva Anestesiol*. 2009;75:251–257.
55. Kaufmann AM, Cardoso ER. Aggravation of vasogenic cerebral edema by multiple-dose mannitol. *J Neurosurg*. 1992;77:584–589.
56. Tommasino C. Fluids and the neurosurgical patient. *Anesthesiol Clin N Am*. 2002;20:329–346, vi.
57. Gleich S, Nemergut M, Flick R. Anesthetic-related neurotoxicity in young children: an update. *Curr Opin Anaesthesiol*. 2013;26:340–347.
58. Jevtovic-Todorovic V, Absalom AR, Blomgren K, et al. Anaesthetic neurotoxicity and neuroplasticity: an expert group report and statement based on the BJA Salzburg Seminar. *Br J Anaesth*. 2013;111:143–151.

Position-Related Complications

M. Srilata, Kavitha Jayaram

Department of Anesthesia and Intensive Care, Nizam's Institute of Medical
Sciences, Hyderabad, India

Position-related complications are very common mishaps that are usually preventable. Neurosurgery encompasses different surgeries in a varied number of positions for easy surgical accessibility that pose a wide range of problems to both the anesthetic and surgical teams.[1] Positioning surgical patients involves added risk to the patient as the anesthetized patient is not aware of this compromised position in the intraoperative period. Positioning of anesthetized patients for surgery forms an important job of the entire team to ensure optimal physiology and to prevent adverse sequelae and trauma due to the required position. The complications related to these positions are described in detail in this chapter.

Positioning of the head is an integral part of positioning the neurosurgical patients, both for craniotomies and spine procedures. Adequate knowledge of the surgical site and understanding the physiology of that position to target the surgical site will guide the proper positioning. The following types of approach are commonly followed in modern neurosurgery. These include anterior parasagittal, frontosphenotemporal (pterional), subtemporal, posterior parasagittal, midline suboccipital, and lateral suboccipital. Most of the spine procedures are undertaken either in the prone or lateral position. Craniotomies are undertaken either in supine, semi-lateral, prone, half-prone, three-quarter prone, or sitting position. Other variants include modifications of these positions to suit the surgery and avoiding complications to some extent.

General anesthesia, muscle relaxation, and positive pressure ventilation interfere with venous return, arterial tone, and autoregulatory mechanisms rendering patients under anesthesia especially vulnerable and relatively uncompensated to circulatory effects of changes in position. For these reasons, arterial blood pressure is often particularly labile immediately after initiation of anesthesia and during patient positioning. Hence, interruption in monitoring to facilitate positioning or turning of operating table must be minimized during this dynamic period.

Fixation of the head: In most cases, the head is either fixed using pins or different frames, e.g., Mayfield frame.[2] This maneuver is quite painful and sometimes augments cardiovascular response. This is dangerous especially in patients with unruptured cerebral aneurysms. This can be attenuated with deepening of anesthesia, scalp block, or local infiltration. On the other hand, any movement of the patient with the head fixed may result in complications like scalp injuries, intracranial hematomas, or eye injuries. The pins should be removed before attempting or administration of reversal agents and extubation.

The physiological changes seen with different positions in neurosurgical practice are depicted in Table 1. Different positions and manipulations with their complications are discussed.

SUPINE POSITION (DORSAL DECUBITUS)

Hemodynamic reserve is best maintained in this position because the entire body is close to the level of heart.

Indications: Encountered for cranial and anterior cervical spine surgeries and for carotid explorations.

Physiological changes: Because the venous compartment is a low pressure compartment, venous return to the heart depends on the body position. Venous return may be compromised with increase in ventilation perfusion mismatch. This position is also associated with compression injuries like ulnar and peroneal neuropathies. This position encounters the least complications otherwise.[3]

TABLE 1 Physiological Changes Seen with Different Positions

Physiological changes in various positions				
	Supine	**Lateral**	**Prone**	**Sitting**
CVS				
Venous return	↑	↓	↓	↓
Cardiac output	↑	↓	↔	↓
Heart rate	↓	↑↔	↑↔	↑
Systemic BP	↔	↓	↓↔	↓
Systemic vascular resistance	↓	↑	↑	↑
Mean arterial pressure	↓↔	↓	↓↔	↓
RS				
FRC	↓	↓	↑↔	↑
TLC	↓	↓	↑↔	↑
Qs/Qt	↑	↑↑	↓	↓
V/Q mismatch	↑	↑↑	↓	↓
CNS				
Jugular venous flow	↑↔	↑↔	↑↔	↓
Cerebral perfusion pressure	↓↔	↔	↑	↔
Intracranial pressure	↔↑	↑	↑	↓↓
Benefits	Easiest position	Optimal approach to temporal lobe	Optimal posterior approach to spine	Optimal posterior approach to posterior fossa and access to airway
Modification	Lawn chair position reverse Trendelenburg	Park bench	Concorde	Semirecumbent

Abbreviations: CVS, cardiovascular system; BP, blood pressure; RS, respiratory system; FRC, functional residual capacity; TLC, total lung capacity; Qs/Qt, pulmonary shunt; V/Q, ventilation/perfusion; CNS, central nervous system.

Complications: Pressure alopecia in occipital region especially in prolonged surgeries, backache, ulnar neuropathy, and stretch on brachial plexus unless head is in neutral position are minimal except for proper placement of arms, head, and neck. Even after short procedures headache and congestion of the conjunctiva and nasal mucosa are observed.

Variants: Its variants include lawn chair position and reverse Trendelenburg position, the advantages being improvement in ventilation perfusion ratio and increase in venous return with better drainage of cerebrospinal fluid. In the lawn chair position the hips and knees are slightly flexed to avoid stress to the back, hips, and knees. In the reverse Trendelenburg position caution is advised to prevent patient from slipping on the table. Use of shoulder braces increases the incidence of brachial plexus neuropathies especially in the steep head down position. Also, the effect of the hydrostatic gradient on the cerebral arterial and venous pressure should be considered in terms of cerebral perfusion pressure.[4]

Special attention: Placement of arterial transducer at the level of the tragus helps in assessment of cerebral perfusion.

LATERAL POSITION

Indications: Includes craniotomy for temporal lobe, skull base and posterior fossa procedures, and retroperitoneal approach for thoracolumbar spine surgeries.[2]

In this position, the dependent arm rests on a padded arm board and the nondependent arm is supported over the folded bedding or suspended with an armrest or foam cradle. An axillary roll is kept just caudal to the dependent axilla (never in the axilla) to avoid compression injury to the brachial plexus. Compression injuries to the common peroneal and saphenous nerves are avoided by placing adequate support in between the legs.

Physiologic changes: The lateral weight of the mediastinum and disproportionate cephalad pressure of the abdominal contents on the dependent lung favors overventilation of the nondependent lung thereby worsening the ventilation perfusion mismatch.[5,6]

Complications: These may include injury to the dependent eye and ear, stretching of the suprascapular nerve, and brachial plexus injury on the dependent side. Due to outflow obstruction in the dependent arm, venous hypertension is a common finding, even with adequate padding.

Special attention: Monitoring of the pulse either by palpation or by using pulse oximetry is essential in the dependent limb for early detection of neurovascular bundle compression. Frequent visualization of the dependent eye and ear with proper positioning of the head and neck are to be taken care of to avoid devastating complications.

Variants: The park bench position is usually indicated for surgeries in the posterior fossa wherein the upper arm is close to the trunk and the upper shoulder is taped to the table. Complications include stretch injuries to the axilla and decreased perfusion to the dependent arm.[7] Macroglossia is a reported complication with extreme neck flexion in this position.[8]

PRONE POSITION

Indications: This is the approach for posterior fossa, suboccipital region, and spine procedures.

This position requires disconnection of tubings and monitors during positioning. Airway complications include accidental extubation, difficult airway access, and kinking of the endotracheal tube. Head and neck positioning is crucial. The head is turned to one side only if neck mobility is adequate. In most cases, the head is positioned neutrally using surgical pillows, a horseshoe headrest, or Mayfield pins. Various types of pillows are available commercially including mirror systems that facilitate intermittent visual confirmation that eyes are unimpinged.[4] To prevent tissue injury, pendulous structures (genitalia, breast) should be clear of compression.

Physiological changes: The increase in intraabdominal pressure caused by turning the patient prone decreases the venous return more so if lower extremities are flexed below and also increases systemic vascular resistance.[9] Compression of inferior vena cava due to improper positioning along with the abovementioned causes increased predilection to bleeding in spine surgeries.

Oxygenation is improved due to decrease in chest wall compliance, improved perfusion to the lung, and opening up of the previously atelectatic dorsal zones.[10] The effects on hemodynamics and respiration are frame-dependent and so special frames are used to support chest, leaving abdominal wall and pelvis free (Wilsons frame, Relton hall frame, Andrews frame, Jackson table and frame).[11]

Complications: These may include compression of the eyes leading to increased intraocular pressure and retinal artery occlusion leading to blindness, especially in patients with major blood loss and severe hypotension. Improper padding and hyperextension of the arms may lead to brachial plexus stretch injuries. Less common complications include venous air embolism and compression of soft tissue structures like ears, nose, breast, and genitalia.

Special considerations: Care must be taken while shifting from supine to prone and vice versa as most adverse events happen at that time especially if the patient has pins or is morbidly obese. Accidental extubations are common due to pooling of secretions. Invasive lines, monitors, and catheters are to be attended to during the positioning. Frequent assessment of the eyes and record keeping is essential particularly in prolonged surgeries. Use of a check list addressing specific points before and after positioning would help in decreasing the overall mortality and morbidity.[12]

Concorde position: This is a variant of the prone position where the head and neck are hyperflexed. Indications for this position include surgical approach to occipital transtentorial and supracerebellar infratentorial area. Adverse complications include compromised cerebral venous return and decreased flow in the vertebral and carotid arteries leading to cerebral infarction, venous congestion of the head and neck, increased intracranial pressure (ICP), chin necrosis, and quadriplegia.[13]

SITTING POSITION

Indications: Tumors in the posterior fossa and sometimes cervical laminectomy.[14]

Physiological changes: Hemodynamic effects of placing supine patient in sitting position is dramatic. Due to pooling of blood in the lower body under general anesthesia, patients are particularly prone to hypotensive episodes. Incremental positioning, use of intravenous fluids, vasopressors, and adjustment of depth of anesthesia can reduce degree and duration of hypotension. Due to drastic variations in the cardiac output, hemodynamic instability and cardiac disease are relative contraindications to this position.

Ventilation is improved compared with the supine position due to downward shift of diaphragm and ventilation of dependent zones is improved. However, low perfusion pressures secondary to decreased venous return may affect oxygenation.

Complications: This is rarely indicated nowadays for its potential devastating complication of venous air embolism and paradoxical air embolism.[15] Excessive cervical flexion can impede arterial and venous flow causing hypoperfusion or venous congestion of the brain.[4] This may also impede normal respiratory excursion. If transesophageal electrocardiography is in place for monitoring air embolism there is more potential for compression of laryngeal structures and tongue. Other complications include pneumocephalus, paraplegia, quadriplegia, macroglossia, brain stem manipulations leading to bradycardia, and cardiac arrest.

Variants: The semirecumbent position (modified sitting position). In this position, the legs are kept as high as possible to improve both the venous return and hemodynamic stability.

Special consideration: Elastic stockings and active leg compression devices can help to maintain venous return. Head holder support is preferably attached to the back section of the table so that patients back may be adjusted or lowered emergently without first detaching the head holder. To assess the cerebral perfusion pressure the arterial transducer is positioned at the level of the tragus as this gives the arterial pressure at the circle of Willis.

Venous air embolism (VAE): Elevation of the surgical field above the level of the heart as well as the inability of dural venous sinuses to collapse because of their bony attachments means that risk of VAE is a constant concern in this position. A large VAE may decrease cardiac output by creating airlock and decrease left ventricular output and sometimes leads to paradoxical air embolism. Preventive strategies like early detection, routine use of monitoring like transcranial Doppler, maintenance of central venous pressure (CVP), and communication with the surgeon has decreased the incidence of VAE from 50–70% to 12–22%.[14,16,17] Treatment includes irrigation of surgical site with saline, resuming head down tilt or left lateral position, and cardiovascular support.

THREE-QUARTER PRONE POSITION

Also called the semiprone or lateral oblique; one of the most difficult positions to manage. Complications include bleeding, brachial plexus injury, compartment syndrome of the dependent arm, pressure sores, macroglossia, and pudendal nerve injury.

Transferring comatose patients: Neurosurgical patients with low Glasgow coma scale score are transferred unconscious to the operating table. All the staff members should ascertain their tasks and responsibilities in assisting and facilitating the movement. Proper securing of all the lines and catheters including endotracheal tube and continuous monitoring are essential before and after any patient movement thus mitigates or avoids any disastrous incidents.[18]

Pressure sores: These are common general complications following any position. This occurs due to decreased perfusion to the tissues subjected to hard surfaces and unequal distribution of high pressure on a relatively small area of the body leading to ischemia. Prevention is better than cure. Adequate and proper padding while positioning (gel pads, foams), regular monitoring, and early postoperative mobilization helps to overcome this.[19]

Preventive measures: Preventive measures starts with preoperative counseling, documentation of intraoperative positioning, and monitoring, and ends with postoperative monitoring and documentation for early recognition of any peripheral neuropathy. The American Society of Anesthesiologists Task force guidelines emphasize these measures with specific attention to upper limb and lower limb positioning to ensure an improvement in patient care.[20]

1. Identification of at-risk patients for developing neuropathy in the preoperative assessment, e.g., elderly, diabetes and underlying neuropathy.
2. Counseling of the patient regarding a particular position adopted for surgery and its complications in the preoperative evaluation. One should ensure in the preoperative period itself whether the patient can comfortably accept the probable surgical position.

3. Documentation of the preexisting neuropathies, if any.
4. Avoiding hyperflexion, hyperextension, and acute rotation of the head and neck. Cervical collars in C-spine patients requires proper fitting to prevent obstruction of venous drainage from the head.
5. Permissible and optimal head rotation from 0–45° is allowed. Further rotation can be accomplished by placing a roll beneath the opposite shoulder.
6. At the time of neck flexion, thyromental distance of at least two fingers breadth is recommended.
7. Wrapping of the legs with elastic crepe bandage to prevent pooling and stasis of blood.
8. Prone positioning is the most difficult and this requires coordination of the operating staff under the guidance of neuroanesthetists at the time of positioning. Monitoring of the pulse oximetry and blood pressure are vital during prone positioning.
9. Positioning of the arm is crucial especially in supine patients. Avoid abduction of the arm >90° in supine patients. Neutral forearm position for the arms is recommended and safe whenever the arms are tucked at the side or abducted on arm boards. Stretch and compression injuries of the upper extremity nerves like median and radial nerve should be avoided.
10. Lower extremity positioning should stress upon avoidance of prolonged pressure and stretching of the peroneal and sciatic nerves, respectively.
11. Monitoring of ICP and jugular bulb pressure along with CVP are helpful in guiding the position.
12. Proper padding and adequate protection of potential compression sites is recommended.
13. Avoid abdominal compression and compression of the femoral vein and artery during prone positioning to facilitate venous return and decrease surgical bleeding. This also favors improved excursion of the diaphragm with increased ventilation and oxygenation.
14. Monitoring of invasive lines is important in prone patients especially with heart and lung comorbidity and trauma patients.
15. Lateral position requires an axillary roll to be placed under the upper chest to avoid compression of the vital structures like brachial plexus and axillary artery.
16. The head should be positioned above the level of the heart to improve venous drainage from the brain, e.g., using reverse Trendelenburg positioning or with flexion of the table in the supine position.

17. Finally, intraoperative charting and documentation of specific position actions with postoperative assessment of functional integrity of potential neuropathies is a relevant aspect in refining patient care.

Complete knowledge of the physiological alterations associated with different positions, applications, and interventions to prevent and treat complications for a neuroanesthetist can help predict potential problems and improve outcome with decreased morbidity and mortality.

References

1. Susset V, Gromollard P, Ripart J, Molliex S. Controversies in neuroanaesthesia: positioning in neurosurgery. *Ann francaises d'anesthesie de Reanim*. 2012;31:e247–252.
2. Rozet I, Vavilala MS. Risks and benefits of patient positioning during neurosurgical care. *Anesthesiol Clin*. 2007;25:631–653. x.
3. Israelian LA, Shimanskii VN, Otamanov DA, Poshataev VK, Lubnin A. Patient positioning on the operating table in neurosurgery: sitting or lying. *Anesteziol i Reanimatol*. 2013:18–26.
4. Cassorla L, Lee JW. Patient positioning. In: Miller RD, ed. *Miller's Anesthesia*. 7th ed. New York, NY: Churchill Livingstone Inc; 2010:2477–2517.
5. Dunn PF. Physiology of the lateral decubitus position and one-lung ventilation. *Int Anesthesiol Clin*. 2000;38:25–53.
6. Baraka A. Ventilation-perfusion matching during one lung-ventilation in the lateral decubitus position. *Middle East J Anesthesiol*. 2013;22:241–244.
7. Jain V, Davies M. Axillary artery compression in park bench position during a microvascular decompression. *J Neurosurg Anesthesiol*. 2011;23:264.
8. Toyama S, Hoya K, Matsuoka K, Numai T, Shimoyama M. Massive macroglossia developing fast and immediately after endotracheal extubation. *Acta Anaesthesiol Scand*. 2012;56:256–259.
9. Toyota S, Amaki Y. Hemodynamic evaluation of the prone position by transesophageal echocardiography. *J Clin Anesth*. 1998;10:32–35.
10. Gattinoni L, Taccone P, Carlesso E, Marini JJ. Prone position in acute respiratory distress syndrome. Rationale, indications, and limits. *Am J Respir Crit care Med*. 2013;188: 1286–1293.
11. Edgcombe H, Carter K, Yarrow S. Anaesthesia in the prone position. *Br J Anaesth*. 2008;100:165–183.
12. Salkind EM. A novel approach to improving the safety of patients undergoing lumbar laminectomy. *AANA J*. 2013;81:389–393.
13. Hicdonmez T, Kilincer C, Hamamcioglu MK, Cobanoglu S. Paraplegia due to spinal subdural hematoma as a complication of posterior fossa surgery: case report and review of the literature. *Clin Neurol Neurosurg*. 2006;108:590–594.
14. Ganslandt O, Merkel A, Schmitt H, et al. The sitting position in neurosurgery: indications, complications and results. a single institution experience of 600 cases. *Acta Neurochir*. 2013;155:1887–1893.
15. Dilmen OK, Akcil EF, Tureci E, et al. Neurosurgery in the sitting position: retrospective analysis of 692 adult and pediatric cases. *Turk Neurosurg*. 2011;21:634–640.
16. Leslie K, Hui R, Kaye AH. Venous air embolism and the sitting position: a case series. *J Clin Neurosci Official J Neurosurg Soc Australasia*. 2006;13:419–422.

17. Hervias A, Valero R, Hurtado P, et al. Detection of venous air embolism and patent foramen ovale in neurosurgery patients in sitting position. *Neurocir (Astur).* 2014;25.

18. Beckmann U, Gillies DM, Berenholtz SM, Wu AW, Pronovost P. Incidents relating to
the intra-hospital transfer of critically ill patients. An analysis of the reports submit-
ted to the Australian Incident Monitoring Study in Intensive Care. *Intensive Care Med.*
2004;30:1579–1585.

19. Knight DJ, Mahajan RP. Patient positioning in anaesthesia. Continuing education in anaesthesia. *Crit Care & Pain.* 2004;4:160–163.

20. Practice advisory for the prevention of perioperative peripheral neuropathies: an updated report by the American Society of Anesthesiologists Task Force on prevention of
perioperative peripheral neuropathies. *Anesthesiology.* 2011;114:741–754.

Postoperative Vision Loss

Kiran Jangra, Vinod K. Grover

Department of Anaesthesia and Intensive Care, Postgraduate Institute of
Medical Education and Research, Chandigarh, India

OUTLINE

Postoperative vision loss (POVL) is defined as partial or complete loss of vision following nonophthalmic procedures. Though rare, when it occurs it is a devastating complication. The incidence of visual loss postoperatively has been reported as 0.002–0.2%.[1–3] POVL is found to occur after cardiac,[3] spine,[2] orthopedic,[3] endonasal surgeries,[4] and urological procedures.[5]

A few isolated case reports show blindness can occur after transsphenoidal surgeries[6] as well as arteriovenous malformation embolization.[7] The incidence is on the rise, particularly in the setting of spinal fusion surgery and probably due to an increased number of complex spinal procedures.

APPLIED ANATOMY OF VISUAL PATHWAY

The visual pathway is the pathway over which a visual sensation is transmitted from the retina to the brain. This includes a cornea and lens that focuses images on the retina, and nerve fibers that carry the visual sensations from the retina through the optic nerve. Optic nerve fibers travel through the optic chiasma to the lateral geniculate body of the thalamus, and optic radiations terminate in an occipital lobe (Figure 1). Each optic nerve carries the fibers from only the ipsilateral retina, while the optic chiasma contains fibers from both the eyes. These fibers pass through the lateral geniculate body on the same side of the brain then reach the occipital lobe through optic radiations.

Interruptions anywhere in the visual pathway can lead to the blindness.

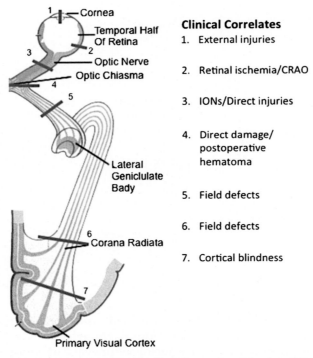

Clinical Correlates

1. External injuries

2. Retinal ischemia/CRAO

3. IONs/Direct injuries

4. Direct damage/ postoperative hematoma

5. Field defects

6. Field defects

7. Cortical blindness

FIGURE 1 **Visual pathway showing site of injuries causing vision loss.** Solid bars indicate level of insults. CRAO: Central retinal artery occlusion; ION: Ischemic ophthalmic neuropathies.

ARTERIAL SUPPLY OF THE OPTIC NERVE

The predominant blood supply of the eye is by the ophthalmic artery (OA), which is the first intracranial branch of the internal carotid artery (Figure 2). The OA gives the posterior ciliary arteries, the central artery of retina, and pial arteries along the optic nerve. The anterior portion of the optic nerve is profusely supplied by various sources, including posterior ciliary arteries and Circle of Zinn–Haller formed by choroidal, posterior ciliary arteries. The posterior segment receives blood supply from the adjacent carotid and hypophyseal arteries. The middle segment of the optic nerve is supplied only by small pial arteries, which are less dense in the middle segment as compared to retrobulbar segment, putting it at risk of ischemia.

CAUSES OF POVL

Vision loss after spinal surgery can be categorized into five groups:

1. External ocular injury (corneal abrasion or sclera injury)
2. Retinal ischemia
3. Ischemic optic neuropathy (INO)
4. Cortical blindness
5. Acute glaucoma
6. Posterior reversible encephalopathy syndrome (PRES)

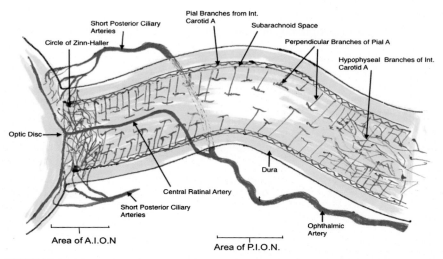

FIGURE 2 **Diagram of vascular supply of the optic nerve.** Multiple arteries richly supply the anterior optic nerve while the midorbital optic nerve is supplied by only the small pial branches. It is the midorbital region of the optic nerve that is involved in PION. A: Artery; AION: Anterior ischemic optic neuropathy; PION: Posterior ischemic optic neuropathy.

External Ocular Injuries

Corneal trauma can be due to direct insult to the eye or due to keratitis. It results in irritation, abrasion, or even laceration. It can be a self-limiting process or it can increase the risk of ocular inflammation and infection. Corneal injuries are extremely painful and usually preventable.

Retinal Ischemia

Central retinal artery occlusion (CRAO) is seen in the conditions where large emboli are injected near the facial vessels[8] or the conditions where the globe is at risk of direct compression. Very rarely, systemic hypotension and impaired venous drainage[9] can also lead to retinal ischemia (Figure 3). Occasionally, retinal arterial thrombosis may occur due to a coagulation disorder. CRAO decreases the blood supply to the entire retina, while branch retinal artery occlusion (BRAO) is a localized injury affecting only a portion of the retina. This complication is usually in major cardiac[3] and vascular surgeries. Improper patient positioning resulting in external compression of the eye can also lead to retinal ischemia during surgeries in prone positioning. External compression of the eye produces sufficient rise in intraocular pressure (IOP) to stop flow in the central retinal artery.[10] Various anomalies such as altered facial anatomy, osteogenesis imperfecta, and exophthalmos increase the vulnerability for external globe compression. Patients of Asian descent tend to have lower nasal bridges, which may increase the risk of external compression.[11] Patients have painless visual loss and abnormal pupil reactivity. Other proposed mechanisms causing retinal ischemia include

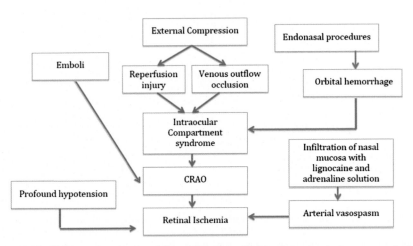

FIGURE 3   Mechanism of retinal ischemia. CRAO: Central retinal artery occlusion.

excitotoxicity,[12] hyperemia and hypoperfusion, and vasospasm (Ligno-caine and adrenaline solution infiltration).[13]

Ischemic Optic Neuropathy

Ischemic optic neuropathy (ION), without warning signs, is the lead-ing cause of sudden visual loss in patients undergoing posterior spinal fusion. Shen et al.[3] found that children below 18 years of age had highest risk of POVL for all procedures, followed by the age group of 50–64 years. Increased risk in children might be due to anatomical and developmental vulnerabilities. ION can be of two types: anterior (AION) and posterior (PION). It can be arteritic or nonarteritic. ION is termed "arteritic" when it is secondary to inflammations of blood vessels, chiefly giant cell arteritis (temporal arteritis). The term nonarteritic is used when it is secondary to occlusive disease or other noninflammatory disorders of blood vessels. Nonarteritic ION, more common than arteritic, is overwhelmingly the type found perioperatively. It has been reported after various neurosur-gical procedures, including instrumental spinal fusion operations[14] and head and neck surgeries.[15]

The etiology of ION is multifactorial. The Postoperative Visual Loss Study Group has published the results of largest case-controlled study to date to determine the risk factors for ION after spinal fusion surgery (Table 1).[16] The consultants and special society members agree that vas-cular risk factors such as hypertension, diabetes, peripheral vascular dis-ease, coronary artery disease, obesity, and tobacco use increase the risk of perioperative vision loss. In addition to vascular factors, preoperative anemia, prolonged surgical duration, significant blood loss, excessive crystalloid use for blood loss replacement, and use of the Wilson frame during prolonged procedures combined with substantial blood loss increase the risk of POVL. Obesity is associated with increased abdominal girth causing elevated central venous pressure (CVP) in the prone posi-tion as well as reducing venous return and cardiac output. The Wilson frame places the patient's head significantly lower than the heart, leading to increased venous pressure in the head.[17] Substantial blood loss causes inflammation, capillary leak, and lower oncotic pressure, which favor interstitial edema formation. The American Society of Anesthesiologists registry[16] consultants considered the procedures to be prolonged when they exceed an average of a 6.5 h duration. Substantial blood loss was defined as an average of 44.7% of estimated blood volume. Various case reports suggest that use of vasopressors such as epinephrine and phen-ylephrine intraoperatively can increase the risk of vision loss.[18,19] How-ever, α-adrenergic receptors are not known to be located in the optic nerve and the blood–brain barrier prevents entry of systemically administered agents, except possibly in the prelaminar zone of the nerve. Therefore, the

TABLE 1   Summary of Practice Advisory for Postoperative Visual Loss[16]

	Parameter studied	Advisory statements
I.	Preoperative patient evaluation and preparation	1. There are identifiable preoperative patient characteristics to predict perioperative ION. 2. Neuroophthalmic evaluation was not useful in identifying patients at risk for POVL. Prolonged procedures, substantial blood loss, or both are anticipated and there is a small, unpredictable risk of POVL.
II.	Intraoperative management Blood pressure management	1. Continuous systemic blood pressure monitoring should be done in high-risk patients. 2. Deliberate hypotensive techniques during spine surgery has not been shown to be associated with the development of POVL and should be determined on a case-by-case basis.
	1. Management of intraoperative fluids	1. CVP monitoring should be considered in high-risk patients. 2. Colloids should be used along with crystalloids to maintain intravascular volume in patients who have substantial blood loss.
	2. Management of anemia	1. Hemoglobin or hematocrit values should be monitored periodically in high-risk patients who experience substantial blood loss. 2. Lower limit of hemoglobin concentration that has been associated with the development of POVL is not documented. 3. Transfusion threshold to prevent POVL cannot be established at this time.
	3. Use of vasopressors	1. There is insufficient evidence to guide for the use of α-adrenergic agonists in high-risk patients during spine surgery. 2. A decision should be made on a case-by-case basis.
	3. Patient positioning	1. No pathophysiologic mechanism by which facial edema can cause perioperative ION. 2. There is no evidence that ocular compression causes isolated perioperative anterior ION or posterior ION. However, direct pressure on the eye should be avoided to prevent CRAO. 3. Head should be positioned at a level at or higher than the heart when possible. 4. Head should be kept in a neutral position (e.g., without significant neck flexion, extension, lateral flexion, or rotation).
III.	Staging of surgical procedures	In high-risk patients with complex spine procedures, surgeries should be staged.

TABLE 1   Summary of Practice Advisory for Postoperative Visual Loss[16]—cont'd

	Parameter studied	Advisory statements
IV.	Postoperative management	1. Vision should be assessed when the patient becomes alert. 2. Urgent ophthalmologic consultation should be obtained. 3. Additional management, including optimizing hemoglobin or hematocrit values, hemodynamic status, and arterial oxygenation. 4. Consider MRI to rule out intracranial causes. 5. There is no role for antiplatelet agents, steroids, or intraocular pressure-lowering agents in the treatment of perioperative ION.

role of vasopressors use in ION remains unclear and no clear inference can be drawn at present.

Theoretical Pathophysiology of ION after Spine Surgery in Prone Position

Elevated venous pressure in the head leading to interstitial edema could result in increased IOP or accumulation of fluid in the optic nerve, or both. Internal "compartment syndrome" may occur in the optic nerve because the central retinal vein exits out of the optic nerve. This damages the optic nerve via direct mechanical compression, venous infarction, or the compression of thread-like pial vessels that feed the optic nerve. A small cup–disc ratio also puts the optic nerve at risk of ischemia.

Cortical Blindness

Cortical blindness can result from global or focal ischemia, cardiac arrest, hypoxemia, intracranial hypertension and exsanguinating hemorrhage, vascular occlusion, thrombosis, intracranial hemorrhage, vasospasm, and emboli.[3] It is usually accompanied by signs of stroke in the parieto–occipital region. The patient may develop agnosia. i.e., the inability to interpret sensory stimuli. The visual field is restored within days, but impairment in spatial perception and in the relationship between sizes and distances may remain.[20]

Acute Glaucoma

Acute angle-closure glaucoma has been described rarely after general anesthesia. Glaucoma usually aggravates in the prone position for a prolonged period.[21] Patients present with headache, cloudy or blurred vision, and a painful red eye accompanied by nausea and vomiting. It should be differentiated from corneal abrasion, which also produces pain but without the papillary signs, increased IOP, and headache.

Posterior Reversible Encephalopathy Syndrome

PRES, also known as reversible posterior leukoencephalopathy syndrome, is the constellation of neurological symptoms including seizures, headaches, altered mental status/function, seizures, loss of vision, and relatively symmetric edema in the subcortical white matter as well as occasionally in the cortices of the occipital and parietal lobes. Though PRES was initially described in 1996[22] and is better known in the obstetric literature, it has also been described in nonobstetric surgery such as a video-assisted thoracoscopic wedge resection,[23] hysterectomy, lumbar fusion,[24] and Chiari malformation.[25] The exact pathophysiology of PRES is still unclear. Two theories of PRES are either that hypertensive episodes surpass the autoregulatory capacity of the cerebral vasculature, causing breakthrough brain edema, or that cytotoxic drugs or diseases cause endothelial injury, leading to edema formation.

DIAGNOSIS

Patients presenting with partial or complete vision loss after surgery should be assessed urgently to diagnose the cause and to start immediate treatment. External corneal injuries present as pain, watering, photophobia, and foreign body sensations. ION and cortical blindness are painless losses of vision. Patients with ION have painless visual loss and abnormal pupil reactivity, which is preserved in cortical blindness. CRAO, secondary to external compression is associated with unilateral loss of vision along with loss of light perception, afferent pupil defect, periorbital and/ or eyelid edema, chemosis, proptosis, ptosis, paresthesias of the supraorbital region, hazy/cloudy cornea, and corneal abrasion. Loss of eye movements, ecchymosis, or other trauma near the eye has also been reported.

Fundoscopic examination shows normal disc (Figure 4(a)) in PION and cortical blindness but AION shows disc edema (Figure 4(b)). BRAO is characterized by cholesterol emboli (bright yellowish, glistening; Figure 4(c)), calcific emboli (white, nonglistening), or migrant pale emboli of platelet and fibrin (dull, dirty white). A cherry-red macula (Figure 4(d)) with a white ground-glass appearance of the retina and attenuated arterioles is a "classic" diagnostic sign in CRAO. The supply of retinal is diminished giving it a pale appearance, while macula supplied by choroidal arteries appears red.

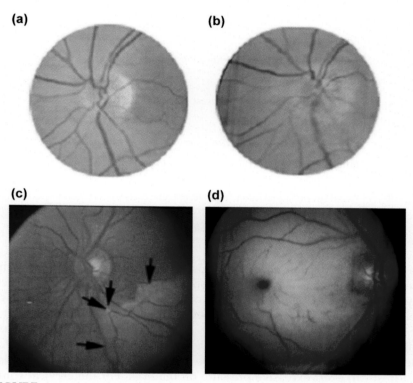

FIGURE 4 **Fundoscopic appearance of optic disc.** (a) normal disc, (b) edematous disc seen in AION, and (c) disc appearance in BRAO. Arrows showing attenuated vessels, (d) disc in CRAO. Macula supplied by choroidal arteries appears as a cherry red spot against ischemic pale retina in CRAO. AION: Anterior ischemic optic neuropathy; BRAO: Branch retinal artery occlusion; CRAO: Central retinal artery occlusion.

Early orbital computed tomography (CT) or magnetic resonance imaging (MRI) showed proptosis and extra ocular muscle swelling, although most cases did not have imaging studies to confirm the diagnosis; orbital hemorrhages and direct ocular insults can be ruled out. A CT/MRI brain scan is required to rule out intracranial pathologies such as cerebral infarction or edema.

PREVENTION

Because blindness is a devastating condition, effort should be made to prevent blindness. Prevention strategies are summarized in Table 2. Corneal injuries can be prevented by the common practice of applying lubricants and taping the patient's eyes shut prior to positioning.[26]

TABLE 2   Strategies to Prevent Postoperative Blindness

1	Keep eye shut by taping.[26]
2	Avoid pressure on the eyes by head rest.
3	Avoid extreme neck rotations.
4	Intermittently examine eyes at least every 20 min.[27]
5	Goggles should be avoided.
6	Mirrors can be used to visualize eyes.
7	Intraoperative optic nerve handling should be minimized. Immediate notification of oculocardiac reflex should be done by the surgeon.
8	Avoid severe hypotension, hypoxia, anemia, excessive crystalloids (as a replacement to blood loss), and prolonged head down position.
9	Complicated spine surgeries should be staged.

To prevent CRAO, the anesthesiologist must avoid compression of the globe. Pressure on the eyes from anesthetic masks is avoidable by selecting a properly fitting mask. In the prone position for surgery, a foam or gel headrest should be used with the eyes properly placed in the opening of the headrest; the position of the head and the eyes should be checked intermittently by palpation or visualization. The horseshoe headrest for the prone-positioned patient must be of appropriate size, as a smaller headrest can exert excessive pressure on the eyes. For the cervical spine surgery prone position, there are greater chances of head movement by the surgeon, leading to change in position and compression of the eye by the horseshoe. A pinhead holder can be used in cervical spine surgeries to minimize such movements. Considering results in rodent models of elevated IOP, it is advisable to examine the eyes after a change in position and the absence of external compression at least every 20 min.[27] A mirror can be positioned underneath to indirectly view the eyes on the transparent headrest. The use of goggles to cover the eyes is not advised when the head is positioned prone in a conventional square foam headrest.[26] During supratentorial surgeries, be vigilant for oculocardiac reflex (OCR). It reflects optic nerve handing or compression on eyeball during the bifrontal base of skull surgeries. Cortical damage can be prevented by maneuvers that decrease the chances of embolization.[28]

TREATMENT

The supportive therapies for all cases of POVL is described in Table 3. Treatment of CRAO[29] includes ocular massage to lower IOP (glaucoma should be ruled out) and thereby dislodging an embolus.

	BRAO	CRAO	IONs	Cortical blindness	Acute glaucoma	PRES
Signs and symptoms	Partial and painless loss of vision Scotomas	Complete blindness Loss of light perception Signs of trauma near the eye Periorbital and eyelid edema Chemosis, proptosis, and ptosis Paresthesias of the supraorbital region Corneal abrasion Loss of eye movements	Painless scotomas partial/complete blindness	Painless Hemianopia Scotomas	Painful red eye Cloudy or blurred vision Headache Nausea Vomiting Often bilateral	Seizures Cortical blindness Homonymous hemianopia, Blurred vision Decreased level of consciousness Headaches Nausea and vomiting Brain stem symptoms Hemiplegia
Light reflex	N or RAPD	A or RAPD	A or RAPD	N	A	N
Fundoscopy	Pale emboli of platelet fibrin (dull, white) Attenuated vessels	Cherry-red macula	AION-optic disc edema Hemorrhages PION-optic disc and fundus initially normal Late-atrophy	Normal	Normal	Papilledema

Continued

TABLE 3   Clinical Features, Diagnosis, and Management of Patients with POVL—cont'd

	BRAO	CRAO	IONs	Cortical blindness	Acute glaucoma	PRES
Radiology	Normal	Proptosis Extraoccular muscle swelling	Normal	Infarct Edema Hemorrhages	Normal	Symmetrical edema in occipital and parieto-occipital cortex and subcortical white matter and posterior frontal lobes
Treatment	Ocular massage-to dislodge emboli Arteriolar dilators Carbogen inhalation (5% CO_2 + 95% O_2) Pentoxyphylline hyperbaric oxygen Embolectomy- Mechanical Nd:YAG laser		No definitive treatment IOP lower agents Mannitol Furesemide Head-up position Lateral canthotomy	Supportive treatment	β-Adrenergic antagonists α-Adrenergic agonists Carbonic anhydrase inhibitor Cholinergic agonists corticosteroids Peripheral iridectomy	Treat causative factor Cerebral decongestants[1]

Abbreviations: BRAO: Branch retinal artery occlusion; CRAO: Central retinal artery occlusion; IONs: Ischemic ocular neuropathy; PION: Posterior ischemic optic neuropathy; PRES: Posterior reversible encephalopathy syndrome; N: Normal; RAPD: Relative afferent pupillary defect; A: Absent; IOP: Intraocular pressure.

Carbogen therapy (5% CO_2, 95% O_2; for 10 min every 2 h for 48 h) in oxygen inhalation have been attempted to enhance dilation and increase oxygen delivery from retinal and choroidal vessels. Hyperbaric oxygen therapy may be beneficial if begun within 2–12 h of symptom onset for 10 min every 2 h for 48 h. Translumenal Nd:YAG laser embolectomy to dislodge the clot and intraarterial or intravenous thrombolysis can be attempted. Pentoxyphylline is a trisubstituted xanthine derivative that works by increasing erythrocyte flexibility, reducing blood viscosity, and increasing microcirculatory flow and tissue perfusion, which has also been used to improve circulation.

There is no definitive treatment of ION. Few case reports have proven the benefit of acetazolamide.[30] Diuretics such as mannitol or furosemide reduce IOP and edema. The benefits of steroids have not yet been proven. Hypotension and anemia should be corrected. Patients should be kept in a head-up position if increased ocular venous pressure is suspected. If visual loss is due to ocular compartment syndrome, immediate decompression (lateral canthotomy) is indicated. A few case reports recommend application of hyperbaric oxygen, use of neuroprotective agents,[31] or drugs that lower IOP, but with no proven efficacy reported.

Acute glaucoma is an emergency, and ophthalmologic consultation should be obtained immediately. Patients are treated with β-adrenergic antagonists, α-adrenergic agonists, carbonic anhydrase inhibitors, cholinergic agonists, and corticosteroids. Peripheral iridectomy should be performed if needed.[32]

To conclude, POVL is a serious complication with serious medicolegal implications. As there is a rapid increase in the number of complex spinal surgeries that increases the incidence of POVL, we must take adequate precautions to prevent POVL.

References

1. Chang SH, Miller NR. The incidence of vision loss due to perioperative ischemic optic neuropathy associated with spine surgery: the Johns Hopkins Hospital Experience. *Spine*. 2005;30:1299–1302.
2. Patil CG, Lad EM, Lad SP, Ho C, Boakye M. Visual loss after spine surgery: a population-based study. *Spine*. 2008;33:1491–1496.
3. Shen Y, Drum M, Roth S. The prevalence of perioperative visual loss in the United States: a 10-year study from 1996 to 2005 spinal, orthopedic, cardiac, and general surgery. *Anesth Analg*. 2009;109:1534–1545.
4. Halvorsen H, Ramm-Pettersen J, Josefsen R, et al. Surgical complications after transsphenoidal microscopic and endoscopic surgery for pituitary adenoma: a consecutive series of 506 procedures. *Acta Neurochir*. 2014;156:441–449.
5. Moslemi MK, Soleimani M, Faiz HR, Rahimzadeh P. Cortical blindness after complicated general anesthesia in urological surgery. *Am J Case Rep*. 2013;14:376–379.
6. Tong H, Wei S, Zhou D, Zhu R, Pan L, Jiang J. Vision deterioration after transsphenoidal surgery for removal of pituitary adenoma. *Zhonghua Wai Ke Za Zhi*. 2002;40:746–748.

7. Kim DJ, Kim DI, Lee SK, Kim SY. Homonymous hemianopia after embolization of an aneurysm-associated AVM supplied by the anterior choroidal artery. *Yonsei Med J.* 2003;44:1101–1105.
8. Park SW, Woo SJ, Park KH, Huh JW, Jung C, Kwon OK. Iatrogenic retinal artery occlusion caused by cosmetic facial filler injections. *Am J Ophthalmol.* 2012;154(4): 653–662.
9. Crockett AJ, Trinidade A, Kothari P, Barnes J. Visual loss following head and neck surgery. *J Laryngol Otol.* 2012;126:418–420.
10. Delattre O, Thoreux P, Liverneaux P, et al. Spinal surgery and ophthalmic complications: a French survey with review of 17 cases. *Spinal Disord Tech.* 2007;20:302–307.
11. Bradish CF, Flowers M. Central retinal artery occlusion in association with osteogenesis imperfecta. *Spine.* 1987;12:193–194.
12. Roth S, Pietrzyk Z. Blood flow after retinal ischemia in cats. *Invest Ophthalmol Vis Sci.* 1994;35:3209–3217.
13. Awad J, Awad A, Wong Y, Thomas S. Unilateral visual loss after a nasal airway surgery. *Case Rep.* 2013;6:119–123.
14. Ho VTG, Newman NJ, Song S, Suzan S, Ksiazek S, Roth S. Ischemic optic neuropathy following spine surgery. *J Neurosurg Anesthesiol.* 2005;17:38–44.
15. Özkiriş M, Akin I, Özkiriş A, Adam M, Saydam L. Ischemic optic neuropathy after carotid body tumor resection. *J Craniofac Surg.* 2014;25(1):58–61.
16. American Society of Anesthesiologists Task Force on Perioperative Visual Loss. Practice advisory for perioperative visual loss associated with spine surgery: an updated report by the American Society of Anesthesiologists Task Force on Perioperative Visual Loss. *Anesthesiology.* 2012;116:274–285.
17. Lorri AL. Perioperative visual loss and anesthetic management. *Curr Opin Anesthesiol.* 2013;26:375–381.
18. Lee LA, Deem S, Glenny RW, et al. Effects of anaemia and hypotension on porcine optic nerve blood flow and oxygen delivery. *Anesthesiology.* 2008;108:864–872.
19. Lee LA, Lam AM. Unilateral blindness after prone lumbar surgery. *Anesthesiology.* 2001;95:793–795.
20. Grover VK, Jangra K. Perioperative vision loss: a complication to watch out. *J Anaesth Clin Pharmacol.* 2012;28:11–16.
21. Singer MS, Salim S. Bilateral acute angle closure glaucoma as a complication of facedown spine surgery. *Spine J.* 2010;10(9):7–9.
22. Hinchey J, Chaves C, Appignani B, et al. A reversible posterior leukoencephalopathy syndrome. *N Engl J Med.* 1996;334:494–500.
23. Eran A, Barak M. Posterior reversible encephalopathy syndrome after combined general and spinal anesthesia with intrathecal morphine. *Anesth Analg.* 2009;108:609–612.
24. Yi JH, Ha SH, Kim YK, Choi EM. Posterior reversible encephalopathy syndrome in an untreated hypertensive patient after spinal surgery under general anesthesia. *Korean J Anesthesiol.* 2011;60:369–372.
25. Hansberry DR, Agarwal N, Tomei KL, Goldstein IM. Reversible encephalopathy syndrome in a patient with a Chiari malformation. *Surg Neurol Int.* 2013;4:130.
26. Grover VK, Kumar KV, Sharma S, Sethi N, Grewal SPS. Comparison of methods of eye protection under general anaesthesia. *Can J Anaesth.* 1998;45:575–577.
27. Roth S. Postoperative vision loss. In: Miller RD, ed. *Textbook of Anesthesia.* 7th ed. New York: Elsevier; 2010:2826.
28. Pugsley W, Klinger L, Paschalis C, Treasure T, Harrison M, Newman S. The impact of microemboli during cardiopulmonary bypass on neuropsychological functioning. *Stroke.* 1994;25:1393–1399.
29. Cugati S, Varma DD, Chen CS, Lee AW. Treatment options for central retinal artery occlusion. *Curr Treat Options Neurol.* 2013;15:63–77.

30. Hayreh SS. Anterior ischaemic optic neuropathy: III, Treatment, prophylaxis, and differential diagnosis. *Br J Ophthalmol.* 1974;58:981–989.
31. Arnold AC, Levin LA. Treatment of ischemic optic neuropathy. *Semin Ophthalmol.* 2002;17:39–46.
32. Emanuel ME, Parrish RK, Gedde SJ. Evidence-based management of primary angle closure glaucoma. *Curr Opin Ophthalmol.* 2014;25(2):89–92.

Postoperative Cognitive Dysfunction

Giuseppina Magni, Federico Bilotta

Department of Anaesthesia and Intensive Care, University of Rome
"Sapienza", Rome, Italy

OUTLINE

DEFINITION

Postoperative delirium (POD) is defined in the Diagnostic and Statistical Manual of Mental Disorders IV as an acute onset fluctuating change in mental status characterized by a reduced awareness of the environment and disturbance of attention. Frequently complicating the course of hospitalized patients, delirium can manifest as a hypoactive status seen in 64% of surgical intensive care unit patients but is often missed or misdiagnosed as depression, a hyperactive status (5–22% of cases), or mixed psychomotor behaviors. It can be associated with hallucinations, delusions, and impairment of memory. Postoperative symptoms typically arise on days 1–3 after surgery, commonly after an initial lucid postoperative phase. **Persistent postoperative cognitive decline (POCD)** is a more subtle condition and diagnosis can be difficult also because there is not a common definition or tested diagnostic criteria. It is commonly intended as an impairment of cognitive functions, including memory, learning, concentration, and speed of mental processing and was first reported in 1955. POCD can affect all age groups but is more frequent and severe in the elderly (>65 years) and may last for days up to months or permanently compromise cognitive abilities. Occurrence of POCD is associated with reduced return to work, social inability, and increased mortality. The pathogenesis of POCD is multifactorial, with the immune response to surgery probably acting as a trigger. Factors that elevate the risk of POCD include old age, preexisting cerebral, cardiac, and vascular disease, alcohol abuse, low educational level, and intra and postoperative complications. The findings of multiple randomized controlled trials indicate that the method of anesthesia does not play a causal role for prolonged cognitive impairment. **Postoperative chronic neurocognitive disorders (POCNCD)** is an insidious and progressive disorder characterized by impairment of memory and at least one other cognitive domain, including language, handling complex tasks, reasoning, or orientation and can be severe enough to interfere with daily function and independence, and cannot be better explained by another diagnosis. Dementia is chronic and associated with irreversible brain pathology. There is an emerging body of evidence that associates dementia with surgery and anesthesia. Anesthetic drugs, notably volatile agents, are known to modulate Alzheimer's pathogenesis in vitro and in animal models, and neuroinflammation, as seen after operation, is a feature of Alzheimer's dementia. However, no link has yet been proven in humans.

In conclusion, postoperative cognitive dysfunction includes a wide variety of conditions—POD, POCD, POCNCD—associated with specific time frame and pre, intra, and postoperative risk factors that also include anesthesia. Current evidence is limited, rapidly evolving and include: adequate clinical surveillance, right from the preoperative period, with accurate screening of individual risk factors and assessment of cognitive status, systematic use of dedicated and structured tests and a dedicated path for high risk patients that can effectively reduce the incidence and related complication.

INTRODUCTION

Anesthesia is supposed to induce a temporary and "fully" reversible loss of neurological and cognitive abilities. It is generally assumed that the effects of anesthetics do not outlast the pharmacological action and that the function of the target organ is restored to its previous state once the agent is eliminated.[1] There is increasing evidence that long-term and even permanent neuronal and neurological changes can follow administration of anesthetics.[2] The initial manifestation of brain damage is a decline in the higher cortical functions of storage, recall of memory, and cognitive processing. Postoperative cognitive disturbances were first described in the mid1950s with a pivotal report—published in 1955 from Bedford—where "adverse cerebral effects of anaesthesia on old people" are described.[3] Postoperative cognitive dysfunction was reported shortly after the introduction of open heart surgery; initially the clinical attention was focused on psychological aspects related to the experimental nature of the surgical procedure and the low probability of a complete recovery or even survival.[4] Therefore, the priority was addressed to minimize postoperative cardiovascular and pulmonary risks. Overtime, the rate of perioperative cardiovascular and respiratory complications and perioperative mortality decreased markedly while the incidence of postoperative cognitive complications remained unchanged.

The American College of Cardiology and the American Heart Association have categorized the neurological complications after cardiac surgery into two groups: type I and type II. Type I includes stroke and transient ischemic attack, coma, and fatal cerebral injury: these deficits are clearly defined and can be diagnosed by clinical neurological examination. Type II includes postoperative impairments in cognition, memory deficits, reduced concentration, and psychomotor disturbances.[5] Postoperative impairment in cognition is commonly categorized into three distinct clinical conditions: POD can appear hours/days after the procedure, persistent POCD can last up to months, and POCNCD that lead to a permanent cognitive impairment as in Alzheimer and dementia. These are separate conditions and can be distinguished by the timing and duration of symptoms (Figure 1).[6]

In this chapter we aim to report available evidence postoperative impairments in cognition—POD, POCD, and POCNCD—and their relationship with anesthesia.

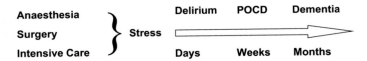

FIGURE 1   Timeline of early and late postoperative cognitive dysfunction after surgery, anesthesia, and intensive care.

ANESTHESIA AND POSTOPERATIVE DELIRIUM

POD is disturbance of consciousness with a reduced ability to focus, sustain, or shift attention with serious implications and increased perioperative morbidity and mortality. In POD there is an acute and changeable alteration of mental state with reduced awareness of the environment and disturbance with spatial or temporal disorientation and memory dysfunction and/or perceptual changes (hallucinations) that cannot be accounted for a preexisting or evolving dementia.[7] Postoperatively, it occurs within 72 h after surgery and fluctuates. It can be characterized by a hyperactive (agitated and combative) or hypoactive status (decreased alertness/ motor activity) or mixed forms with fluctuating mood. Prevalence of POD is 5–15% after elective general and loco regional anesthesia, with considerably higher rates after emergency surgery but can be as high as up to 50–60% in elderly patients undergoing emergency hip surgery.[8,9] Occurrence of POD is associated with a cascade of events culminating in increased dependence, higher mortality, and more persistent cognitive impairment.[10,11]

As part of the assessment for POD, it is important to define the patient's baseline level of cognitive function in the preoperative phase. If the patient is not displaying symptoms of delirium on admission, baseline cognitive functioning can be assessed at that time with use of the mini-mental state examination (MMSE).[12] The MMSE is a simple and easy test and should be part of the preoperative evaluation. For the diagnosis of POD the Diagnostic and Statistical Manual of Mental Disorders DSM-5 or the International Classification of Disease and Related Health Problems ICD-10, are the gold standards and also apply in acutely ill and hospitalized patients.[13] At large, the use of dedicated and structured test should be systematically implemented in the postoperative evaluation right from admission to postanesthesia care unit. Use of the confusion assessment method (CAM) algorithm at the bedside increases the likelihood of making the correct diagnosis. The CAM has been validated in a number of settings, has high sensitivity and specificity, and can be administered in approximately in 2–5 min.[14–16] The nursing delirium screening scale is a simple and effective diagnostic tool as easily repeatable in the intensive care unit (ICU) as in the ward.[17] The assessment of preoperative risk factors related to PD is of great importance and allows for selection of patients at increased risk in whom a dedicated perioperative path is indicated. Risk factors for PD include preoperative, intraoperative, and postoperative.

PREOPERATIVE RISK FACTORS

Age is a major preoperative risk factor: age >70 years is associated with an odds ratio of 3.3 for PD and age >80 is associated with an odds ratio of 5.2.[18] Type of surgery: orthopedic, abdominal aortic aneurysm, and cardiac thoracic surgery are principally linked to an increased risk.[18,19] The European System for Cardiac Operative Risk Evaluation is a clinical risk factor index, based on 18 variables, that predicts perioperative survival in cardiac surgery patients and is also useful to estimate the risk for POD[20]. The importance of genetic profile for POD is not yet completely clear: a polymorphism for apolipoprotein E is possibly a risk factor for POD as it is associated with chronic neurodegenerative disorders (i.e., dementia).[21] In chronic obstructive pulmonary disease the underlying mechanism is probably based on chronic hypoxia that facilitates mitochondrial dysfunction and promotes brain dysfunction and cognitive decline. Patients with COPD have worse performance than controls in a number of neuropsychological tests including executive functions, attention, nonverbal reasoning, and problem solving ability.[22] In obstructive sleep apnea the causative mechanisms are possibly related to the imbalance between brain oxygen requirement and oxygen supply ("respiratory encephalopathy").[23] The use of continuous positive pressure ventilation during the night time may be an effective approach for treatment.[24] Psychiatric and neurodegenerative disorders and history of alcohol or illicit drug abuse are associated with an increased risk for PD.[25,26] There are several clinical factors associated with an increased risk for PD that are suitable for preoperative correction: fluid fasting time, electrolytes, low serum albumin, malnutrition, anemia, glycemic abnormalities, and preoperative premedication with benzodiazepines[27–31]. Preoperative fluids fasting time is independently associated with an increased incidence of POD. Electrolyte abnormalities and especially hyponatremia, a frequent complication of renal disease and chronic diuretic therapy, is often detected in elderly patients and should be corrected preoperatively. Serum albumin concentration is related with cognitive performance and can be considered as a predictor and a precipitating factor for POD. Serum albumin elicits drug and hormone binding activity along with an antioxidant and oxygen radical trapping that prevents toxic cognitive impairment. Furthermore, low levels of albumin in the brain and cerebrospinal fluid (CSF) are associated with increased formation of amyloid β-peptide fibrils and the risk for chronic neurodegenerative disorders including Alzheimer's disease (AD). Therefore, quantifying nutritional intake can be really important in elderly undergoing surgery: preoperative nutritional status is also a predictor of the risk for POD. The Malnutrition Universal Screening Tool is a five-step screening tool, that provides an effective approach to assess adequacy of nutrition and can be used to derive a malnutrition risk score.[32] It consists of three components: body mass index, history of unexplained weight loss, and acute illness effect. Anemia can severely impact on brain metabolism and oxygen transport, and should be aggressively treated in the preoperative period.[33] It is important to emphasize that the avoiding premedication with benzodiazepines is associated with reduced risk for POD[31].

INTRAOPERATIVE RISK FACTORS

POD has been associated with surgery-related risk factors such as severe bleeding (greater than 1000 cc) leading to acute anemia and postoperative hematocrit <30 requiring postoperative blood transfusions.[34]

Several drugs, including atropine and ketamine, and the use of propofol compared with sevoflurane are associated with a higher incidence of POD.[35,36] Intraoperative tight glucose control seems not to be recommended because it increases the risk of POD after cardiac surgery.[37] Particularly in elderly patients it is extremely relevant to prevent intraoperative hypotension and hypocapnia: intraoperative mean arterial pressure and partial pressure of carbon dioxide are among the physiologic variables related to the occurrence of PD because they induce a significant reduction of cerebral blood flow.[38]

Depth of anesthesia measured by BIS (too low and too high) is associated with an increased risk of POD.[39] The incidence of POD in surgical patients whose depth of anesthesia was monitored by BIS was 16.7%, compared with 21.4% in the control group (P = 0.036).[40] Similar results reported that BIS-guided anesthesia reduced anesthetic exposure and decreased the risk of postoperative delirium by 35%. For every 1000 elderly patients undergoing major surgery, the use of a BIS value between 40 and 60 prevented 83 patients from delirium.[41]

POSTOPERATIVE RISK FACTORS

Several clinical conditions, including severe pain, administration of benzodiazepine and anticholinergic drugs, sensory deprivation, delayed ambulation, and inadequate nutritional status are associated with risk of developing PD and should be aggressively prevented.[42] Moreover, low cardiac output requiring inotrope infusion, new onset atrial fibrillation, persistent hypoxia or hypercapnia, and ICU admission are associated with an increased risk of POD.[43]

PRECIPITATING FACTORS

In the postoperative period several factors, such as sleep deprivation, bladder and central venous catheterization, more than three medications added before the onset of delirium, anticholinergic drugs, alcohol or drug withdrawal, infections, and pain can precipitate POD and should be prevented and treated. Nursing surveillance and accurate staff communication can play a critical role in this process.[42]

ETIOLOGY AND PATHOGENESIS

A variety of neurotransmitter systems has been implicated in the pathogenesis of POD: serum anticholinergic activity, norepinephrine, melatonin, and lymphokines have been associated with delirium.[42,44] Delirium has been hypothesized to occur as a result of the inflammatory response associated with the stress of surgery: chemokines have been found to be elevated in the early postoperative period of patients who developed delirium after cardiac surgery. As chemokines are able of disrupting blood–brain barrier integrity in vitro, this finding suggest a possible relationship of these inflammatory mediators to delirium pathogenesis.[45]

PREVENTION AND TREATMENT

There is no single intervention that can avoid POD. Treatment and prevention require awareness of the diagnosis, reduction or elimination of modifiable risk factors, early diagnosis and treatment, early detection of coexisting or postoperative medical problems and excellent cooperation among anesthesiologist, nursing staff, and other medical specialists. The prevention/intervention are focused on the postoperative management of risk factors for POD: visual and hearing impairment, cognitive impairment, sleep deprivation, immobility, and dehydration.[46] Interventions as maintaining oxygen saturation at >90%, systolic blood pressure at >90 mmHg, and the hematocrit at >30% are effective as tight monitoring of fluid and electrolyte status.[47] Pain control, careful review of the patient's medications, regulation of bowel and bladder function, adequate nutritional intake, early mobilization and rehabilitation, appropriate environmental stimulation, and normalization of the patient's sleep–wake cycle are also key measures.[46] Evidence on pharmacological prevention of POD are lacking; a metaanalysis of 38 randomized controlled trials supports a possible role of α-agonists as adjuvants during ICU sedation and in pediatric patients receiving general anesthesia.[48, 49] Pharmacological treatment is not first-line approach: antipsychotic medication can be used when

POD interferes with the patient's ability to cooperate, places the patient in danger of harm, or excessively increases metabolic demands. The drug of choice remains haloperidol administered at a dose of 0.5–1 mg intravenously every 10–15 min until the behavior is controlled.[50]

ANESTHESIA AND PERSISTENT POSTOPERATIVE COGNITIVE DYSFUNCTION

A landmark article in the field of POCD was published in the Lancet in 1998 by investigators at the International Study of Postoperative Cognitive Dysfunction (ISPOCD-1).[51] This study examined 1218 patients at least 60 years of age at 13 European hospitals from eight countries that presented for major abdominal, noncardiac thoracic, or orthopedic surgery under general anesthesia. POCD was reported in 25.8% of patients 1 week after surgery and in 9.9% of patients 3 months after surgery compared with a control group that did not have surgery and had an incidence of cognitive changes of 3.4% at 1 week and 2.8% at 3 months. Increasing age, duration of anesthesia, education, a second operation, and postoperative respiratory infection were found to be significant factors associated with POCD. Type of anesthesia (general or locoregional) is not associated with differences in the rate of POCD. The use of regional or general anesthesia in patients >60 years scheduled for major noncardiac surgery did not represent a specific tool in the incidence of POCD at 3 months after surgery. The ISPOCD-2 study reported, in 438 elderly patients, no significant differences in POCD after general anesthesia and local anesthesia at 3 months follow up (14.3% and 13.9%; p = 0.93)[52].

Relevant risk factors for POCD are:

- Advanced age (>60 years);
- Poorer level of education;
- Severity and duration of surgery.

Age is a relevant issue: in patients who had undergone major surgery. POCD has been detected at discharge from the hospital in 36.6% of surgical patients aged 18–39, 30.4% of those aged 40–59, and 41.4% of those aged 60 and up. Three months later, 12.7% of the patients over age 60 still had POCD: the risk of developing dementia in the following 3–7 years is reported to be nearly doubled in elderly patients. POCD at hospital discharge has also been associated with increased mortality in the first 3 months and 1 year following surgery.[53] Despite an established association with poor short and long-term outcome and with an increased morbidity and mortality, POCD frequently goes unrecognized. Estimates of the incidence of POCD vary with the type of surgery; prevalence of POCD is more limited in minor surgery and day-case surgery (reported in about 6.6%), where the physiological stress response is less intense while highest risk is reported in major vascular, orthopedic, and cardiac surgery.[54,55] In cardiac surgery, the incidence of POCD is reported as high as 50–80% at hospital discharge reduced to 20–50% at 6 weeks, and to 10–30% at 6 months after operation.[56] Several possible mechanisms for POCD have been suggested that include brain hypoperfusion and hypoxia.[57] However, in the ISPOCD-1 study, no correlation was found between hypoxemia or hypotensive episodes and POCD.[51] Other explanations included surgical stress-associated inflammatory reactions, alterations in hormonal homeostasis, and direct anesthetic agent toxicity.[58,59]

Neuropsychological testing is required to detect POCD: the z-score is considered the most rigorous and was used in the landmark International Study on Postoperative Cognitive Dysfunction (ISPOCD-1) study. A z-score is a dimensionless unit that indicates how far an individual's performance in a test deviates, in terms of standard deviation, from the average performance of a control population.[60] POCD is defined as a z-score of 2 or more. Patients can be also screened for cognitive impairment using the MMSE performed before and after anesthesia.[12] This test quantitatively assesses cognitive impairment on a scale from 0–30 (lower scores indicate worse impairment) based on answers to a variety of questions and is suggested as one method to identify patients within suspected cognitive impairment. A decrease in MMSE >2 points is considered clinically significant. The MMSE is a useful screening tool for POCD in hospitalized elderly patients and might recognize patients in whom medical treatment can effectively prevent the progression to dementia.[61]

POCD and Drugs

Ample preclinical and clinical evidence demonstrate the relationship between opioids and POCD and this might extend to hypnotics.[62–64] There is conflicting evidence that anesthetic agents cause systemic inflammation resulting in POCD; in animals studies, isoflurane or i.v. (intravenous) anesthesia administration without surgery, was not associated with cytokine activation and behavioral changes or POCD.[65,66] Volatile agents may enhance neuronal apoptosis, and may increase neurodegenerative processes.[67,68] Furthermore, sevoflurane-induced burst-suppression causes cerebral vasodilatation, which impairs cerebral blood flow autoregulation and might ultimately lead to hypoperfusion.[69] In mice, high doses of isoflurane (2%) are associated with better cognitive performance after anesthesia than lower isoflurane doses (1%) suggesting that detrimental effects might be limited to lower doses.[70] In humans, deeper isoflurane anesthesia titrated with BIS (median BIS 38.9) resulted in better postoperative information processing compared with a higher (mean BIS 50.7) BIS regimen.[71] Moreover, BIS-guided depth of anesthesia combined with cerebral oxygen saturation monitoring was considered as an effective approach to reduce postoperative cognitive impairment.[72] In two studies comparing propofol with sevoflurane and desflurane a higher incidence of POCD was detected in patients after propofol-based anesthesia.[73,74] These results suggest that there might be a protective effect of halogenates-based anesthesia, possibly mediated by anesthetic "pre and postconditioning."

Prevention

Prevention of POCD is the most effective way to reduce related complications. However, predisposing factors, such as age, chronic illness, and preexisting cognitive impairment, cannot be modified. Preventative measures recommended with elective surgical patients include[75-78]:

- Preoperative assessment of cognitive function;
- Preoperative measurement of hemoglobin and electrolytes, with appropriate correction;
- BIS-guided depth of anesthesia;
- Prevention of dehydration secondary to prolonged fasting;
- Administration of prescribed medication on the day of surgery;
- Intervention to aid orientation;
- Adequate sleeping;
- Physical rehabilitation;
- Sedation strategies: Avoid benzodiazepine use in elderly patients.

In conclusion, POCD can occur in all age groups after surgery, but is more common in elderly patients undergoing major surgery. Even though there is a well-known association with poor short and long-term outcome, and with perioperative morbidity and mortality, POCD frequently goes unrecognized.[79] However, its implication should not be overlooked and greater attention should be addressed to prevent, recognize, and treat POCD.

ANESTHESIA AND POSTOPERATIVE CHRONIC NEUROCOGNITIVE DISORDERS

POCNCDs such as dementia and AD are possibly related to anesthesia in terms of triggering and acceleration of the disease.[80] AD is a progressive disorder characterized by cognitive and neurological functional decline, encompassing multiple cognitive domains that cannot be explained by alternative diagnosis.[81] Guidelines included decreased levels of amyloid-beta (Aβ) and increased total tau or phosphorylated tau in the CSF among the diagnostic criteria.[82] The amyloid cascade hypothesis states that some forms of the Aβ peptide are neurotoxic and cause abnormal phosphorylation of tau, leading to intracellular tau forming paired helical filaments which result in neurofibrillary tangles. This cascade results in mitochondrial damage, abnormal calcium balance, apoptosis and neurodegeneration.[83] Increased Aβ peptide levels in CSF are followed by amyloid accumulation, cerebral atrophy, and impaired cerebral glucose metabolism that proceed over a decade before symptoms occur.[84,85] Strong evidence for this theory has been derived by clinical, genetic, biomarker, and autopsy studies.[86–92] The ratio of total tau to Aβ is currently used as a diagnostic adjunct for AD.[93]

Anesthetic effect: Surgery and anesthesia could influence cognition by altering cerebral perfusion and autoregulation and with possible pharmacological mechanisms.[94] Some surgical specialties (cardiac, thoracic, orthopedic, etc.) are associated with a higher risk of POCNCD although it is unclear if this is due to induced changes in cerebral physiology or directly related to the procedure itself.[95,96] In spite of strong preclinical evidence, clinical data on the relationship between anesthesia and AD are inconsistent.[97–99] In vitro and animal studies demonstrate that halothane and isoflurane increase cytotoxicity of amyloid peptides and sevoflurane and isoflurane can cause neuronal apoptosis as propofol increases tau phosphorylation in the mouse hippocampus.[100–103] General anesthesia modifies central cholinergic transmission through nicotinic and muscarinic receptors, and cholinergic dysfunction has been implicated in the clinical symptoms of dementia.[104] The role of neuroinflammation has also been widely studied. In mice, surgery leads to the production of tumor necrosis factor α, which subsequently disrupts the blood–brain barrier, causing an infiltration of inflammatory macrophages in the brain parenchyma, specifically the hippocampus.[66] The levels of the inflammatory cytokines interleukin (IL)-1β and IL-6 are increased in mice after instrumentation and surgery than in those receiving anesthesia without surgical instrumentation, demonstrating that the inflammation and cognitive deficits may largely be a result of surgery rather than effects of anesthesia itself.[105] The effects of general anesthesia on biological markers have also provided relevant insights demonstrating AD biomarkers in the CSF after surgery; unfortunately, the small size of the studies and the uncertain correlation with cognitive deficits dictate prudence in the interpretation of the results.[106,107] Even if a consensus statement in 2009 ruled that benefits of anesthesia may outweigh its potentially toxic effects, is interesting to note that anesthesiologists die from Parkinson disease at a significantly higher rate than matched internists.[108,109]

TESTING FOR DEMENTIA

As mentioned above—see the section on POD—the MMSE is a useful perioperative screening tool especially in patients with existing cognitive deficits that are at increased risk for POD and POCD.[61] Originally designed as a screening tool for dementia, MMSE tests global cognitive functions, including orientation, recall, attention, calculation, language manipulation, and constructional praxis. The maximum total score is 30 and a score of 24 is suggestive, but not diagnostic, of dementia or delirium. The MMSE is a short test that can be used by nonspecialists and has been extensively studied in different populations but it is not adequately sensitive for mild cognitive deficit and POCD, as it can be influenced by age, education, language, motor, and visual impairments.[110,111]

CONCLUSIONS

In conclusion, postoperative cognitive dysfunction includes a wide variety of conditions—POD, POCD, and POCNCD—associated with specific time frame and pre, intra, and postoperative risk factors that also include anesthesia. Current evidence is limited and rapidly evolving, and includes adequate clinical surveillance, right from the preoperative period, with accurate screening of individual risk factors and assessment of cognitive status, systematic use of dedicated and structured tests and a dedicated path for high risk patients that can effectively reduce the incidence and related complication. Long-term prospective studies or randomized controlled trials are necessary to clarify the possible associations between anesthesia, surgery, and the various forms of perioperative cognitive impairment and how to prevent and minimize the related impact.

References

1. Hanning CD. Postoperative cognitive dysfunction. *Br J Anaesth*. 2005;95:82–87.
2. Hussain M, Berger M, Eckenhoff RG, Seitz DP. General anesthetic and the risk of dementia in elderly patients: current insights. *Clin Intervention Aging*. 2014;9:1619–1628.
3. Bedford PD. Adverse cerebral effects of anaesthesia on old people. *Lancet*. 1955;269: 259–263.
4. Boshes B, Priest WS, Yacorzynski GK, Zaks MS. The neurologic, psychiatric and psychologic aspects of cardiac surgery. *Med Clin N Am*. 1957;41:155–169.
5. Eagle KA, Guyton RA, Davidoff R, et al. ACC/AHA guidelines for coronary artery bypass graft surgery: executive summary and recommendations. *Circulation*. 1999;100:1464–1480.
6. Lloyd DG, Ma D, Vizcaychipi MP. Cognitive decline after anaesthesia and critical care. *Contin Educ Anaesth Crit Care Pain*. 2012;12(3):105–109.
7. Diagnostic and Statistical Manual of Mental Disorders. 4th ed. (DSM-IV–TR; www.dsmivtr.org/).
8. Deiner S, Silverstein JH. Postoperative delirium and cognitive dysfunction. *Br J Anaesth*. 2009;103:41–46.
9. Bruce AJ, Ritchie CW, Blizard R, Lai R, Raven P. The incidence of delirium associated with orthopedic surgery: a meta-analytic review. *Int Psychogeriatr*. 2007;19:197–214.
10. Chaput AJ, Bryson GL. Postoperative delirium: risk factors and management: continuing professional development. *Can J Anaesth*. 2012;59:304–320.
11. Martin BJ, Buth KJ, Arora RC, Baskett RJ. Delirium: a cause for concern beyond the immediate postoperative period. *Ann Thorac Surg*. 2012;93:1114–1120.
12. Folstein MF, Folstein SE, McHugh PR. "Mini-Mental State". A practical method for grading the cognitive state of patients for the clinician. *J Psychiatr Res*. 1975;12:189–198.

13. *The ICD-10 Classification of Mental and Behavioural Disorders.* Geneve: World Health Organization; 1993.
14. Inouye SK, van Dyck CH, Alessi CA, Balkin S, Siegal AP, Horowitz RI. Clarifying confusion: the confusion assessment method. *Ann Intern Med.* 1990;113:941–948.
15. Inouye SK. The dilemma of delirium: clinical and research controversies regarding diagnosis and evaluation of delirium in hospitalized elderly medical patients. *Am J Med.* 1994;97:278–288.
16. Ely EW, Margolin R, Francis J, et al. Evaluation of delirium in critically ill patients: validation of the confusion assessment method for the intensive care unit (CAM-ICU). *Crit Care Med.* 2001;29(7):1370–1379.
17. Gaudreau JD, Gagnon P, Harel F, Tremblay A, Roy MA. Fast, systematic, and continuous delirium assessment in hospitalized patients: the nursing delirium screening scale. *J Pain Symptom Manage.* 2005;29(4):368–375.
18. Marcantonio ER, Goldman L, Mangione C, et al. A clinical prediction rule for delirium after elective non cardiac surgery. *JAMA.* 1994;271:134–139.
19. Balasundaram B, Holmes J. Delirium in vascular surgery. *Eur J Vasc Endovasc Surg.* 2007;34:131–134.
20. Euroscore. Homepage. Internet Available at: www.euroscore org.
21. Van Munster BC, De Rooij SE, Korevaar JC. The role of genetics in delirium in the elderly patient. *Dement Geriatr Cogn Disord.* 2009;28:187–195.
22. De Carolis A, Giubilei F, Caselli G, et al. Chronic obstructive pulmonary disease is associated with altered neuropsychological performance in young adults. *Dement Geriatr Cogn Disord Extra.* 2011;1(1):402–408.
23. Flink BJ, Rivelli SK, Cox EA, et al. Obstructive sleep apnea and incidence of postoperative delirium after elective knee replacement in the non-demented elderly. *Anesthesiology.* 2012;116:788–796.
24. Lombardi C, Rocchi R, Montagana P, Silani V, Parati GF. Obstructive sleep apnea syndrome: a cause of acute delirium. *J Clin Sleep Med.* 2009;5:569–570.
25. Hohman TJ, Beason-Held LL, Resnick SM. Cognitive complaints, depressive symptoms, and cognitive impairment: are they related? *J Am Geriatr Soc.* 2011;59:1908–1912.
26. Litaker D, Locala J, Franco K, Bronson DL, Tannous Z. Preoperative risk factors for postoperative delirium. *Gen Hosp Psychiatry.* 2001;23:84–89.
27. Bekkar AY, Weeks EJ. Cognitive function after anaesthesia in the elderly. *Best Pract Res Clin Anaesthesiol.* 2003;17:259–272.
28. Radtke FM, Franck M, MacGuill M, et al. Duration of fluid fasting and choice of analgesic are modifiable factors for early postoperative delirium. *Eur J Anaesthesiol.* 2010;27:411–416.
29. Schlanger LE, Bailey JL, Sands JM. Electrolytes in the Aging. *Chronic Kidney Dis.* 2010;17:308–309.
30. Llewellyn DJ, Langa KM, Friedland RP, Lang IA. Serum albumin concentration and cognitive impairment. *Curr Alzheimer Res.* 2010;7:91–96.
31. Taipale PG, Ratner PA, Galdas PM, et al. The association between nurse-administered midazolam following cardiac surgery and incident delirium: an observational study. *Int J Nurs Stud.* 2012;49:1064–1073.
32. Ahmed T, Haboubi N. Assessment and management of nutrition in older people and its importance to health. *Clin Interv Aging.* 2010;5:207–216.
33. Peters R, Burch L, Warner J, Beckett N, Poulter R, Bulpitt C. Haemoglobin, anaemia, dementia and cognitive decline in the elderly, a systematic review. *BMC Geriatr.* 2008;8:18.
34. Marcantonio ER, Goldman L, Orav EJ, Cook EF, Lee TH. The association of intraoperative factors with the development of postoperative delirium. *Am J Med.* 1998;105(5):380–384.
35. Bilotta F, Doronzio A, Stazi E, et al. Early postoperative cognitive dysfunction and postoperative delirium after anaesthesia with various hypnotics: study protocol for a randomised controlled trial—the PINOCCHIO trial. *Trials.* 2011;12:170.

IX. MISCELLANEOUS

36. Nishikawa K, Nakayama M, Omote K, Namiki A. Recovery characteristics and post-operative delirium after long duration laparoscope-assisted surgery in elderly patients: propofol-based vs. sevoflurane-based anesthesia. *Acta Anaesthesiol Scand.* 2004;48:162–168.

37. Saager L, Duncan AE, Yared JP, et al. Intraoperative tight glucose control using hyper-insulinemic normoglycemia increases delirium after cardiac surgery. *Anesthesiology.* 2015;122:1214–1223.

38. Siepe M, Pfeiffer T, Gieringer A, et al. Increased systemic perfusion pressure during cardiopulmonary bypass is associated with less early postoperative cognitive dysfunction and delirium. *Eur J Cardiothorac Surg.* 2011;40:200–207.

39. Monk TG, Saini V, Weldon BC, Sigl JC. Anesthetic management and one-year mortality after noncardiac surgery. *Anesth Analg.* 2005;100:4–10.

40. Radtke FM, Franck M, Lendner J, Krüger S, Wernecke KD, Spies CD. Monitoring depth of anaesthesia in a randomized trial decreases the rate of postoperative delirium but not postoperative cognitive dysfunction. *Br J Anaesth.* 2013;110(1):98–105.

41. Chan MT, Cheng BC, Lee TM, Gin T, CODA trial group. BIS-guided anesthesia decreases postoperative delirium and cognitive decline. *J Neurosurg Anesthesiol.* 2013;25(1):33–42.

42. Inouye S. Delirium in older persons. *N Engl J Med.* 2006;354:1157–1165.

43. Roach GW, Kanchuger M, Mangano CM, et al. Adverse cerebral outcomes after coronary bypass surgery. Multicenter study of perioperative Ischemia research group and the Ischemia research and education Foundation investigators. *N Engl J Med.* 1996;335(25):1857–1863.

44. Steiner LA. Postoperative delirium. Part 1:pathophysiology and risk factors. *Eur J Anaesthesiol.* 2011;28:628–636.

45. Rudolph JL, Ramlawi B, Kuchel GA, et al. Chemokines are associated with delirium after cardiac surgery. *J Gerontol.* 2008;63(2):184–189.

46. Inouye S, Bogardus Jr ST, Charpentier PA, et al. A multicomponent intervention to prevent delirium in hospitalized older patients. *N Engl J Med.* 1999;340(9):669–676.

47. Benjamin D, Robertson MD, Timothy J, Robertson MD. Postoperative delirium after hip fracture. *J Bone Jt Surg Am.* 2006;88(9):2060–2068.

48. Zhang H, Lu Y, Liu M, et al. Strategies for prevention of postoperative delirium: a systematic review and meta-analysis of randomized trials. *Crit Care.* 2013;17(2):R47.

49. Pickard A, Davies P, Birnie K, Beringe R. Systematic review and meta-analysis of the effect of intraoperative α^2-adrenergic agonists on postoperative behaviour in children. *Br J Anaesth.* 2014;112(6):982–990.

50. Brown TM, Boyle MF, Delirium. ABC of psychological medicine. *BMJ.* 2002;325:644.

51. Moller JT, Cluitmans P, Rasmussen LS, et al. Long-term postoperative cognitive dysfunction in the elderly ISPOCD 1 study. ISPOCD investigators. International Study of Post-Operative Cognitive Dysfunction. *Lancet.* 1998;351(9106):857–861.

52. Rasmussen LS, Johnson T, Kuipers HM, et al. ISPOCD2 (International Study of Postoperative Cognitive Dysfunction) Investigators. Does anaesthesia cause postoperative cognitive dysfunction? A randomised study of regional versus general anaesthesia in 438 elderly patients. *Acta Anaesthesiol Scand.* 2003;47(3):260–266.

53. Monk TG, Weldon BC, Garvan CW, et al. Predictors of cognitive dysfunction after major non cardiac surgery. *Anesthesiology.* 2008;108:18–30.

54. Rasmussen LS. Postoperative cognitive dysfunction: incidence and prevention. *Best Pract Res Clin Anaesthesiol.* 2006;20(2):315–330.

55. Newman S, Stygall J, Hirani S, Shaefi S, Maze M. Postoperative cognitive dysfunction after non cardiac surgery: a systematic review. *Anesthesiology.* 2007;106:572–590.

56. Newman MF, Kirchner JL, Phillips-Bute B, et al. Neurological Outcome Research Group and the Cardiothoracic Anesthesiology Research Endeavors Investigators. Longitudinal assessment of neurocognitive function after coronary-artery bypass surgery. *N Engl J Med.* 2001;344(6):395–402.

57. Li M, Bertout JA, Ratcliffe SJ, Eckenhoff MF, Simon MC, Floyd TF. Acute anemia elicits cognitive dysfunction and evidence of cerebral cellular hypoxia in older rats with systemic hypertension. *Anesthesiology.* 2010;113:845–858.
58. Rasmussen LS, O'Brien JT, Silverstein JH, Johnson TW, Siersma VD, Canet J. Is perioperative cortisol secretion related to post-operative cognitive dysfunction? *Acta Anaesthesiol Scand.* 2005;49:1225–1231.
59. Hudson AE, Hemmings HC. Are anaesthetics toxic to the brain? *Br J Anaesth.* 2011;107:30–37.
60. Collie A, Darby DG, Falleti MG, Silbert BS, Maruff P. Determining the extent of cognitive change after coronary surgery: a review of statistical procedures. *Ann Thorac Surg.* 2002;73:2005–2011.
61. De Marchis GM, Foderaro G, Jemora J, et al. Mild cognitive impairment in medical inpatients: the Mini-Mental State Examination is a promising screening tool. *Dement Geriatr Cogn Disord.* 2010;29(3):259–264.
62. Kofke WA, Garman RH, Janosky J, Rose ME. Opioid neurotoxicity: neuropathologic effects in rats of different fentanyl congeners and the effects of hexamethonium-induced normotension. *Anesth Analg.* 1996;83:141–146.
63. Kofke WA, Attaallah AF, Kuwabara H, et al. The neuropathologic effects in rats and neurometabolic effects in humans of large-dose remifentanil. *Anesth Analg.* 2002;94:1229–1236.
64. Silbert BS, Scott DA, Evered LA, Lewis MS, Kalpokas M, Maruff P, et al. A comparison of the effect of high and low-dose fentanyl on the incidence of postoperative cognitive dysfunction after coronary artery bypass surgery in the elderly. *Anesthesiology.* 2006;104:1137–1145.
65. Wan Y, Xu J, Ma D, Zeng Y, Cibelli M, Maze M. Postoperative impairment of cognitive function in rats: a possible role for cytokine-mediated inflammation in the hippocampus. *Anesthesiology.* 2007;106:436–443.
66. Terrando N, Monaco C, Ma D, Foxwell BM, Feldmann M, Maze M. Tumor necrosis factor-alpha triggers a cytokine cascade yielding postoperative cognitive decline. *Proc Natl Acad Sci USA.* 2010;107:47.
67. Eckenhoff RG, Johansson JS, Wei H, et al. Inhaled anesthetic enhancement of amyloid-beta oligomerization and cytotoxicity. *Anesthesiology.* 2004;101:703–709.
68. Dong Y, Zhang G, Zhang B, et al. The common inhalational anesthetic sevoflurane induces apoptosis and increases beta-amyloid protein levels. *Arch Neurol.* 2009;66(5):620–631.
69. Reinsfelt B, Westerlind A, Ricksten SE. The effects of sevoflurane on cerebral blood flow autoregulation and flow-metabolism coupling during cardiopulmonary bypass. *Acta Anaesthesiol Scand.* 2011;55:118–123.
70. Valentim AM, Alves HC, Olsson IA, Antunes LM. The effects of depth of isoflurane anesthesia on the performance of mice in a simple spatial learning task. *J Am Assoc Lab Anim Sci.* 2008;47:16–19.
71. Farag E, Chelune GJ, Schubert A, Mascha EJ. Is depth of anesthesia, as assessed by the bispectral index, related to postoperative cognitive dysfunction and recovery? *Anesth Analg.* 2006;103:633–640.
72. Ballard C, Jones E, Gauge N, et al. Optimised anaesthesia to reduce postoperative cognitive decline (POCD) in older patients undergoing elective surgery, a randomised controlled trial. *PLoS One.* 2012;7(6):e37410.
73. Schoen J, Husemann L, Tiemeyer C, et al. Cognitive function after sevoflurane- vs propofol-based anaesthesia for on-pump cardiac surgery: a randomized controlled trial. *Br J Anaesth.* 2011;106(6):840–850.
74. Royse CF, Andrews DT, Newman SN, et al. The influence of propofol or desflurane on postoperative cognitive dysfunction in patients undergoing coronary artery bypass surgery. *Anaesthesia.* 2011;66:455–464.

75. Sanguineti VA, Wild JR, Fain MJ. Management of postoperative complications: general approach. *Clin Geriatr Med.* 2014;30(2):261–270.
76. Juliebo V, Bjoro K, Krogseth M, Skovlund E, Ranhoff AH, Wyller TB. Risk factors for preoperative and postoperative delirium in elderly patients with hip fracture. *J Am Geriatr Soc.* 2009;57(8):1354–1361.
77. Wang Y, Sands LP, Vaurio L, Mullen EA, Leung JM. The effects of postoperative pain and its management on postoperative cognitive dysfunction. *Am J Geriatr Psychiatry.* 2007;15(1):50–59.
78. Wang W, Wang Y, Wu H, et al. Postoperative cognitive dysfunction: current developments in mechanism and prevention. *Med Sci Monit.* 2014;20:1908–1912.
79. Milisen K, Foreman MD, Wouters B, et al. Documentation of delirium in the nursing and medical records of elderly hip fracture patients. *J Gerontol Nurs.* 2002;28:23–29.
80. Vanderweyde T, Bednar MM, Forman SA, Wolozin B. Iatrogenic risk factors for Alzheimer's disease: surgery and anesthesia. *J Alzheimers Dis.* 2010;22(3):91–104.
81. McKhann GM, Knopman DS, Chertkow H, et al. The diagnosis of dementia due to Alzheimer's disease: recommendations from the National Institute on Aging-Alzheimer's Association workgroups on diagnostic guidelines for Alzheimer's disease. *Alzheimers Dement.* 2011;7(3):263–269.
82. Dubois B, Feldman HH, Jacova C, et al. Advancing research diagnostic criteria for Alzheimer's disease: the IWG-2 criteria. *Lancet Neurol.* 2014;13(6):614–629.
83. Hardy JA, Higgins GA. Alzheimer's disease: the amyloid cascade hypothesis. *Science.* 1992;256(5054):184–185.
84. Jack Jr CR, Knopman DS, Jagust WJ, et al. Hypothetical model of dynamic biomarkers of the Alzheimer's pathological cascade. *Lancet Neurol.* 2010;9(1):119–128.
85. Sperling RA, Aisen PS, Beckett LA, et al. Toward defining the preclinical stages of Alzheimer's disease: recommendations from the National Institute on Aging-Alzheimer's Association workgroups on diagnostic guidelines for Alzheimer's disease. *Alzheimers Dement.* 2011;7(3):280–292.
86. Bateman RJ, Xiong C, Benzinger TL, et al. Clinical and biomarker changes in dominantly inherited Alzheimer's disease. *N Engl J Med.* 2012;367(9):795–804.
87. Knopman DS, Parisi JE, Salviati A, et al. Neuropathology of cognitively normal elderly. *J Neuropathol Exp Neurol.* 2003;62(11):1087–1095.
88. Savva GM, Wharton SB, Ince PG, Forster G, Matthews FE, Brayne C. Age, neuropathology, and dementia. *N Engl J Med.* 2009;360(22):2302–2309.
89. Fagan AM, Mintun MA, Mach RH, et al. Inverse relation between in vivo amyloid imaging load and cerebrospinal fluid Abeta42 in humans. *Ann Neurol.* 2006;59(3):512–519.
90. Aizenstein HJ, Nebes RD, Saxton JA, et al. Frequent amyloid deposition without significant cognitive impairment among the elderly. *Arch Neurol.* 2008;65(11):1509–1517.
91. Clark CM, Xie S, Chittams J, et al. Cerebrospinal fluid tau and beta-amyloid: how well do these biomarkers reflect autopsy-confirmed dementia diagnoses? *Arch Neurol.* 2003;60(12):1696–1702.
92. Green AJ, Harvey RJ, Thompson EJ, Rossor MN. Increased tau in the cerebrospinal fluid of patients with frontotemporal dementia and Alzheimer's disease. *Neurosci Lett.* 1999;259(2):133–135.
93. Maddalena A, Papassotiropoulos A, Müller-Tillmanns B, et al. Biochemical diagnosis of Alzheimer disease by measuring the cerebrospinal fluid ratio of phosphorylated tau protein to beta-amyloid peptide42. *Arch Neurol.* 2003;60(9):1202–1206.
94. van Harten AE, Scheeren TW, Absalom AR. A review of postoperative cognitive dysfunction and neuroinflammation associated with cardiac surgery and anaesthesia. *Anaesthesia.* 2012;67(3):280–293.
95. Chen PL, Yang CW, Tseng YK, et al. Risk of dementia after anaesthesia and surgery. *Br J Psychiatry.* 2014;204(3):188–193.

96. Lee TA, Wolozin B, Weiss KB, Bednar MM. Assessment of the emergence of Alzheimer's disease following coronary artery bypass graft surgery or percutaneous transluminal coronary angioplasty. *J Alzheimers Dis*. 2005;7(4):319–324.
97. Bohnen N, Warner MA, Kokmen E, Kurland LT. Early and midlife exposure to anesthesia and age of onset of Alzheimer's disease. *Int J Neurosci*. 1994;77:181–185.
98. Seitz DP, Shah PS, Herrmann N, Beyene J, Siddiqui N. Exposure to general anesthesia and risk of Alzheimer's disease: a systematic review and meta-analysis. *BMC Geriatr*. 2011;11(1):83.
99. Sprung J1, Jankowski CJ, Roberts RO, et al. Anesthesia and incident dementia: a population-based, nested, case-control study. *Mayo Clin Proc*. 2013;88(6):552–561.
100. Culley DJ, Baxter M, Yukhananov R, Crosby G. The memory effects of general anesthesia persist for weeks in young and aged rats. *Anesth Analg*. 2003;96:1004–1009.
101. Culley DJ, Baxter MG, Yukhananov R, Crosby G. Long-term impairment of acquisition of a spatial memory task following isoflurane-nitrous oxide anesthesia in rats. *Anesthesiology*. 2004;100:309–314.
102. Xie Z, Culley DJ, Dong Y, et al. The common inhalation anesthetic isoflurane induces caspase activation and increases amyloid beta-protein level in vivo. *Ann Neurol*. 2008;64:618–627.
103. Whittington RA, Virág L, Marcouiller F, et al. Propofol directly increases tau phosphorylation. *PLoS One*. 2011;6(1):e16648.
104. Ma J, Shen B, Stewart LS, Herrick IA, Leung LS. The septohippocampal system participates in general anesthesia. *J Neurosci*. 2002;22(2):RC200.
105. Cibelli M, Fidalgo AR, Terrando N, et al. Role of interleukin-1beta in postoperative cognitive dysfunction. *Ann Neurol*. 2010;68(3):360–368.
106. Palotás A, Reis HJ, Bogáts G, et al. Coronary artery bypass surgery provokes Alzheimer's disease-like changes in the cerebrospinal fluid. *J Alzheimers Dis*. 2010;21(4):1153–1164.
107. Tang JX, Baranov D, Hammond M, Shaw LM, Eckenhoff MF, Eckenhoff RG. Human Alzheimer and inflammation biomarkers after anesthesia and surgery. *Anesthesiology*. 2011;115(4):727–732.
108. Baranov D, Bickler PE, Crosby GJ, Culley DJ, Eckenhoff MF, Eckenhoff RG. Consensus statement: first international Workshop on anesthetics and Alzheimer's disease. *Anesth Analg*. 2009;108(5):1627–1630.
109. Peretz C, Alexander BH, Nagahama SI, Domino KB, Checkoway H. Parkinson's disease mortality among male anesthesiologists and internists. *Mov Disord*. 2005;20:1614–1617.
110. Nilsson FM. Mini Mental State Examination (MMSE)—Probably one of the most cited papers in health science. *Acta Psychiatr Scand*. 2007;2007(116):156–157.
111. Mitchell AJ. A meta-analysis of the accuracy of the Mini-Mental State Examination in the detection of dementia and mild cognitive impairment. *J Psychiatr Res*. 2009;43:411–431.

Trigeminocardiac Reflex

Hemanshu Prabhakar[1], Bernhard J. Schaller[2]

[1]Department of Neuroanaesthesiology and Critical Care, All India Institute of Medical Sciences, New Delhi, India; [2]University of Southampton, Southampton, UK

DEFINITION

The trigeminocardiac reflex (TCR) is a reproducible brain stem reflex originating as a result of stimulation of the trigeminal nerve (anywhere along its course) and manifests as a sudden development of cardiac dysrhythmia up to asystole, arterial hypotension, apnea, and gastric hypomotility.[1] However, under general anesthesia, the classically described symptoms may not be appreciated, other than cardiac dysrhythmia and arterial hypotension. It is then defined by reduction in the mean arterial pressure and the heart rate by more than 20% of its baseline values coinciding with the stimulation of the trigeminal nerve.

First described as the Kratschmer's reflex in cats and rabbits,[2] this reflex is now being increasingly studied. This intraoperative phenomenon not only occurs during neurosurgical procedures but also during maxillofacial,[3] ophthalmic,[4] nasal,[5] dental,[6] and skull-base surgeries.[7] Interestingly, the reflex can be elicited by stimulation of any of the three divisions of the fifth cranial nerve, that is, ophthalmic, maxillary, or mandibular nerves.

PATHOPHYSIOLOGY

The physiological mechanism of the TCR is that following stimulation of the sensory nerve endings of the trigeminal nerve, signals are sent to the sensory nucleus of the trigeminal nerve via the Gasserion ganglion. This afferent pathway continues along the short internuncial nerve fibers in the reticular formation to connect with the efferent pathway in the motor nucleus of the vagus nerve. Depressor fibers of the vagus nerve end in the myocardium, leading to autonomic changes (Figure 1).[8,9]

The Flowchart Below Explains the Pathway

Sensory nerve endings of trigeminal nerve→Gasserian ganglion→ Trigeminal nerve→Superficial medullary dorsal horn and sensory nucleus of trigeminal nerve→via short internuncial neurons to vagal motor nucleus →vagus nerve→depressor fibers from vagus ending in myocardium.

It is suggested that the parasympathetically mediated bradycardia, sympathetically-mediated vasoconstriction, and the central inhibition of the respiratory rhythm (apnea) must be modulated by the trigeminal

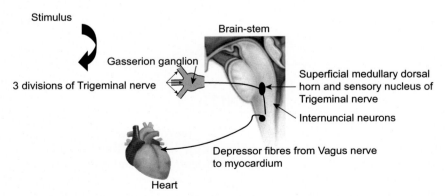

FIGURE 1   Schematic diagram showing the mechanism of the trigeminocardiac reflex.

system within the brainstem.[1] It must be remembered that the autonomic nervous system activation is central to the occurrence of TCR.[1] It is suggested that the coactivation of the sympathetic and parasympathetic systems may be involved in the occurrence of the TCR.[9] It is known that the autonomic influences on heart are generally weak. Parasympathetic fibers primarily innervate the atria and the conducting tissues, whereas sympathetic fibers are more widely distributed throughout the heart. Therefore, vagal effects frequently have a rapid onset and resolution; whereas, sympathetic influences generally have a gradual onset and dissipation. It has been suggested that myelination status of the nerve may not be an important risk factor and phenotypic heterogeneity could be the basis of susceptibility for simultaneous autonomic nerve activation.[9]

VARIANTS

The occurrence of the TCR may either be due to (1) peripheral or (2) central stimulation of the fifth nerve.[10,11] Stimulation of the trigeminal nerve or any of its branches anywhere along the course of its distribution can elicit the TCR.

Meng and colleagues[12] suggest that during percutaneous radiofrequency thermocoagulation, a pressor response is found rather than a depressor. In our center also, we often encounter pressor responses during Gasserion ganglion rhizolysis or thermocoagulation. It is suggested that the TCR triggered by peripheral stimulation via spinal nucleus of the trigeminal nerve to the Kolliker–Fuse nucleus is different from the TCR triggered by central stimulation via nucleus of solitary tract to the lateral parabrachial nucleus.[13]

CAUSE

Any surgical procedure in and around the area of distribution of the trigeminal nerve can produce the TCR. Some of the surgeries where this response has been observed are ophthalmic surgery,[4] craniofacial surgery,[3] skull-base surgery,[7] dental surgery,[3] trigeminal rhizolysis,[14] and any other procedure on the head.

SIGNS AND SYMPTOMS

As mentioned in the earlier section, the classical features for the diagnosis of the TCR include:

1. Bradycardia
2. Arterial hypotension
3. Apnea
4. Gastric hypermotility

A nonspecific feature may include the electrocardiographic changes such as T wave inversion, and shortening of the QT interval[9,15] that follow the occurrence of the TCR.

DIAGNOSIS

The occurrence of this reflex may easily be diagnosed based on its classical features and the hemodynamic values, such as a drop of more than 20% to the base rate both of the mean arterial pressure and of the heart rate.

However, it must be noted that events of TCR may occur without warning signals[10]. Sudden intense stimulation of the central part of the fifth cranial nerve may produce asystole without warning signs of bradycardia or hypotension[10]. Similar findings have also been reported by Schaller and colleagues[16] in their retrospective study of patients undergoing cerebellopontine surgery.

PREDISPOSING FACTORS

Various predisposing factors have been postulated as predisposing patients to the TCR. These factors include hypercapnea, hypoxemia, light plane of anesthesia, children (with high resting vagal tone), narcotics such as alfentanyl and sufentanil, preoperative use of beta-blockers and calcium channel blockers, and acidosis.[1] Some of the intraoperative factors such as light plane of anesthesia, hypercarbia, hypoxia, and acidosis should be promptly corrected as the potentiate TCR.[1]

TREATMENT

One of the first steps following the occurrence of the TCR is to inform the surgeon. Cessation of stimulus immediately reverses the phenomenon. Administration of anticholinergics such as atropine or glycopyrrolate may be required in some cases where bradycardia is severe or persists despite cessation of the stimulus. Preemptive administration of atropine or glycopyrrolate for the prevention of the TCR may be ineffective as demonstrated by some authors.[11,14] It has been observed that atropine blocks cholinergic fibers but does not totally prevent either bradycardia or hypotension in animals possibly because their trigeminal depressor response includes both activation of vagal cardioinhibitory fibers and inhibition of adrenergic vasoconstriction after electrical stimulation of the spinal trigeminal tract and trigeminal nuclear complex.[17] In most cases, the patient responds to the above treatment. However, at times, the TCR may be refractory to the conventional methods of treatment. In such cases, use of vasopressors such as epinephrine and other immediate cardiac life support may be required.[18]

A prophylactic measure for prevention of the TCR has been suggested with local anesthetic infiltration or block of the nerve/nerves which convey afferent stimulus.[19]

Considering the fact that TCR may occur without prior signals, the vigilant role of the anesthetist and knowledge of TCR cannot be over emphasized.

CLINICAL RELEVANCE

As the TCR may occur without prior hemodynamic changes,[10] it is important to identify warning signs that may precede the TCR. At the same time, it is also essential to understand the clinical outcome of such a response. The results of a prospective study suggest that serum biomarkers on ischemia may be useful as surrogate markers to prevent occurrence of TCR.[20] The role of electrophysiological monitoring during the TCR has also been suggested by Gharabaghi et al.[21] Their preliminary results indicate that intraoperative monitoring of auditory evoked potential changes related to the TCR predict postoperative hearing function and serve as a valuable prognostic tool. Further studies may, however, be needed to evaluate the possible role of electrophysiological monitoring in detection and prevention of the TCR, but it underlines that the intraoperative occurrence of the TCR can have substantial impact on the postoperative functional outcome. In their work on the TCR, on the other hand, Schaller and colleagues have suggested that the TCR may be an "oxygen-conserving reflex".[1] Therefore, especially the duration of bradycardia and hypotonia might be an important on which of both sides the pendulum strikes.

It is generally believed that appropriate detection and management of the TCR depends upon the tumor characteristics, surgical maneuver, and changes in auditory evoked potentials which in turn will lead to successful clinical application of this entity.[21] There is another school of thought where the possible role of serum biomarkers in the occurrence of the TCR is being considered by the investigators. Schaller and colleagues[22] believe that serum biomarkers for ischemia may be useful as surrogate markers to prevent the occurrence of the TCR. The same authors also suggest that radiological indicators of potential anoxic cerebral damage may also be of clinical importance.[22]

With the present knowledge on the TCR, we can say that as patient characteristics do not influence the occurrence of this reflex, one should anticipate the consequences of TCR in all patients undergoing surgeries on the head.

References

1. Schaller B, Cornellius JF, Prabhakar H, et al. The trigeminocardiac reflex: an update of the current knowledge. *J Neurosurg Anesthesiol*. 2009;21:187–195.
2. Kratschmer F. Uber Reflexe von der Nasenschleimhaut auf Athmung und Kreislauf. [about reflexes of the nasal mucosa on breathing and circulation] *Sher Akad Wis Wien*. 1870;62:147–170.
3. Bohluli B, Bayat M, Sarkarat F, Moradi B, Tabrizi MH, Sadr-Eshkevari P. Trigeminocardiac reflex during Le Fort I osteotomy: a case-crossover study. *Oral Surg Oral Med Oral Pathol Oral Radiol Endod*. 2010;110:178–181.
4. Simon JW. Complications of strabismus surgery. *Curr Opin Ophthalmol*. 2010;21:361–366.
5. Yorgancilar E, Gun R, Yildirim M, Bakir S, Akkus Z, Topcu I. Determination of trigeminocardiac reflex during rhinoplasty. *Int J Oral Maxillofac Surg*. 2012;41:389–393.
6. Arakeri G, Arali V. A new hypothesis of cause of syncope: trigeminocardiac reflex during extraction of teeth. *Med Hypotheses*. 2010;74:248–251.
7. Koerbel A, Gharabaghi A, Samii A, et al. Trigeminocardiac reflex during skull base surgery: mechanism and management. *Acta Neurochir (Wien)*. 2005;147:727–732.
8. Lang S, Lanigan DT, van der Wal M. Trigeminocardiac reflexes: maxillary and mandibular variants of the oculocardiac reflex. *Can J Anaesth*. 1991;38:757–760.
9. Khurana H, Dewan P, Ali Z, Prabhakar H. Electrocardiaographic changes due to vagosympathetic coactivation during the trigeminocardiac reflex. *J Neurosurg Anesthesiol*. 2009;21:270.
10. Prabhakar H, Anand N, Chouhan RS, Bithal PK. Sudden asystole during surgery in the cerebellopontine angle. *Acta Neurochir (Wien)*. 2006;148:699–700.
11. Prabhakar H, Rath GP, Arora R. Sudden cardiac standstill during skin flap elevation in a patient undergoing craniotomy. *J Neurosurg Anesthesiol*. 2007;19:203–204.
12. Meng Q, Zhang W, Yang Y, Zhou M, Li X. Cardiovascular responses during percutaneous radiofrequency thermocoagulation therapy in primary trigeminal neuralgia. *J Neurosurg Anesthesiol*. 2008;20:131–135.
13. Schaller B, Sandu N, Filis A, Buchfelder M. Cardiovascular responses during percutaneous radiofrequency thermocoagulation therapy in primary trigeminal neuralgia: an explanation of the trigeminocardiac reflex? *J Neurosurg Anesthesiol*. 2008;20:270.
14. Rath GP, Dash HH, Prabhakar H, Pandia MP. Cardiorespiratory arrest during trigeminal rhizolysis. *Anaesthesia*. 2007;62:971–972.
15. Schaller BJ, Filis A, Buchfelder M. Trigemino-cardiac reflex in humans initiated by peripheral stimulation during neurosurgical skull-base operations. Its first description. *Acta Neurochir (Wien)*. 2008;150:715–718.
16. Schaller B, Probst R, Strebel S, Gratzl O. Trigeminocardiac reflex during surgery in the cerebellopontine angle. *J Neurosurg*. 1999;90:215–220.
17. Kumada M, Dampney RAL, Reis DJ. The trigeminal depressor response: a novel vasodepressor response originating from the trigeminal system. *Brain Res*. 1977;119:305–326.
18. Prabhakar H, Ali Z, Rath GP. Trigemino-cardiac reflex may be refractory to conventional management in adults. *Acta Neurochir (Wien)*. 2008;150:509–510.
19. Blanc VF. Trigeminocardiac relexes (editorial). *Can J Anaesth*. 1991;38:696–699.
20. Filis A, Schaller B, Buchfelder M. Trigemino-cardiac reflex in pituitary surgery. A prospective pilot study. *Nervenarzt*. 2008;79:669–675.
21. Gharabaghi A, Acioly MA, Koerbel A, Tatagiba M. Prognostic factors for hearing loss following the trigeminocardiac reflex. *Acta Neurochir (Wien)*. 2007;149:737–738.
22. Schaller BJ, Filis A, Buchfelder M. Detection and prevention of the trigeminocardiac reflex during skull base surgery. *Acta Neurochir (Wien)*. 2007;149:331.

CHAPTER

43

Venous Air Embolism

Hemanshu Prabhakar, Parmod K. Bithal

Department of Neuroanaesthesiology and Critical Care, All India Institute
of Medical Sciences, New Delhi, India

OUTLINE

DEFINITION

Venous air embolism (VAE) is defined as entrainment of air in the venous circulation during any surgical procedure that may produce systemic effects.

Historically, VAE was reported as early as 1667 when death was reported in animals following air entrainment into the veins. It was not until 1846 that the term "embolism" was coined by Virchow.[1] As knowledge of VAE became evident, more authors reported this complication during clinical

© 2016 Elsevier Inc. All rights reserved.

practice. The reported incidence of VAE in literature ranges from 25% to 60%. However, with advanced monitoring systems such as transesophageal echocardiography and intracardiac transvenous echocardiography, incidence may be higher.[2]

VAE can occur during any surgical procedure but is observed commonly in neurosurgical practice. Laparoscopies for gastrointestinal surgeries, urology, gynecological, ophthalmic, cardiac, thoracic, and orthopedic procedures, carry a risk of VAE. However, it is the neurosurgical procedures that report maximally the occurrence of VAE. Some of the common neurosurgeries that carry a high incidence of VAE include posterior fossa surgery, craniosynostosis, surgery performed in the sitting position, spine surgeries, and peripheral nerve repairs.[3] There have been reports that even application and removal of skull pins may also cause VAE[4]. Other than occurring during the intraoperative period, VAE may also occur during "awake" procedures such deep brain stimulation.[5]

Many centers routinely use hydrogen peroxide at the end of neurosurgical procedures to act as hemostatic and for debridement. Reports are now available showing that hydrogen peroxide, per se, may produce oxygen embolism which could be dangerous.[6] Interestingly, there are studies that show that during surgery, the greatest chance of VAE occurs during manipulation or dissection of the muscles.[7]

VARIANT

Paradoxical air embolism (PAE) may be considered a variant of VAE which occurs due to right to left shunting at the atrial level as in case of patent foramen ovale (PFO) and in the presence of arteriovenous malformations. The air then enters the cerebral circulation to produce neurological signs and symptoms. The air may enter the coronary circulation producing cardiac arrhythmias and/or cardiac ischemia.

As the reported incidence of PFO is 20–30%, the calculated risk of PAE is 5–10%.[1] An echocardiography during the Valsalva maneuver is useful in detecting PFO.[8] A systematic review by Fathi and colleagues[9] suggests that the rate of clinical and transesophageal detected PAE is reported between 0% and 14%.

PATHOPHYSIOLOGY

It is considered that whenever a sufficient gradient exists between the right atrium and the upper area of incision or point of entrance of air, there occurs a possibility of venous air embolism. However, the sequelae of VAE depend on the rate and volume of air absorbed. This in turn depends on the size of the vessel and the pressure gradient. As well as resulting in mechanical occlusion of vessels, VAE has been shown to produce changes in the pulmonary vasculature as a result of hypoxia and sympathetic stimulation. This leads to increased microvascular permeability, release of endothelin 1, platelet aggregation, and release of toxic free radicals result in development of systemic inflammatory response and pulmonary edema.[1] Cerebral and myocardial ischemia may ensue later. Electrocardiographic changes, arrhythmias and cardiovascular collapse may be observed in extreme situations. It has been suggested that during VAE-induced hypotension, sympathetic activation through baroreceptors may be depressed by vagal afferents originating from cardiopulmonary receptors.[10] Another physiological change noted as a result of VAE is platelet dysfunction leading to thrombocytopenia.[11] There are also reports of development of pulmonary edema secondary to VAE that could be considered severe pulmonary sequelae of VAE.[12]

SIGNS AND SYMPTOMS

The various signs and symptoms resulting from VAE may be related to the respiratory, cardiovascular, and central nervous systems. They are as follows:

1. Gasping respiration, in awake patients. Acute dyspnea, tachypnea, coughing, breathlessness, light headedness, and wheezing;
2. Increased central venous pressure and pulmonary airway pressure;
3. Arrhythmias;
4. Electrocardiogram (ECG) changes: ST–T changes;
5. Hypotension;
6. Abnormal heart sounds;
7. Tachycardia or bradycardia;
8. Decreased peripheral resistance;
9. Change in cardiac output;
10. Cyanosis;
11. Jugular venous distention;
12. May proceed to shock if hypotension persists;
13. Altered sensorium;
14. Cerebral edema and hyperemia resulting in coma.

The threshold for detection of some physiological responses in animal studies after injection of air are tabulated (Table 1).

TABLE 1   Threshold for Detection of Various
Physiological Responses after Injection of Air in Animals

Physiological responses	Volume of air (mL/kg/min)
1. Initial gasp	0.36
2. Central venous pressure	0.4
3. Pulmonary artery pressure	0.42
4. Heart rate	0.42
5. Peripheral resistance	0.52
6. Cardiac output	0.52
7. ECG changes	0.6
8. Blood pressure	0.69
9. First change in heart sounds	1.7

FACTORS AFFECTING VAE

Following factors contribute to the occurrence of VAE.

1. Position of body: there is an increased chance of air embolism in the sitting position compared with horizontal (supine, prone, or lateral positions).
2. Depth of ventilation.
3. Volume of air entering: a larger volume of air of approximately 5 mL/kg may produce and air-lock in the right ventricle outlet and cause sudden cardiovascular collapse.
4. Rate of air entry: it has been suggested that a pressure reduction of 5 cm H_2O across a 14G cannula can transmit approximately 100 mL of air per second.[13]
5. Central venous pressure: hypovolemia is a predisposing factor for the occurrence of VAE and PAE.[14]

DIAGNOSIS

In earlier days, VAE was often diagnosed clinically following aspiration of air from the central venous catheters or intraoperative hemodynamic instability. With advanced monitoring devices, detection and management of VAE has become simple. The various monitors that are used in clinical practice are mentioned below[15]:

1. Precordial Doppler: most sensitive, noninvasive, and nonquantitative. Its placement on the left parasternal area is as

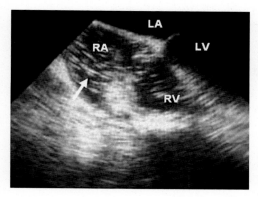

FIGURE 1 Intraoperative transesophageal echocardiography showing venous air embolism in the right atrium (bold white arrow). Abbreviations: RA, right atrium; RV, right ventricle; LA, left atrium; LV, left ventricle.

sensitive to clinical venous air embolism as right parasternal placement.[16] However, intravenous mannitol administration mimics venous air embolism as detected by Doppler.

2. Transesophageal Doppler: overcomes chest configuration problems faced with precordial Doppler.
3. End-tidal carbon dioxide (a sudden decrease of >2–5 mmHg): convenient, sensitive, noninvasive, semiquantitative, and nonspecific, to be judged cautiously during systemic hypotension.
4. End-tidal nitrogen: specific for air, changes occur 30–90 s earlier than end-tidal carbon dioxide.[17] The presence of a leak in the circuit or cuff gives a false positive diagnosis. Moreover, it is no longer manufactured now and is of historical importance only.
5. Pulmonary artery catheter/pressure: insensitive, detects pulmonary artery hypertension caused by the mechanical obstruction and reflex vasoconstriction from local hypoxemia due to air embolus. It is invasive.
6. Transesophageal echocardiography: most sensitive, invasive, nonquantitative (Figure 1). It is also an expensive piece of equipment.
7. Central venous pressure: increases during VAE.
8. Central venous catheter: air aspirated from the catheter placed in the right atrium is confirmatory of VAE.
9. Electrocardiogram: changes such as bradycardia, premature ventricular contractions, ST–T wave depression, variable P waves, and heart blocks.
10. Airway pressure: airway constriction following VAE results in decreased ventilatory compliance.
11. Arterial blood pressure: a systemic arterial hypotension is one of the late signs of VAE.
12. Transcranial Doppler: highly sensitive (sensitivity: 91.3%; specificity: 93.8%; accuracy: 92.8%). A contrast-enhanced transcranial Doppler has been shown to be highly sensitive and specific for detection of patent foramen ovale compared with contrast-enhanced transesophageal echocardiography.[18]

TABLE 2   Threshold for Air Detected by Various Monitors

Monitors	Volume of air detected (mL/kg)
1. Transesophageal echocardiography	0.01–0.19
2. Precordial Doppler	0.02–0.24
3. End-tidal carbon dioxide	0.5
4. Pulmonary artery catheter	0.25
5. Pulse oximetry	0.7–1.5
6. Esophageal stethoscope	0.75
7. Arterial blood pressure	>1.0
8. "Mill wheel" murmur	>2.0

The threshold for detection of air by some of these monitors is tabulated (Table 2).

There are other monitoring methods also such as the Doppler monitoring of carotids and middle cerebral arteries and the Bispectral Index and Spectral Entropy.[1,19] It has been shown that air in the jugular veins can be detected using Doppler monitoring. Similarly VAE may lead to changes in the Bispectral Index values, if other causes have been ruled out.[1]

TREATMENT

The steps to be followed in the event of occurrence of VAE are as follows:

1. Early detection.
2. Inform the surgeon.
3. Irrigate surgical field with saline.
4. Rapid aspiration from the central line.
5. Discontinue nitrous oxide (if being administered), deliver 100% oxygen.
6. Vasopressors if required to maintain hemodynamics.
7. Change of position, if seated or prone; Durant's maneuver—partial left lateral position with head low.
8. Compression of jugular veins.
9. Hyperbaric oxygen therapy has also shown promising results, especially in cases of cerebral arterial gas embolism.
10. The possible role of perfluorocarbons in reabsorption of air embolus has also been studied. However, this modality remains experimental so far.[20]

PREVENTION

1. Adequate patient positioning. Avoid positions that elevate surgical site above the level of heart, as far as possible.
2. Central venous catheters should be placed in all surgeries where one in anticipating VAE.
3. Maintain a good hydration of the patient.
4. Application of positive end expiratory pressure (PEEP) remains controversial.[21,22] It has also been demonstrated that levels of PEEP up to 10 cm H_2O do not alter the interatrial pressure difference.[23]
5. Military antishock trouser in children.
6. Use of compression stockings.

References

1. Smith DS. Anesthetic management for posterior fossa surgery. In: Cottrell JE, Young WL, eds. *Neuroanesthesia*. 5th ed. Mosby Elsevier; 2010:203–217.
2. Schafer ST, Lindemann J, Brendt P, Kaiser G, Peters J. Intracardiac transvenous echocardiography is superior to both precordial Doppler and transesophageal echocardiography techniques for detecting venous air embolism and catheter-guided air aspiration. *Anesth Analg*. 2008;106:45–54.
3. Mirski MA, Lele AV, Fitsimmons L, Young TJK. Diagnosis and treatment of vascular air embolism. *Anesthesiology*. 2007;106:164–177.
4. Prabhakar H, Ali Z, Bhagat H. Venous air embolism arising after removal of Mayfield skull clamp. *J Neurosurg Anesthesiol*. 2008;20:158–159.
5. Deogaonkar A, Avitsian R, Henderson JM, Schubert A. Venous air embolism during deep brain stimulation surgery in an awake supine patient. *Stereotact Funct Neurosurg*. 2005;83:32–35.
6. Prabhakar H, Rath GP. Venous oxygen embolism with use of hydrogen peroxide during craniotomy in supine position. *J Clin Neurosci*. 2008;15:1072.
7. Bithal PK, Pandia MP, Dash HH, Chouhan RS, Mohanty B, Padhy N. Comparative incidence of venous air embolism and associated hypotension in adults and children operated for neurosurgery in the sitting position. *Eur J Anaesthesiol*. 2004;21:517–522.
8. Black S, Muzzi DA, Nishimura RA, Cucchiara RF. Preoperative and intraoperative echocardiography to detect right-to-left shunt in patients undergoing neurosurgical procedures in sitting position. *Anesthesiology*. 1990;72:436–438.
9. Fathi AR, Eshterhardi P, Meier B. Patent foramen ovale and neurosurgery in sitting position: a systematic review. *Br J Anaesth*. 2009;102:588–596.
10. Abiki M, Ogura S, Seki K, et al. Role of vagal afferents in hypotension induced by venous air embolism. *Am J Physiol*. 1994;266:R790–795.
11. Schafer ST, Sandalcioglu IE, Stegen B, Neumann A, Asgari S, Peters J. Venous air embolism during semi-sitting craniotomy evokes thrombocytopenia. *Anaesthesia*. 2011;66:25–30.
12. Arora R, Chablani D, Rath GP, Prabhakar H. Pulmonary oedema following venous air embolism during transsphenoidal pituitary surgery. *Acta Neurochir (Wien)*. 2007;149: 1177–1178.
13. Flanagan JP, Gradisar IA, Gross RJ, Kelly TR. Air embolus: a lethal complication of subclavian venipuncture. *N Engl J Med*. 1969;281:488–489.
14. Pfitzner J, McLean AG. Venous air embolism and active lung inflation at high and low CVP: a study in upright anaesthetized sheep. *Anesth Analg*. 1987;66:1127–1134.

15. Albin MS. Air embolism. In: Albin MS, ed. *Textbook of Neuroanesthesia with Neurosurgical and Neuroscience Perspectives*. The McGraw Hill Companies Inc.; 1997:1009–1025.
16. Schubert A, Deogaonkar A, Drummond JC. Precordial Doppler probe placement for optimal detection of venous air embolism during craniotomy. *Anesth Analg.* 2006;102:1543–1547.
17. Matjasko J, Petrozza P, Mackenzie CF. Sensitivity of end-tidal nitrogen in venous air embolism detection in dogs. *Anesthesiology.* 1985;63:418–423.
18. Stendel R, Gramm HJ, Schroder K, Lober C, Brock M. Transcranial Doppler ultrasonography as a screening technique for detection of a patent foramen ovale before surgery in the sitting position. *Anesthesiology.* 2000;93:971–975.
19. Chazot T, Liu N, Tremelot L, Joukovsky P, Fischler M. Detection of gas embolism by bispectral index and entropy monitoring in two cases. *Anesthesiology.* 2004;101:1053–1054.
20. Eckmann DM, Lomivorotov VN. Microvascular gas embolization clearance following perfluorocarbon administration. *J Appl Physiol.* 2003;94:860–868.
21. Meyer PG, Cuttaree H, Charron B, Jarreau MM, Peri AC, Sainte-Rose C. Prevention of venous air embolism in paediatric neurosurgical procedures performed in the sitting position by combined use of MAST suit and PEEP. *Br J Anaesth.* 1994;73:795–800.
22. Schmitt HJ, Hemmerling TM. Venous air emboli occur during release of positive end-expiratory pressure and repositioning after sitting position surgery. *Anesth Analg.* 2002;94:400–403.
23. Zasslow MA, Pearl RG, Larson CP, Silverberg G, Shuer LF. PEEP does not affect left atrial–right atrial pressure difference in neurosurgical patients. *Anesthesiology.* 1988;68:760–763.

CLINICAL SCENARIOS

Clinical Scenario 1

Hemanshu Prabhakar

Department of Neuroanaesthesiology and Critical Care, All India Institute
of Medical Sciences, New Delhi, India

A 24-year-old male, weighing 70 kg, was admitted to the hospital with complaints of severe occipital headache and vomiting over the past four days. He had a progressive decrease in vision in both eyes over the past 15 days. His past medical and surgical history was unremarkable. He was conscious with normal motor and sensory examination of the central nervous system. All routine investigations were found to be within the normal range. Noncontrast computed tomography (NCCT) of the head revealed a gross hydrocephalus with obstruction at the level of the fourth ventricle. Magnetic resonance imaging (MRI) scan revealed a fourth ventricular space–occupying lesion, causing hydrocephalus.

The patient was scheduled for midline suboccipital craniectomy and tumor excision in the sitting position. The patient was positioned in the sitting position after induction of general anesthesia and placement of the flexometallic tube size 8.5. General measures for the sitting position were taken, such as appropriate neck flexion, keeping a two-finger gap between the chin and the sternum, proper padding of the pressure points, and proper support of both the upper and lower limbs.

Intraoperative, there were transient episodes of hypotension following blood loss, which were managed with adequate fluid and blood replacement. The surgery lasted 7 h, and the patient was shifted to the intensive care unit for mechanical ventilator support and further management. On spontaneous recovery from neuromuscular blockade, an examination revealed paraparesis while the sensorium remained intact. An NCCT of the head revealed mild brain stem edema along with an operative site cavity. Over the next few hours, he became quadriparetic. Methyl prednisone infusion was started. A T2-weighted MRI showed a hyperintense signal extending from C3 to D2 along with a mid expansion of the cord.

Over the next few days, the patient's strength in his upper limbs recovered to normal, but he remained paraplegic at the end of 3 months follow up.

Clinical Scenario 2

Hemanshu Prabhakar

Department of Neuroanaesthesiology and Critical Care, All India Institute
of Medical Sciences, New Delhi, India

A 38-year-old man, weighing 75 kg, was scheduled for a posterior fossa surgery in the sitting position. His past medical and surgical history was unremarkable. Besides routine intraoperative monitoring, a transesophageal echocardiographic (TEE) monitor probe (HDI-1500, ATL Ultrasound; Philips, Bothell, WA) was placed to obtain a four-chamber view. A Mayfield clamp was used to stabilize the head of the patient in a sitting position. The patient had an uneventful surgical and anesthetic course. At the end of surgery, the patient was positioned supine gradually, and skull pins were removed. Immediately after the Mayfield clamp was removed, the patient developed tachycardia as the heart rate increased from 94 beats per minute (bpm) to 170 bpm and systolic blood pressure decreased from 145 to 68 mmHg. At the same time, the end-tidal carbon dioxide ($EtCO_2$) dropped suddenly from 38 to 22 mmHg. The monitor of the TEE showed continuous air emboli entering the right atrium. It was then noticed that there was injury at one of the pin insertion sites. The surgeon immediately applied bone wax to the bony edges and sutured the scalp as air was being aspirated via the central venous catheter placed in the right subclavian vein. Nearly 20 mL of air could be aspirated before the patient showed signs of improvement. The $EtCO_2$ increased to 33 mmHg and the heart rate and systolic blood pressure settled to 101 bpm and 122 mmHg, respectively. No further air entrainment was visible on the TEE monitor. The trachea was extubated and the patient had an uneventful stay in the intensive care unit.

http://dx.doi.org/10.1016/B978-0-12-804075-1.00045-6

Clinical Scenario 3

Hemanshu Prabhakar

Department of Neuroanaesthesiology and Critical Care, All India Institute
of Medical Sciences, New Delhi, India

A 45-year-old male, weighing 52 kg and presenting with a diagnosed case of craniopharyngioma, was apparently well two months previously when he developed a progressive decrease in vision (right eye > left eye). He was unable to visualize on the lateral side. Upon examination, his right-side pupil was not reacting to light. There was no history of vomiting, headache, seizures, motor or sensory deficits, or difficulty in walking. His past medical and surgical history was unremarkable. Under general anesthesia, a craniotomy was performed for tumor excision. After an uneventful anesthetic and surgical course, he was shifted to the intensive care unit with a tracheal tube in situ. On the first postoperative day, his trachea was extubated as the postoperative computerized tomography scan was normal and all the extubation criteria were fulfilled. One week after surgery, his condition deteriorated and he became drowsy and lethargic. His urine output decreased to <500 mL per 24 h; however, his central venous pressure was 14 cmH$_2$O. His blood investigation showed severe dyselectrolytemia (Serum Na$^+$–117 meq/lt, Serum K$^+$–2.6 meq/lt). A 3% NaCl infusion at the rate of 30 mL/h along with KCl supplement was started to correct the electrolyte imbalance. The electrolyte levels improved gradually over a period of 1 day (Serum Na$^+$–122 meq/lt, Serum K$^+$–3.7 meq/lt) along with improvement in his sensorium and general condition.

Clinical Scenario 4

Hemanshu Prabhakar

Department of Neuroanaesthesiology and Critical Care, All India Institute
of Medical Sciences, New Delhi, India

A 25-year-old male who suffered from a road traffic accident was brought to the emergency department with facial abrasions and a history of loss of consciousness. Upon examination, he was conscious and oriented (Glasgow Coma Scale (GCS) results: eye response: 4; verbal response: 5; motor response: 6) with a pulse rate of 110/min, blood pressure (BP) rate of 130/70 mmHg, and a respiratory rate of 20/min. Respiratory, cardiovascular, and systemic examinations were normal. A computed tomography (CT) scan of the head revealed a mild frontal depressed fracture with extradural hematoma of 10 mm thickness. Chest X-ray revealed no abnormalities. Patient was admitted and kept under observation.

After 1 h, deterioration in the patient's conscious level was noted with GCS E3V5M5, anisocoria, and labored breathing with a respiratory rate of 36/min with oxygen saturation (SpO_2) 91% on oxygen supplementation. Respiratory system examination revealed bilateral equal air entry with fine crepitations in the basal lung areas. His BP recorded was now 80/50 mmHg. An emergency chest X-ray was ordered and an emergency ultrasound of the chest was performed. Ultrasonography revealed pleural sliding with increased B lines (>15 per field). Chest X-ray showed bilateral diffuse infiltrates. The emergency CT scan revealed an increase in the size of epidural hematoma (volume 35°cc^3). Immediately, the patient was shifted to the operation theater and anesthesia was induced with fentanyl 3 µg/kg, propofol 2 mg/kg, and vecuronium 0.1 mg/kg. Mechanical ventilation of lungs was started with tidal volume 10 mL/kg and respiratory rate 15 breaths per minute. The airway pressures were 27 cm H_2O. With 100% oxygen, the oxygen saturation remained 88%. Pink frothy sputum was observed in the tracheal tube. A positive end-expiratory pressure (PEEP) of 8 cm H_2O was applied and injection of morphine 7.5 mg with furosemide 40 mg BD started. Immediate surgical evacuation of extradural hematoma was performed and the patient shifted to neurointensive care unit (NICU) for further monitoring and management.

In the NICU, SpO_2 decreased to 85% with 100% oxygen. PEEP was increased to 12 cm H_2O and an intraventricular catheter was placed to monitor intracranial pressure and the effect of PEEP on intracranial dynamics. Morphine 7.5 mg thrice daily and furosemide 40 mg twice daily were continued. During the next 12 h, the patient's saturation improved and the fraction of inspired oxygen concentration (FiO_2) reduced to 40% with PEEP of 5 cm H_2O. Patient remained conscious with a full score of GCS. The chest X-ray cleared. Patient was tracheally extubated and shifted to the ward after 8 h.

Clinical Scenario 5

Hemanshu Prabhakar

Department of Neuroanaesthesiology and Critical Care, All India Institute
of Medical Sciences, New Delhi, India

A 32-year-old male patient, weighing 76 kg was admitted to the neu-rosurgical intensive care unit (ICU) with a history of quadriparesis following a road traffic accident. On further workup, he was found to have sustained a cervical cord injury at the C5–6 level. He was managed conservatively in the ICU for 3 weeks, and was transferred to the high dependency unit thereafter. On day 32 of his injury, a call was received by the neurointensivist as the patient was complaining of acute anxiety, severe pounding headache, heavy sweating and flushing of the skin over the face, neck, and shoulders, goose bumps, blurring of vision, stuffy nose, and a feeling of tightness in his chest. The patient was undergoing a physical therapy session when his symptoms developed. On physical examination, his room air saturation was 98%, heart rate was 62 beats per min, and blood pressure was 180/110 mmHg.

Suspecting an episode of autonomic dysreflexia, the patient's head was raised to 90° and all his clothing loosened. Immediate release nifedipine capsule 10 mg was given to the patient to bite and swallow, for acute management of the hypertension. Simultaneously, a search for the instigating cause of the dysreflexia was begun. The patient elicited a history of regular bowel habits. He had an indwelling catheter for urination, but complained that there was no urine output in the last 3–4 h. The catheter was closely examined to rule out any kinks or twists. Gentle bladder irrigation was then performed with 30 mL saline at room temperature. Following bladder irrigation, the urine output increased and around 250 mL urine was drained immediately. The patient's symptoms settled markedly following bladder emptying.

His heart rate and blood pressure were monitored every 5 min thereafter, for 2 h. The patient remained comfortable and his vitals were within normal limits. He was kept under close observation for around 4 h. Following this, the patient and the physical therapist were counselled regarding the symptoms of autonomic dysreflexia, and the prevention strategies to mitigate further episodes, if they occur.

Clinical Scenario 6

Hemanshu Prabhakar

Department of Neuroanaesthesiology and Critical Care, All India Institute
of Medical Sciences, New Delhi, India

A 40-year-old male, weighing 68 kg, with a history of injuries from a road traffic accident was brought to the emergency department in an unconscious state. He was tachypneic (respiratory rate 33 breaths per minute), with a heart rate (HR) at 100 beats/min, blood pressure (BP) at 160/100 mmHg, and with a maintained saturation of 80% on 100% oxygen. Air entry was grossly diminished on the right side of the chest. He was immediately intubated tracheally and an intercostal drain was placed. There was a gush of air, and soon, saturation improved. His Glasgow Coma Scale (GCS) was E2M3V3; a computed tomography (CT) head scan was done after initial stabilization. The CT scan revealed a large extradural hematoma with midline shift, and a decision for evacuation was taken. As he was being prepared for surgery, the ECG on the monitor started showing 4 mm ST segment changes. A 12-lead ECG was done, which revealed ST segment depression in leads V2–V4 with few ventricular ectopics, though his vitals remained stable with HR 90 beats/min, noninvasive BP 170/106 mmHg, and SpO$_2$ 98% on ventilator.

Troponin I was tested, which was negative. Arterial blood gas revealed no electrolyte abnormalities. Because the surgery was urgent, high-risk consent was taken and the patient was shifted to OT. Intraoperatively, ST depression was persistent in leads V1–V4 with few ventricular ectopics. There were no changes in hemodynamics. There was around 600 mL of blood loss during surgery, and the rest of the surgical and anesthetic course was uneventful.

After the surgery, the patient was shifted to the intensive care unit (ICU) for ventilator support. The 12-lead ECG was repeated in the ICU, which did not show any abnormality. The ST-T wave changes had reverted back.

A repeat Troponin I test was done 6 h later, which was again negative. The patient remained hemodynamically stable in the postoperative period. The patient was kept in the ICU for 1 day and then tracheally extubated when his GCS improved.

The ECG changes were transient and related to head injury only.

Clinical Scenario 7

Hemanshu Prabhakar

Department of Neuroanaesthesiology and Critical Care, All India Institute
of Medical Sciences, New Delhi, India

An 11-year-old child weighing 26 kg presented in the neurosurgical outpatient department with sudden onset and gradually progressive weakness in all four limbs. A clinical and radiological examination supported the diagnosis of atlantoaxial dislocation. The surgical plan was to decompress the cervicomedullary junction anteriorly and to fix the spine by posterior approach.

The patient was operated under general anesthesia, first in the supine position for foramen magnum decompression and thereafter in the prone position in the same sitting. In the prone position, the patient's head was supported by a horseshoe. The patient's baseline hemoglobin was 12 gm%. Intraoperative blood loss was 1500 mL, which was replaced with 3.5 L of crystalloids, 4 units of packed red blood cells, 2 units of fresh frozen plasma, and 2 units of platelet concentrates. Intraoperatively, hemodynamics remained stable. Postoperatively, the patient was conscious and moving all four limbs. The trachea was extubated after confirming return of airway reflexes and adequate tidal volume. Immediately after extubation, unilateral vision loss was detected on routine examination by the attending anesthesiologist. Urgent ophthalmological consultation was sought. Ophthalmic examination showed eyelid edema, chemosis, ptosis, paresthesia of the supraorbital region, afferent pupil defect, and complete blindness in the right eye with absent light perception and loss of eye movements. A fundoscopic examination showed a cherry-red spot. Diagnosis of the central retinal artery occlusion was made. The patient was managed by an external ocular massage, intraoclular pressure decreasing agents such as acetazolamide and mannitol, and in a 30° head-up position with tight monitoring of blood pressure and hematocrit. Twelve hours after starting the treatment, the patient's vision started improving. At discharge on the 10th postoperative day, finger counting was present in the patient.

Clinical Scenario 8

Hemanshu Prabhakar

Department of Neuroanaesthesiology and Critical Care, All India Institute
of Medical Sciences, New Delhi, India

A 56-year-old, right-handed female presented to the neurosurgical emergency with chief complaints of sudden onset severe headache followed by multiple episodes of vomiting in past 24 h. Patient was a known hypertensive with a history of irregular medication. There was no history of any other comorbid illness.

On examination, she appeared confused and disoriented and had marked neck rigidity. The rest of the neurological examination was unremarkable with no localizing signs. Her hemodynamic status was stable. A noncontrast computed tomographic (NCCT) scan of the head revealed a small intracerebral hematoma in the right temporal lobe with diffuse subarachnoid hemorrhage (Fischer Grade 4).

On cerebral digital subtraction angiography, a right internal carotid artery (ICA) bifurcation aneurysm measuring 4.0 × 3.5 mm was seen, which was coiled under general anesthesia in the same sitting. The postembolization NCCT head scan was unremarkable, with no evidence of fresh bleeding or hydrocephalus. The patient was admitted in the neurosurgical intensive care unit (NICU) and started on oral nimodipine 60 mg every 4 h. Euvolemia was maintained using normal saline infusion. Hypertensive therapy was started with norepinephrine infusion to keep Mean blood pressure at least 10–15% above the baseline.

A routine transcranial Doppler (TCD) examination of cerebral arteries was performed daily in conjunction with repeated neurological examination.

The patient remained asymptomatic for 2 days. On the third day after surgery, the patient appeared drowsy along with left-sided weakness in both of her limbs (upper limb more than lower limb).

A TCD examination revealed increased velocity in the right middle cerebral artery (MCA), suggestive of cerebral vasospasm. Cerebral

http://dx.doi.org/10.1016/B978-0-12-804075-1.00051-1

angiography showed severe diffuse vasospasm in the right ICA territory. Chemical angioplasty with intraarterial nimodipine (4 mg) was performed, with significant increase in blood flow in the vasospastic arterial territory.

Postprocedure, the patient showed an improvement in left-sided weakness, which worsened again after 2 days. A repeat chemical angioplasty with intraarterial nimodipine (4 mg) and intraarterial milrinone (8 mg over 30 min) was done with complete resolution of angiographic vasospasm.

Postprocedure, the patient was kept on continuous intravenous infusion of milrinone (0.5–1.5 µg/kg/min). The infusion was started at a dose of 0.5 µg/kg/min and gradually increased to 1.5 µg/kg/min until day 14 after the initial bleeding.

Daily TCD examination revealed stable MCA velocities. The patient recovered fully without neurological deficits and was discharged from the NICU on day 15.

CHAPTER

52

Clinical Scenario 9

Hemanshu Prabhakar

Department of Neuroanaesthesiology and Critical Care, All India Institute
of Medical Sciences, New Delhi, India

An 18-year-old female patient, weighing 45 kg, was scheduled for a craniotomy and excision of a midbrain ependymoma in the prone position. Her clinical, biochemical, and coagulation parameters were normal. In the operating theater, standard monitors (electrocardiograph (ECG), noninvasive blood pressure, and pulse oximeter) were attached. General anesthesia was induced with fentanyl and thiopentone, and intubation was facilitated with vecuronium. Anesthesia was maintained with oxygen, air, isoflurane, fentanyl, and atracurium, with controlled ventilation to achieve normocarbia. The patient was positioned prone on a Mayfield frame. General measures for the prone position were taken with appropriate padding of pressure points, eye protection, and adequate neck flexion by two-finger breadth between sternum and mentum. Intraoperative monitoring included heart rate, ECG, oxygen saturation by pulse oximetry, Respiratory rate, end-tidal carbon dioxide, central venous pressure (via the basilic vein), invasive blood pressure, airway pressure, volume of intravenous fluids infused, urine output, nasopharyngeal temperature, arterial blood gas, blood glucose, and blood loss. In the intraoperative period, there was a gradual increase in the airway pressures over a period of time from 18 to 35 mmHg. The surgeon also observed brain bulge in the patient, which was attended to with mannitol and steroids. Despite confirmation of adequate air entry bilaterally and no added sounds, airway pressures reached 38 cm H_2O. The entire circle system was assessed until the patient end but in vain. Examination of the patient's face revealed protruded edematous tongue. Sternomental space was reassessed and was adequate. Fiber optic examination of the endotracheal tube (ETT) showed gross flexion at the level of the oropharynx due to increased warmth and laxity of the tube. The position of the ETT was readjusted into the retro-mandibular space, and the length of the intraoral portion was reduced to avoid tube kink. After these measures were taken, the airway pressures came down to 19 cm of H_2O. The rest of the surgical and anesthetic course was uneventful.

Clinical Scenario 10

Hemanshu Prabhakar

Department of Neuroanaesthesiology and Critical Care, All India Institute
of Medical Sciences, New Delhi, India

A 32-year-old female, weighing 56 kg presented with persistent head-ache (5 months), decreased bilateral vision (left eye more than right eye), and diplopia for 2 months. A brain magnetic resonance imaging (MRI) scan revealed a sellar mass of size $1.2 \times 0.8 \times 0.9$ cm which extended into the suprasellar region. Her pituitary hormone profile showed mild elevated prolactin levels of 31 µg/L (normal <20 µg/L), decreased thyroid-stimulating hormone level of 0.131 mIU/L (normal range 0.4–4 mIU/L), with free T_4 levels of 9.26 pmol/L (normal range 7.5–21 pmol/L), and decreased adrenocorticotropic hormone level of 7 pg/mL (normal range 10–46 pg/mL). Her visual field test did not show any field defect. She was started on hydrocortisone replacement therapy (30 mg) and levothyroxine (100 µg) daily. Her other investigations were within normal range and surgery was planned to excise the mass lesion. The patient underwent transsphenoidal resection of a pituitary tumor and the surgery was uneventful. A postoperative MRI scan showed complete resection of tumor. In the postoperative period, the patient was comfortable with stable vitals. Urine output was in the range of 40–60 mL/h and her investigations were within normal range (hemoglobin, 12.5 gm/dL; blood glucose, 115 mg/dL; blood urea, 25 mg/dL; serum creatinine, 0.9 mg/dL; serum sodium, 139 mmol/L; serum potassium, 4.7 mmol/L). However, on postoperative day 2, the patient started complaining of increased thirst and her urine output increased to 300–500 mL/h. On investigation, serum sodium was found to be elevated (152 mmol/L), plasma osmolality was increased (302 mOsm/kg), and her urine was dilute with a specific gravity of 1.002. A diagnosis of diabetes insipidus was made and patient managed accordingly.

Index

'*Note*: Page numbers followed by "f" indicate figures, "t" indicate tables, and "b" indicate Boxes.'

Printed in the United States
By Bookmasters